Progress of Lens Biochemistry Research

Documenta Ophthalmologica
Proceedings Series volume 8

Editor H. E. Henkes

Dr. W. Junk bv Publishers The Hague 1976

Progress of Lens Biochemistry Research
Volume in honour of
Prof. Dr. med. J. Nordmann

edited by O. Hockwin

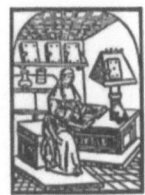

Dr. W. Junk bv Publishers The Hague 1976

ISBN-13: 978-90-6193-148-5   e-ISBN-13: 978-94-010-1571-4
DOI: 10.1007/978-94-010-1571-4

CONTENTS

PREFACE

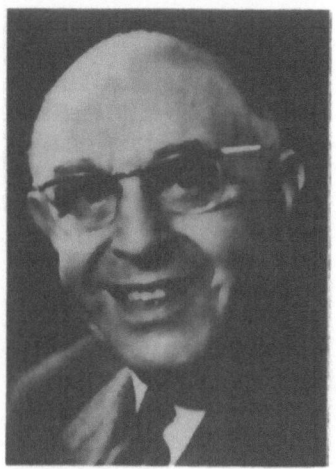

On August 25, 1976 Prof. Dr. med. JEAN NORDMANN, Emeritus Professor of Strasbourg University, will celebrate his 80th anniversary.

The task of paying tribute to Professor NORDMANN's many services to ophthalmology in a way worthy of the occasion is so difficult that we decided to concentrate on the focal point of his life's work.

In this issue scientists engaged in lens research from all over the world offer reports of their latest findings together with their best wishes and felicitations as a birthday gift to the Nestor of lens research. They thereby express their gratitude to Professor NORDMANN, who, with the lifelong indefatigable enthusiasm of a scientist, has most successfully persued the problems of lens metabolism.

It is our sincerest hope that we may look forward to many more years in which to take advantage of Professor NORDMANN's superior knowledge.

Among the contributions to this festive donation we miss the works of some authors who have always held Professor NORDMANN's special interest. The editor has received several letters of longstanding friends who would have liked to submit a manuscript but had been unable to meet the deadline: Professor NORDMANN may rest assured that they, too, belong to the great number of congratulators from our field of research.

We have been able to make this dedication thanks to Professor HENKES who readily agreed to publish our contributions in Documenta Ophthalmologica.

Dr. Junk publishers have done their utmost to ensure prompt publication.

OTTO HOCKWIN, Bonn

INTRA-NUCLEAR INCLUSIONS IN THE LENS FIBRES OBSERVED IN THE GALACTOSE-INDUCED CATARACT IN THE YOUNG RAT

A. BRINI, M.E. STOECKEL, A. PORTE & J. KLETHI

(Strasbourg, France)

ABSTRACT

Electron microscopy of young rat lenses with early changes due to galactose diet point to an early alteration of the nucleo-plasmatic relationship. Peculiar alterations of the nuclei are seen in the lens fibres during their maturation.

The galactose-induced cataract can be provoked within 3 to 6 days in the young rat or rabbit, simply with a galactose diet. The early lesions are localized along the equator; they are detected with the slit lamp, after dilatation of the pupil, and usually form a crown of superficial vesicles and of flat opacities. The latter are proximal to the vesicles and appear later. The ultrastructure of these lesions is well known (BRINI et al., 1961, 1963; KUWABARA et al., 1969). The vesicle-like appearance is due to a dilatation of the intercellular spaces (KUWABARA et al., 1969) preceding swelling and necrosis of fibres. This picture is evidence of an early osmotic alteration which is generally thought to be related to the accumulation of galactitol – a result of reduction of abnormally stored galactose – in·the lens (KINO-SHITA et al., 1962). This explanation does not account, however, for the precise localization of the lesions in the fibres at a certain stage of differentiation. The diversified metabolic alterations which were described in several tissues during human galactosemia and in galactose-fed animals also suggest a more complex pathogenesis (see SEGAL, 1972).

According to our electron microscopic observations on the young rat on a galactose diet, an early alteration of the nucleo-plasmatic relationship is indicated: e.g., peculiar alterations of the nuclei are seen in the lens fibres during their maturation.

MATERIAL AND METHODS

Twelve Wistar rats were put on a 50% galactose diet soon after weaning. Lens alterations were detected with the slit lamp. The lenses were removed between the third day (when the first lesions were observed) and the tenth day. They were cut meridionally under fixative (glutaraldehyde 5%, phosphate buffer 0.1 M, pH 7.4). Post-fixation with osmic acid was performed in some cases. The tissue was embedded in araldite-epon. Semi-thin sections were controlled with light microscopy after toluidine blue, hemalun-eosin or Feulgen staining. Ultra-thin sections were treated with uranyl-acetate and lead citrate and studied with a Siemens Elmiskop IA.

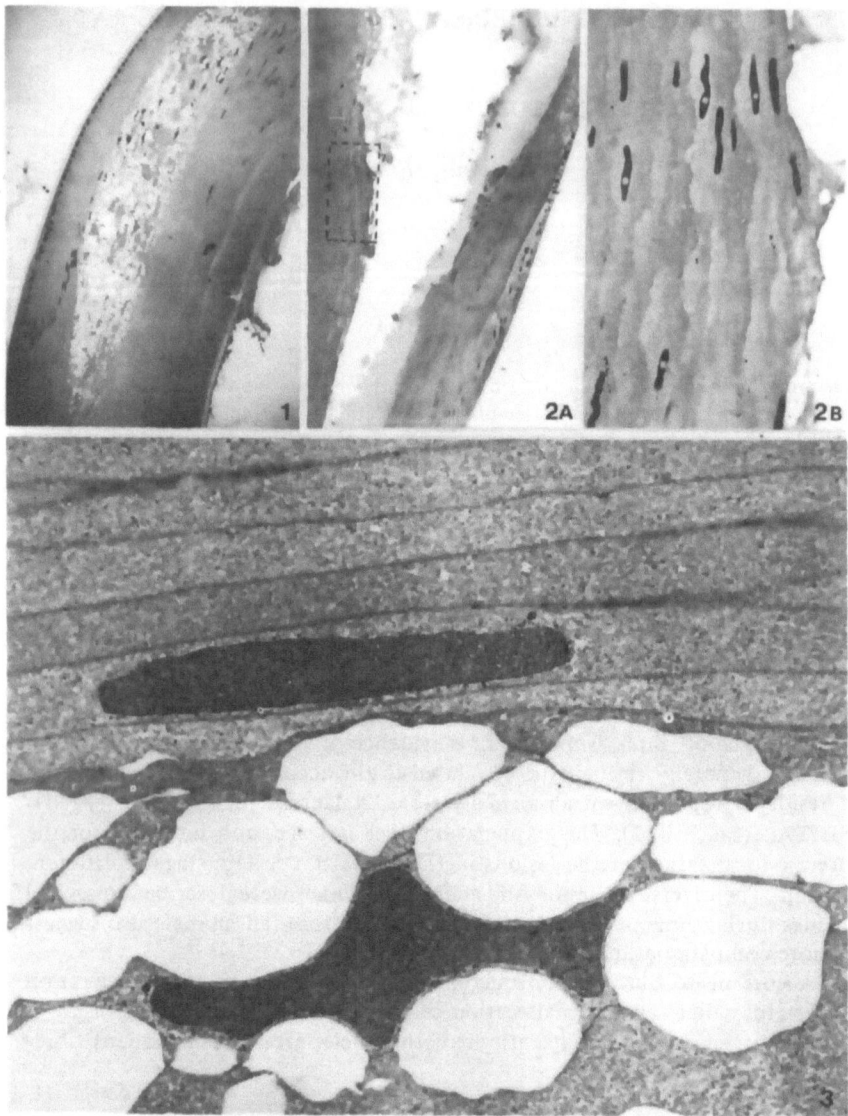

Fig. 1. 3 days galactose diet. Semi-thin sagittal section, Hemalun-eosine stained. Equatorial vesicular area. X 80.

Fig. 2. 9 days galactose diet. Semi-thin section, hemalun-eosin stained.
A. Same orientation as in fig. 1. More advanced stage of cataract (tear in the necrotic area is an artefact). The nuclei which contain inclusions are proximal to the lesion. X 80.
B. Detail of fig. 2A (framed area) showing poorly stained spherical intranuclear inclusions. X 500.

Fig. 3. 3 days galactose diet. Equatorial area. Top: superficial layers with normal appearance; bottom: 'vesicles' by dilatation of the intercellular spaces. X 5,750.

RESULTS

On light microscopy control sections, the lesions first appear as an area of clear vesicles strictly localized along the equator (Fig. 1). Electron microscopy shows that these 'vesicles' are actually dilatations of the intercellular spaces (Fig. 3) at the level of the young fibres, which are still interlinked by desmosomes and tight junctions, most of the latter being of the gap junction or nexus-type (PORTE et al., 1975). These alterations are not observed in the epithelium or at a distance from the equator. In the more differentiated fibres, which are proximal to the vesicle area, only nuclear alterations, as yet irregular, are observed. Later, the vesicle area presents a downright degenerative appearance, with swelling and vacuolization of the fibres and disappearance of the cellular outlines. The alterations of the nuclei in the fibres beneath the lesions are then obvious and constant (Fig. 2).

They appear as spherical inclusions, which stain slightly with eosin, and are Feulgen-negative. Several inclusions may be present in the same nucleus (Fig. 4). With electron microscope (Figs. 3-6), these inclusions appear devoid of chromatin and constituted of very fine fibrillary material obviously different from the much coarser material of the fibre cytoplasm. They are surrounded by chromatin, have no limiting membranes and cannot be considered as cytoplasmic invaginations. They are independent of the nucleoles, which normally appear diversified in this area (fragmentation and mottled appearance, spherical or annular condensation). Besides the typical inclusions, all the nuclei of the fibres in this part of the lens exhibit diffuse areas where granular chromatin becomes scarce, and within which fine fibrillar material accumulates.

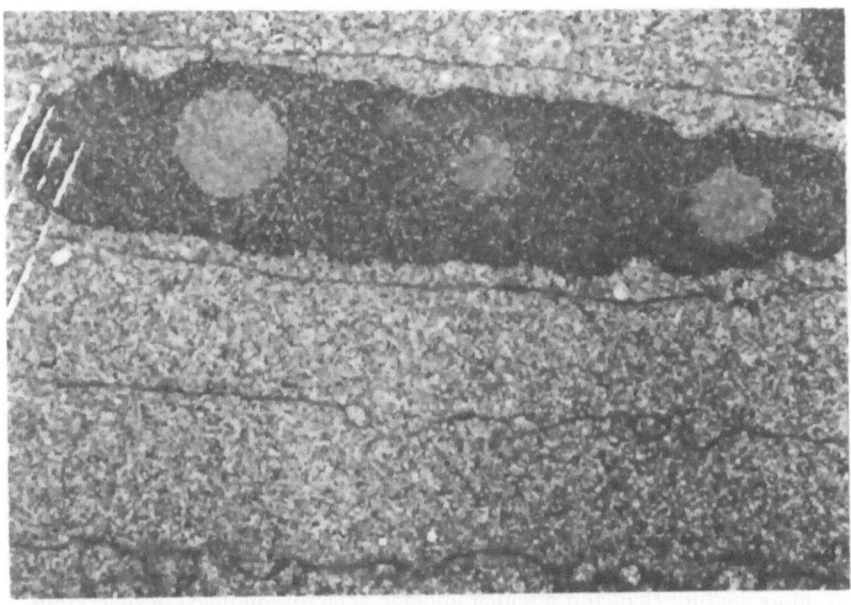

Fig. 4. 6 days galactose diet. Nucleus with 3 inclusions. X 7,200.

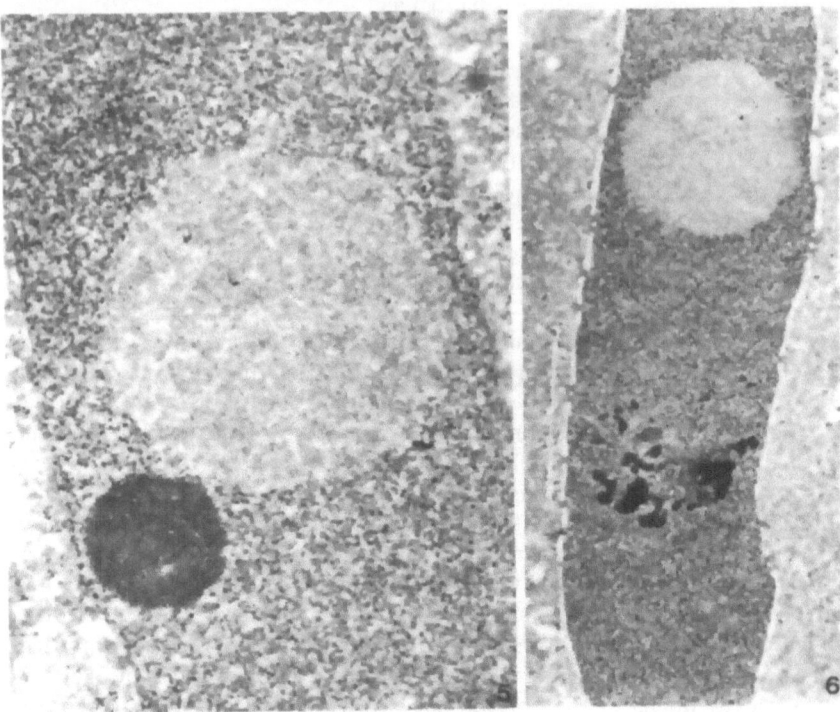

Fig. 5. 6 days galactose diet. Fine fibrillar appearance of the intra-nuclear inclusion contrasting with the greater granularity and density of the chromatin. Dense spherical nucleolus close to the inclusion. X 22,000.

Fig. 6. 9 days galactose diet. Inclusions in a nucleus, the nucleolus of which has a reticular appearance. X 10,500.

DISCUSSION

A degradation of the DNA in the lens fibres preceding the disappearance of the nuclei seems well established (MODAK & BOLLUM, 1970). The intra-nuclear alterations of the lens fibres in the galactose-induced cataract could be interpreted as an intensification of this degradation. Indeed, the inclusions are formed in areas of chromatin rarefaction, perhaps by a condensation of unmasked nucleo-plasmic proteins. This interpretation needs to be checked by a more precise ultrastructural cytochemical study. Some relationship between the fine fibrillar material of the inclusions and the altered chromatin cannot be excluded. At any rate, it seems obvious that the alterations of the nuclei cannot be linked with an osmotic disorder; there is neither vesiculation of the intercellular spaces nor any swelling of the fibres in this area.

The fibres with intranuclear inclusions contain but scarce ribosomes and are more mature than those which undergo galactose-induced degeneration. Possibly an alteration of the nucleoprotein components which is well tolerated by the mature fibre may have a more pronounced effect on younger fibres which are in an active elongation phase and have a higher level of protein synthesis. This might explain the localization of the degenerative lesions in the fibres. A somewhat similar reasoning could be applied to the osmotic disorders: the young fibres which show intercellular vesiculation are probably more sensitive to the galactose-induced energy deficiency.

REFERENCES

BRINI, A. & A. PORTE. Structure et formation des fibres dans le cristallin normal. Leurs modifications dans la cataracte au galactose. Etude au microscope électronique chez le rat. *Bull. Soc. Fr. Ophtalm.* 5: *340-343* (1961).

BRINI, A., A. PORTE & M.E. STOECKEL. Modifications ultrastructurales du cristallin dans certaines cataractes expérimentales et humaines. *Bull. et Mém. Soc. Fr. Ophtalm.* 67: *193-206* (1963).

KINOSHITA, J.H., L.O. MEROLA, K. SATOH & E. DIKMAK. Osmotic changes caused by the accumulation of dulcitol in the lenses of rats fed with galactose. *Nature* 194: *1085* (1962).

KUWABARA, T., J.H. KINOSHITA & D.G. COGAN. Electron microscopic study of galactose-induced cataract. *Invest. Ophthal.* 8: *133-149* (1969).

MODAK, S.P. & F.J. BOLLUM. Terminal lens cell differenciation. III. Initiator activity of DNA during nuclear degeneration, *Exptl Cell Res.* 62: *421-432* (1970).

PORTE, A., A. BRINI & M.F. STOECKEL. Fine structure of the lens epithelium, *Ann. Ophth.* 7: *623-634* (1975).

SEGAL, S. Disorders of galactose metabolism, in The metabolic basis of inherited disease. Ed. by J.B. Stanbury, J.B. Wyngaarden & D.S. Fredrickson. McGraw-Hill (1972).

Keywords:

Rat
Galactose-cataract
Electron microscopy
Lens fiber inclusions

Authors' address:

Consultations externes
Clinique Ophtalmologique
Hospices Civils de Strasbourg
1 place de l'Hopital
F-67005 Strasbourg Cedex
France

ELECTRON MICROSCOPIC STUDY OF CATARACTOUS LENSES
OF DIABETIC SAND RATS (PSAMMOMYS OBESUS)*

TOICHIRO KUWABARA, M.D. & SHIGEKUNI OKISAKAA, M.D.

(Bethesda, Maryland/Boston, Mass.)

SCHMIDT-NIELSEN et al. (1964) described Egyptian sand rats as developing a diabetes mellitus-like syndrome when fed with standard laboratory rat chow instead of a leafy vegetable diet. This animal model had provided a unique opportunity for the investigation of biochemical and cytological aspects of diabetes by several authors (MIKI et al., 1966, HACKEL et al., 1967, LEBOVITZ et al., 1974, ZIEGLER et al., 1975).

Although SCHMIDT-NIELSEN et al. (1964) pointed out that cataracts of the lens was one of the earliest changes in the diabetic sand rat, detailed cytologic study of the cataract has not been reported. The present study deals with histologic and fine structural examination of the cataractous lenses of diabetic Egyptian sand rats.

MATERIALS AND METHODS

Egyptian sand rats (*psammomys obesus*) were raised in the Elliott P. Joslin Research Laboratory, Department of Medicine, Harvard Medical School, Boston, Massachusetts. The eyes examined in this communication were obtained from the sand rats studied in a series of projects, one of which was reported by MIKI et al. (1966). Adult animals were fed with Purina laboratory rat chow with free access to 5% saline. The animals invariably became obese within two weeks, their blood glucose level reaching 250-400 mg/100 ml during the experimental period of 4-10 weeks. The earliest cataractous change was observed on the 4th week with the high caloric diet. Twelve animals which developed cataracts on or before the 4th week were divided into three groups. On the 4th, 6th, and 10th week one group each was killed by decapitation.

The excised whole lens of one eye was fixed in a 4% glutaraldehyde solution in 0.15 M phosphate buffer (pH 7.2) at room temperature for 24 hours. Small pieces of lens tissue were obtained from the anterior, bow and posterior zones and post fixed in 1% osmium tetroxide in the same buffer solution. Small pieces of the posterior retina were also excised for electron microscopy. The specimens were dehydrated in ethanol and embedded in an epoxy resin. Sections cut at 0.5 μm were stained with toluidine

* Part of this investigation was supported by Public Health Service Research Grant EY 01421 from the National Eye Institute.

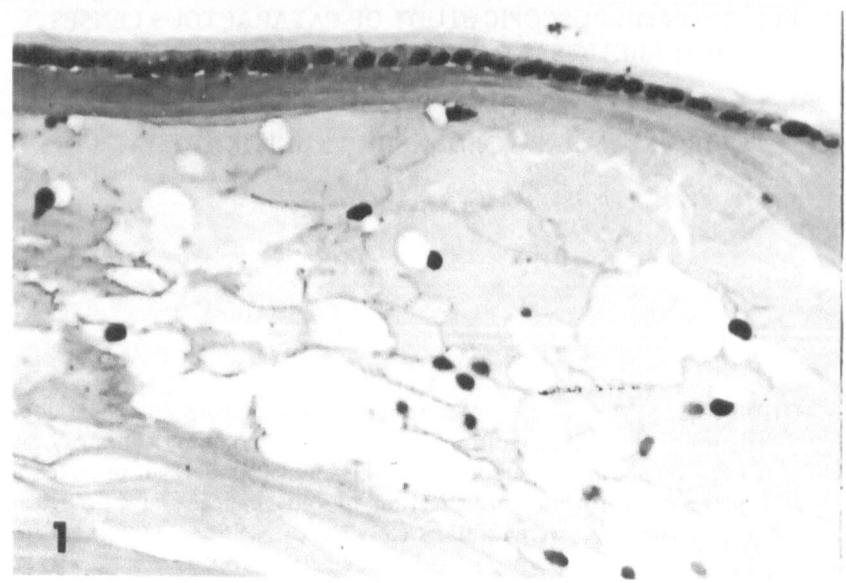

Fig. 1. 4 week feeding. Anterior portion. Superficial cortical cells are markedly swollen. Pyknotic nuclei are present in the swollen cells. Some cells are liquefied. Paraffin section, hematoxylin-eosin stain. 250X.

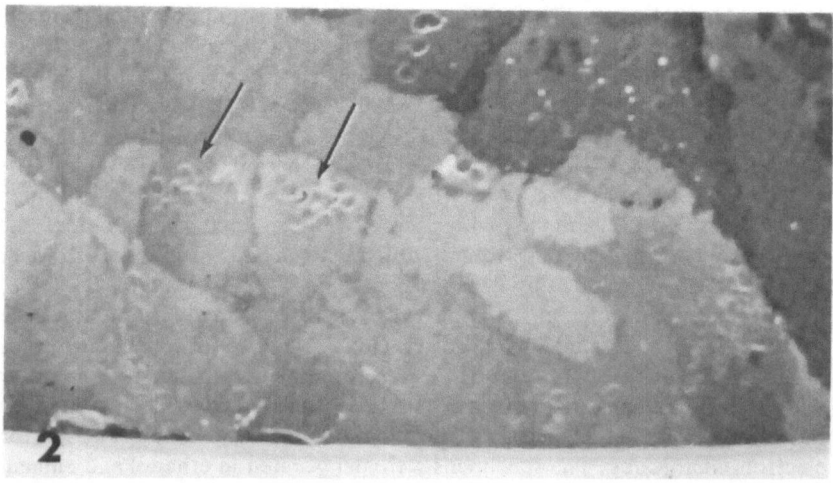

Fig. 2. 4 week feeding. Posterior portion. Superficial cortical cells are markedly swollen. Some cells are hyperchromatic. Degenerated protein forms clusters (arrows). Epon section, toluidine blue stain. 400X.

blue and examined by light microscopy, and ultra-thin sections were examined by electron microscopy following staining with uranyl acetate and lead citrate. The other eye of the same animal was fixed in 7% neutral formalin for histologic study. Portions of the retina of this eye were examined by the trypsin digestion technique. 4 adult sand rats which had been fed with a mixture of vegetables and whose blood glucose levels were below 100 mg/100 ml were used as the normal control. No opacity was noticed in the lens of these normal animals.

RESULTS

Animals examined in this study had an acute ketotic-type diabetic syndrome for more than four weeks. The hyperglycemia which was present in all those animals was associated with an increased amount of insulin in the serum during the early disease condition. Degeneration of the beta cells of the pancreatic islands and fatty degeneration of the liver cells were histologically noted in all diabetic animals. The retinal tissue was generally normal except for those of two 10 week fed animals which showed segmental degeneration and dilatation of the large retinal artery.

Early changes

Faint opacity was grossly noted in the equatorial cortex around the end of the third week, but these earliest cataractous lenses were not examined in this study. The lenses at the fourth week showed marked opacity in the cortex and often in the whole lens. Histologic examination revealed that superficial cortical lens cells were markedly swollen and that the bow configuration of the bow nuclei was disorganized. Pyknotic nuclei were present in the swollen cells (Fig. 1). Degenerated and liquefied cells were electron lucent, finely vacuolated, and their cell membranes were broken in several locations. Many epithelial cells showed increased density of the cytoplasm and contained increased numbers of ribosomes and rough endoplasmic reticulum. Some epithelial cells were markedly swollen or vacuolated. The posterior lens cells were also swollen and contained degenerated substance (Fig. 2). The degeneration was more pronounced in the deeper cortical cells. The degeneration process progressed into a larger area of the cortex with further feeding. Lenses examined on the 6th week showed marked liquefaction in the whole cortex. The liquefied lens fibers had lost cell membranes and a large area was filled with granular substances of varying size and density. The liquefied substance appeared to flow into the intercellular spaces between the surviving lens fibers.

Later changes

Localized proliferation of cells was frequently noted in severely cataractous lenses during 6-10 week's feeding. Also, the epithelial cells often migrated toward the posterior surface instead of forming the bow configuration by elongation of the cell. A few nucleated spindle shaped cells formed small mounds inside the capsule at both the anterior and posterior zones. The

9

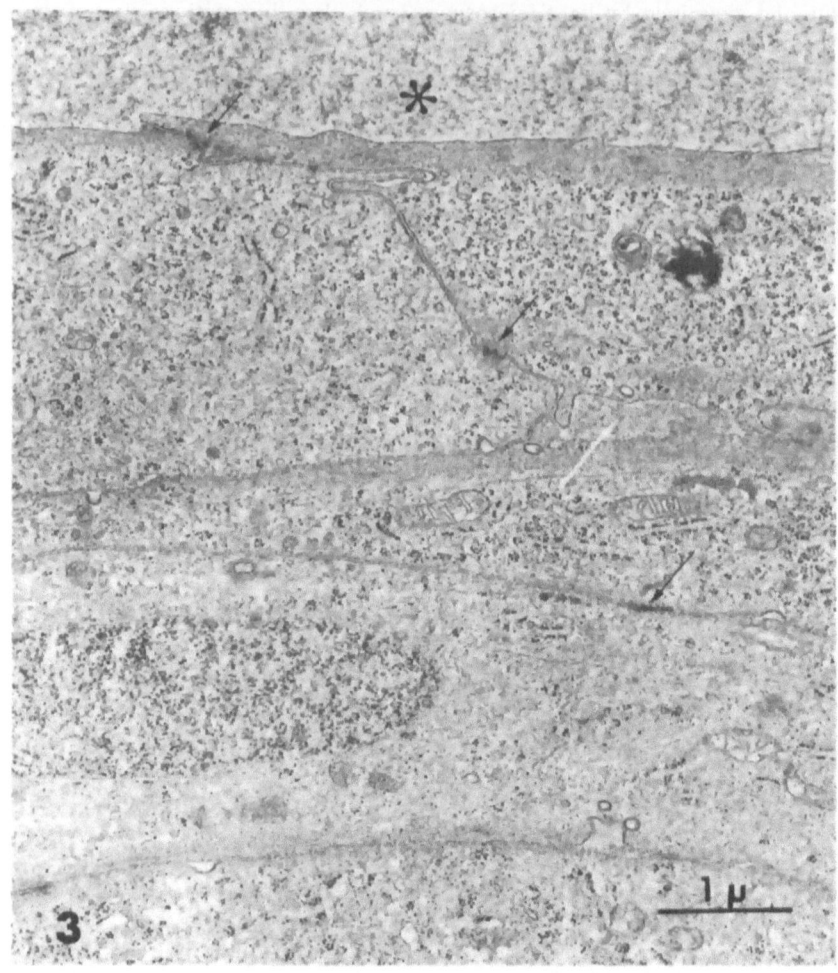

Fig. 3. 6 week feeding. Accumulating cells in the posterior portion. Cortical cells of this lens are markedly liquefied (*). The proliferating lens cells contain ribosomes, mitochondria and microtubules and are well attached to each other by junctions (arrows). The liquefied substance accumulates between the cells (white arrow). 17,500X.

cytologic appearance of the proliferating cells was similar to that of the elongating cells at the bow area (Fig. 3). The cytoplasm consisted mainly of fine granular substances which were similar to the normal lens protein granules, and contained slightly more microorganelles than normal. A moderate number of microtubules was present in these short cells. The cells, though not directly attached to the capsule, were well attached to each other at several junctions. Occasionally, small intercellular spaces were formed and the liquefied substance accumulated. Also some surviving cells in the superficial cortex, especially at the posterior equatorial zone, which had elongated to become the mature fibers showed markedly irregular interdigitations (Fig. 4). These cells became stubby and often contained fine vesicles and membranous microorganelles. Also, large intercellular spaces were formed between these cells.

At the later stage of the cataract, the proliferating cells began to form abnormal capsule materials. These changes were most frequently seen within the epithelium in the anterior portion and in the islands of proliferating cells in other locations. The proliferated lens cells formed an excessive PAS staining positive substance (Fig. 5). Electron microscopically, the newly formed substance was a loose fibrous tissue which had no firm attachment to the cells. The proliferated lens cells were separated from the original capsule (Fig. 6). The loose fibrous tissue became more compact and banded collagen fibers were formed (Fig. 7). The anterior capsule was somewhat thicker than normal. The proliferated cells at this stage were irregular in shape and well attached to each other. Desmosomes and gap junctions were regularly present between the cells. The cytoplasmic appearance resembled that of the epithelial cell. The major part of the lens substance, including the lenticular nucleus, was markedly liquefied. Also small patches of calcification were formed in the degenerated cortex. Some totally liquefied lenses were ruptured at the later stage.

The structure of the control normal lenses was identical to that of the albino rat (KUWABARA et al., 1969).

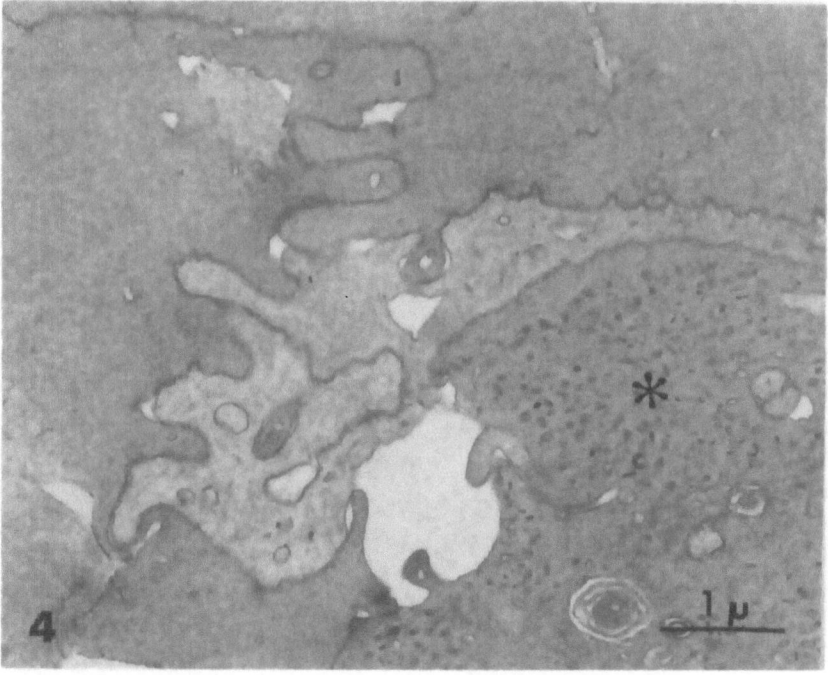

Fig. 4. 6 week feeding. Posterior portion. Surviving cortical cells show markedly inter-digitated cell membranes. These cells often accumulate fine vesicles (*). Large intercellular spaces are common. 16,000X.

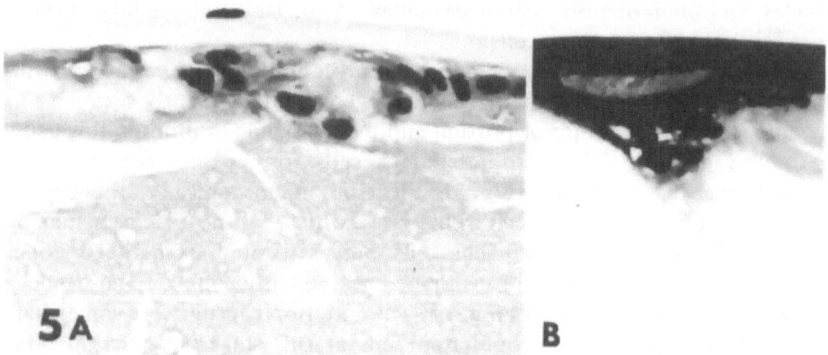

5A   B

Fig. 5. 10 week feeding. Anterior portion. A. The epithelial cells are irregular in arrangement and amorphous nodular substance is accumulated. Paraffin section, hematoxylin-eosin staining. 400X. B. PAS staining shows thickened capsule and nodular PAS positive substances. The cortical lens substance is liquefied. 400X.

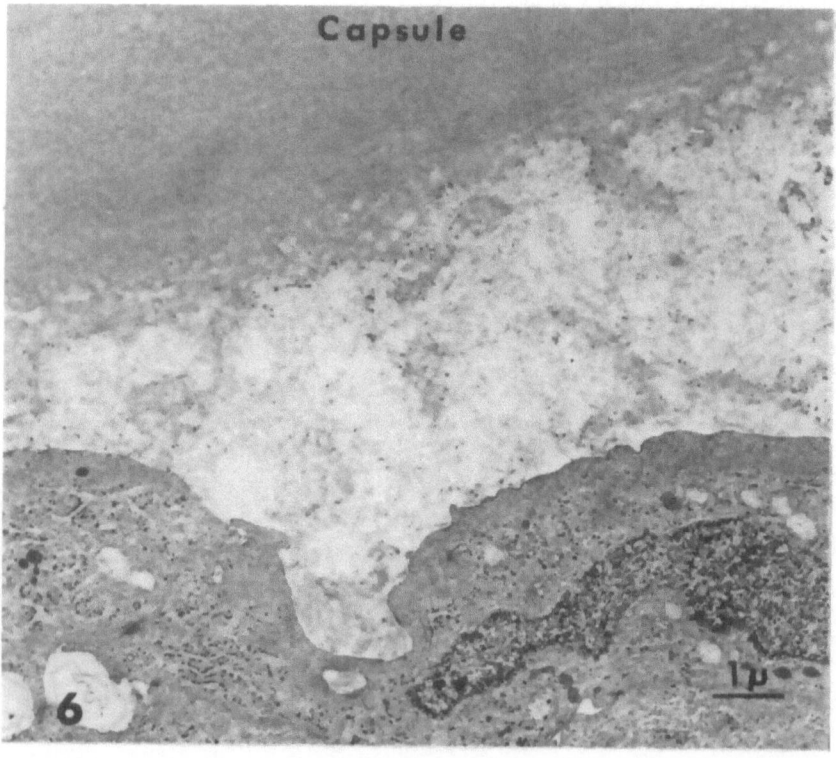

Fig. 6. 10 week feeding. Anterior portion. The capsule is thickened and separated from the epithelial cells which show irregular shape. The space between the capsule and the epithelium is occupied by the loose fibrous tissue. 8,700X.

12

DISCUSSION

A diabetes mellitus-like syndrome is induced in the Egyptian sand rat by changing its diet from the natural leafy vegetable to the high caloric laboratory chow. The serum glucose level of the animal elevated from the normal 100 mg/100 ml to 200-400 mg. In this hyperglycemic condition, cataractous change occurs at a relatively early stage. The appearance of the cataractous lens of this diabetic animal is strikingly similar to that of experimentally induced galactose cataract (KUWABARA et al., 1969). Swelling of the cortical lens cells becomes apparent in the 4th week of high caloric feeding in the sand rat, whereas the similar change occurs on the third day of the galactose feeding in the albino rat. Subsequent pathologic process in the diabetic sand rat and galactose fed albino rat was identical except for the time courses. The pathologic process in the sand rat is considerably slower than that of the galactose fed rat. In addition, cell proliferation is considerably more extensive in the sand rat.

Migration and proliferation of lens cell are common phenomena in cataractous lenses of various causes. COGAN & DONALDSON (1951) emphasized this phenomenon as the main pathogenesis of the posterior cataract formation following the radiation injury. Galactose induced rat cataracts

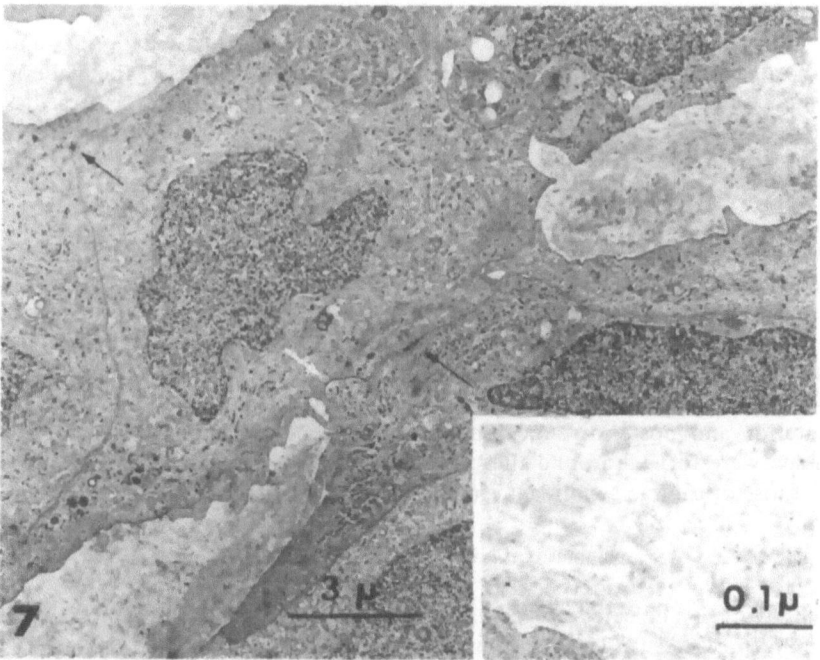

Fig. 7. 10 week feeding. Anterior portion. Irregular epithelial cells are well attached to each other. Desmosomes (arrows) and a gap junction (white arrow) are present. The loose fibrous tissue is formed around the abnormal epithelial cells. 5,700X. The insert shows banded fibers in the loose fibrous tissue. 124,000X.

13

also show these changes (VON SALLMAN & GRIMES, 1969; KUWABARA et al., 1969). Also, proliferation of the capsule is observed in the cataract of Down's syndrome (COGAN & KUWABARA, 1962) and in experimental cataracts induced by suckling mouse cataract agent (FRIEDLAENDER et al., 1976). The epithelial cells in the damaged lens which have lost their elongating ability, proliferate to form islands and aberrant capsules. It is noteworthy to mention that the proliferating cells are unable to elongate, though they contain a moderate number of microtubules. PIATIGORSKY (1975) has emphasized the importance of microtubules in the elongation of lens cells, but the present findings suggest the presence of other factors for elongation of the lens cell. Formation of banded fibers in the sub-capsular tissue has been demonstrated by HENKIND & PROSE (1967) in an anterior polar cataract.

These late changes in the sand rat lenses may be secondary reactions to the degeneration of lens cells which is induced by hyperglycemia. Although the pathologic course is rapid, the young anterior lens cells which have survived the initial damage seem to produce these secondary changes.

Accumulation of a sugar alcohol has been demonstrated as the pathogenesis of galactose induced cataract by KINOSHITA et al. (1962). In a few sand rats studied a high sorbitol accumulation in the lenses has been observed (KINOSHITA, 1967). The retention of sorbitol in the lenses leads to marked swelling. Thus the biochemical changes that occur in the lens of a sand rat appear similar to those in diabetic rats.

Since the biochemical and clinical findings of the diabetic Egyptian sand rat are similar to those of diabetes mellitus, the pathogenesis of the diabetic cataract in the human and the sand rat may be identical. The sand rat has proved to be a good animal model in the study of diabetic cataract.

SUMMARY

A diabetes mellitus-like syndrome was induced in the Egyptian sand rat (*psammomys obesus*) by changing its diet from the natural leafy vegetable to laboratory chow. Cataractous changes were developed in all experimental animals after about three week's feeding of the high caloric diet. The first lenticular change was marked swelling and then degeneration of the cortical cells. The surviving lens cells proliferated and formed islands in the anterior and posterior subcapsular region. Nodular masses of the fibrous tissue were formed around the proliferating cells. These changes are similar to those of cataracts in diabetes mellitus of the human.

ACKNOWLEDGEMENT

This work is dedicated to Professor Jean Nordmann. Dr. J.H. Kinoshia has kindly provided us with his unpublished data on the sand rat. The authors are grateful for his criticism on this work.

14

REFERENCES

COGAN, D.G. & DONALDSON, D.D. Experimental radiation cataracts. I. Ctaracts in the rabbit following single x-ray exposure. *AMA Arch. Ophthalmol.* 45: *508-522* (1951).

COGAN, D.G. & KUWABARA. T. Pathology of cataracts in mongoloid idiocy: A new concept of the pathogenesis of cataracts of the coronary cerulean type. *Doc. Ophthalmol.* 16: *73-80* (1962).

FRENKEL, G. & KRAICER, P.F. Evaluation of tests for latent diabetes in the sand rat and rat. *Acta Endocrinol.* 72: *727-736* (1973).

FRIEDLAENDER, R.P., BARILE, M.F. & KUWABARA, T. Ocular pathology induced by the suckling mouse cataract agent (SMCA). *Invest. Ophthalmol.* 15:640-647(1976).

HACKEL, D.B., LEBOVITZ, H.E., FROHMAN, L.A., MIKAT, E. & SCHMIDT-NIELSEN, K. Effect of caloric restriction on the glucose tolerance and plasma insulin of the sand rat. *Metabolism* 16 *1133-1139* (1967).

HAMAI, Y., FUKUI, H.N. & KUWABARA, T. Morphology of hereditary mouse of cataract. *Exp. Eye Res.* 18: *537-546* (1974).

HENKIND, P. & PROSE, P. Anterior polar cataract. Electron-microscopic evidence of collagen. *Am. J. Ophthalmol.* 63 *768-771* (1967).

KINOSHITA, J.H. Cataracts in galactosemia. *Invest. Ophthalmol.* 4: *786-799* (1965).

KINOSHITA, J.H. Elevation of sorbitol content in diabetic sand rats. Unpublished data, 1967.

KINOSHITA, J.H., MEROLA, L.O., SATOH, K. & DIKMAK, E. Osmotic changes caused by the accumulation of dulcitol in the lenses of rats fed with galactose. *Nature* 194: *1085-1087* (1962).

KUWABARA, T. The maturation of the lens cell: a morphologic study. *Exp. Eye Res.* 20: *427-443* (1975).

KUWABARA, T., KINOSHITA, J.H. & COGAN, D.G. Electron microscopic study of galactose-induced cataract. *Invest. Ophthalmol.* 8: *133-149* (1969).

LEBOVITZ, H.E., WHITE, S., MIKAT, E. & HACKEL, D.B. Control of insulin secretion in the Egyptian sand rat (psammomys obesus). *Diabetologia* 10: *679-684* (1974).

MIKI, E., LIKE, A.A., SOELDNER, J.S., STEINKE, J. & CAHILL, G.F., Jr. Acute ketotic type diabetic syndrome in sand rats with special reference to the pancreas. *Metabolism* 15: *749-760* (1966).

PIATIGORSKI, J. Lens elongation in vitro and microtubules. *Annals N.Y. Acad. Sc.* 253: *333-347* (1975).

SCHMIDT-NIELSEN, K., HAINES, H. & HACKEL, D.B. Diabetes mellitus in the sand rat induced by standard laboratory diets. *Science* 143: *689-690* (1964).

ZIEGLER, M., HAHN, H.-J., ZEIGLER, B., KOHLER, E. & FIEDLER, H. Paradoxical glucagon response after stimulation with glucose and arginine in isolated pancreatic sand rat islets. *Diabetologia* 11: *63-69* (1975).

Keywords:

Cataract
Sugar cataract
Egyptian sand rat
Sand rat
Diabetes
Electron microscopy

Authors' addresses:

Dr T. Kuwabara*
Building 6, Room 213
National Eye Institute
Bethesda, Maryland, USA
Dr S. Okisaka
Joslin Diabetes Foundation
Research Laboratory
Boston, Massachusetts, USA

* Requests for reprints to be addressed to Dr Kuwabara

RNA SYNTHESIS IN THE LENSES OF NORMAL CHICKS AND IN TWO STRAINS OF CHICKS WITH HYPERPLASIA OF THE LENS EPITHELIUM

D.E.S. TRUMAN, R.M. CLAYTON, A.G. GILLIES & H.J. MACKENZIE

(Edinburgh, U.K.)

ABSTRACT

Comparisons of the synthesis of RNA in the lens of chicks with normal morphology (N) and two strains of chick with hyperplasia of the lens epithelium (Hy-1 and Hy-2) indicate that the rates of synthesis of ribosomal RNA, t-RNA and the fraction of RNA of 6-14S, which includes some of the mRNA, are under independent genetic control. RNA synthesis is responsive to the culture conditions of the lenses and this response is itself affected by the genotype of the lenses.

INTRODUCTION

Two strains of chick, Hy-1 and Hy-2, characterized by hyperplastic lens epithelium forming a folded multilayered structure, have been described previously (CLAYTON, 1975). The epithelium has a high growth rate and an abnormal propensity for fibre differentiation in Hy-1 and these characteristics have been shown to be an intrinsic property of the cells. These strains also exhibit differences from normal in the rate of incorporation of uridine into RNA (CLAYTON et al., 1976a). This paper describes further studies on the RNA metabolism of the lenses of these strains of chick together with one of normal morphology (N) suggesting that the selection for growth rate has operated at a number of levels affecting RNA metabolism in different ways. Studies on protein metabolism in these strains are presented in another paper (CLAYTON et al., 1976b).

MATERIAL AND METHODS

Birds

Day old chicks of the Hy-1 and Hy-2 strains and of the N or normal control strain were obtained from Sterling Poultry Products Ltd., Ratho, Midlothian and the Poultry Research Centre, Edinburgh.

Culture of lenses

Eyes were removed from birds after decapitating them and were dissected out under sterile conditions and explanted directly into medium 199 (Flow Laboratories Ltd) to which was added 10 per cent foetal calf serum (FCS) and 200 i.u./ml of penicillin. Incubation was at 37 ° in 5 per cent CO_2 in air. ^{3}H-uridine was made up in identical medium, making use of 10 x concentrated medium 199 to achieve the correct final concentration. The isotope concentration was 230 μCi/ml.

Preparation of polysomes and supernatant fraction

The method used was that described previously (CLAYTON *et al.*, 1974).

Measurement of radioactivity

For measurements on homogenates, supernatant fraction and suspensions of polysomes, samples were precipitated with trichloroacetic acid (TCA) to a final concentration of 5 per cent, filtered onto discs of Whatman glass fibre (GFA-1) and the filters were washed with 5 per cent TCA, absolute ethanol and ether. After drying they were placed in vials with a scintillant containing 12.5 g PPO and 0.75 g dimethyl POPOP in 2.5 l toluene.

When RNA samples had been fractionated by electrophoresis on poly-acrylamide gels, the gels were cut into 1 mm slices which were solubilised by heating overnight at 50 ° in 0.5 ml of a 10 per cent (v/v) solution of 100 vol H_2O_2. The scintillant then used contained 25 g PPO and 1.5 g dimethyl POPOP in 3 l toluene and 2 l 2-methoxyethanol. Scintillation chemicals were obtained from Koch-Light Laboratories Ltd., Colnbrook, Bucks, U.K.

RNA isolation and fractionation

The method used was that of WILLIAMSON, *et al.*, (1971).

RESULTS

Uridine incorporation into total RNA

When lenses from chicks of the three strains under study were incubated in the presence of ^{3}H-uridine for 1 hr and then transferred to fresh medium without label, the time course of incorporation into RNA was as shown in Fig. 1. With lenses from day old birds, strain Hy-1 showed greatest initial incorporation and this continued at a high rate for a period of 24 hr after the end of the pulse of radioactivity. Lenses from birds of strain N, a slow-growing control, showed a lower initial rate of incorporation, which also declined with time, so that after 24 hr the incorporation was only about 36 per cent of strain Hy-1. The other hyperplastic strain, Hy-2, showed an initial incorporation slightly less than N, but declining less with time and giving a final incorporation intermediate between Hy-1 and N.

Lenses of week-old birds of all strains showed a somewhat lower rate of incorporation than at one day old, but the difference between the strains was also less. Again strain Hy-2 was intermediate between N and Hy-1.

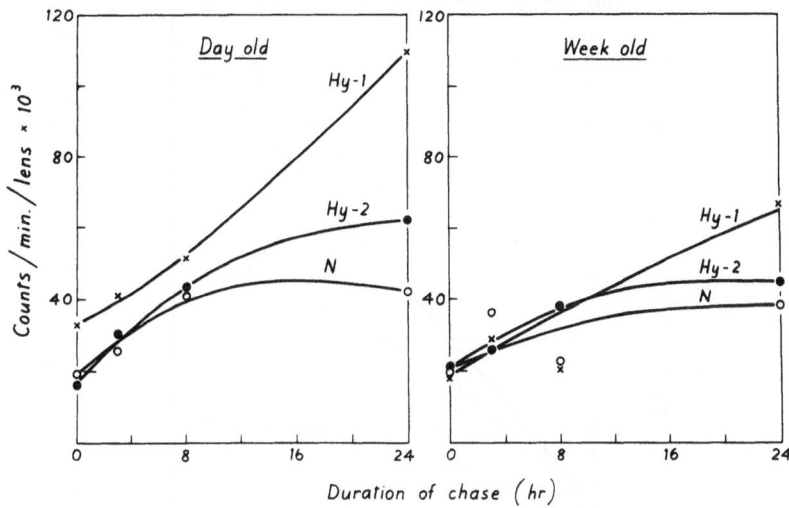

Fig. 1. Time course of incorporation into total RNA following labelling for 1 hr with ³H-uridine.

Table I.

| | Incorporation counts/min/lens × 10³ | | |
	Mean	Std. deviation	Std. error
N	75.13	5.26	1.17
Hy-1	87.62	6.66	1.49
Hy-2	48.61	1.36	0.30

Variability of incorporation

An attempt to estimate the variability of behaviour of individual lenses was made by incubating twenty lenses of each strain in the presence of ³H-uridine and then measuring the incorporation into each lens separately. The labelling period was 2 hr after a pre-incubation period of 2 hr. The results are shown in Table 1.

Incorporation into transfer RNA (tRNA)

The pattern of incorporation of ³H-uridine into tRNA following a 1 hr pulse with the label, using lenses from day-old chicks, is shown in Fig. 2. Here again there is a high and persistent rate of incorporation into tRNA in strain Hy-1, a much lower rate in strain N lenses and an intermediate rate in strain Hy-2. At the end of 24 hr the N lenses showed less than 30 per cent of the level of incorporation into RNA shown by the Hy-1 lenses.

19

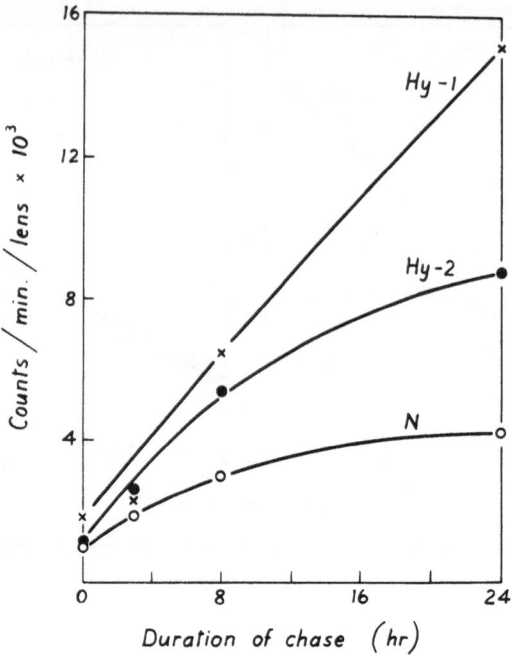

Fig. 2. Time course of incorporation into tRNA of day-old chick lenses following labelling for 1 hr with ³H-uridine.

Incorporation into polysomal RNA

The time course of uridine incorporation into polysomal RNA, following a 1 hr pulse label, in the day old chick lenses is somewhat similar to that into total RNA, though in the case of polysomal RNA there is a decline in the rate of incorporation even into the Hy-1 strain. The relationship between the strains at the end of 24 hr is quite similar with regard to incorporation into polysomal RNA and into total RNA in day old lenses, but with one week old birds the relationship between N and Hy-2 strains is different when polysomal RNA is considered. The N lenses show a relatively high initial rate of incorporation, greater than either Hy-1 or Hy-2 lenses, but the rate of incorporation then declines with time and after 24 hr some radio-activity may be lost by turnover so that the incorporation into N lenses may be less than Hy-2 at this stage. In the lenses from week old birds, incorporation into polysomal RNA in strain Hy-1 is markedly less than in day old, but is still greater than in the other strains.

Fractionation of polysomal RNA

RNA isolated from polysomal preparations was further fractionated by electrophoresis on polyacrylamide gels which, after scanning for UV absorption, were sliced for the measurement of radioactivity. The result obtained with strain N lenses after a 24 hr chase following a 1 hr pulse is shown in

20

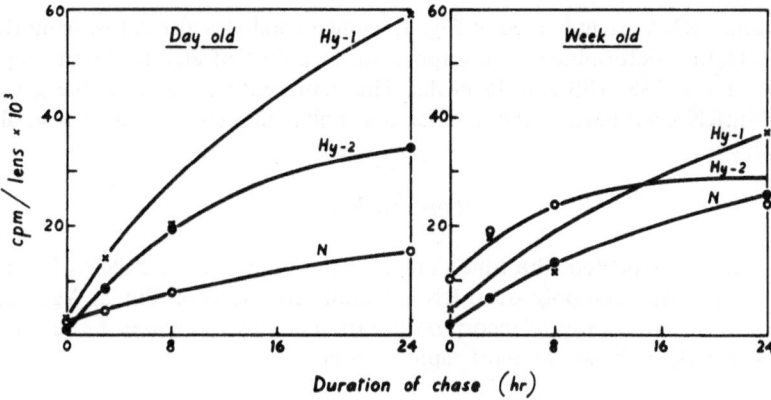

Fig. 3. Time course of incorporation into polysomal RNA following labelling for 1 hr with ³H-uridine.

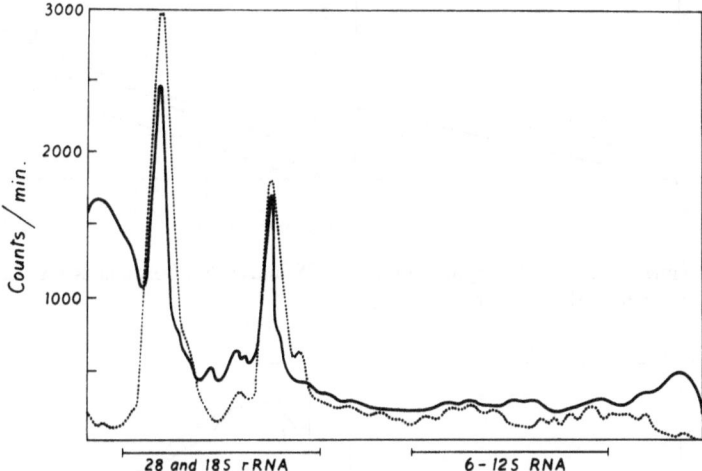

Fig. 4. Fractionation of polysomal RNA from lenses of strain N by electrophoresis on polyacrylamide gel. Incubation was for 24 hr after labelling for 1 hr with ³H-uridine. Solid line, optical density; dotted line, radioactivity.

Fig. 4. The trace of optical density results mainly from unlabelled carrier RNA added during isolation of the RNA and shows in addition to the main 28S and 18S peaks a small amount of 4-5S RNA at the end of the gel furthest from the origin and a peak of material near the origin which is clearly of high molecular weight. The curve of radioactivity, which is derived from incorporation into the incubated lenses also shows peaks corresponding to 28S and 18S RNA and also two low and polydisperse peaks in the region between 6 and 14S. Other gels showed a similar pattern. For comparisons between the strains the total radioactivity in the slices cut from the 18 to 28S region of the gel was taken to represent incorporation into

21

ribosomal RNA, as indicated in Fig. 4, while a total was also taken from the 6-14S region, determined by interpolation in a plot of electrophoretic mobility of the 28S, 18S and 4S peaks. This represents a region of the gel in which mRNA has been found in chick lens polysomes (WILLIAMSON et al., 1972).

Ribosomal RNA

As would be expected, the time course of incorporation into rRNA is similar to that into total polysomal RNA. Results are shown in Fig. 5. Week old lenses show lower rates of incorporation than do day old lenses, but at both ages strain Hy-1 shows the most rapid incorporation.

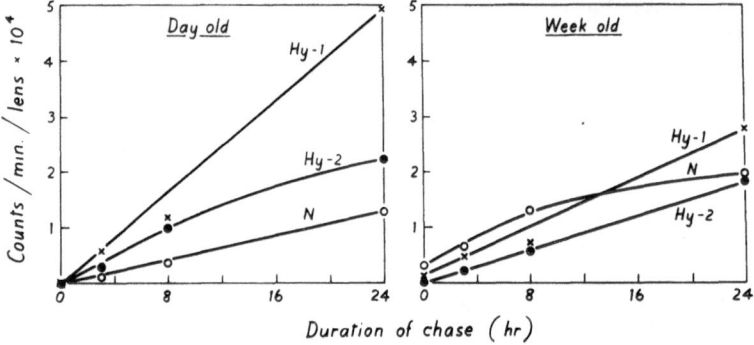

Fig. 5. Time course of incorporation into 28S and 18S ribosomal RNA following labelling for 1 hr with ^{3}H-uridine.

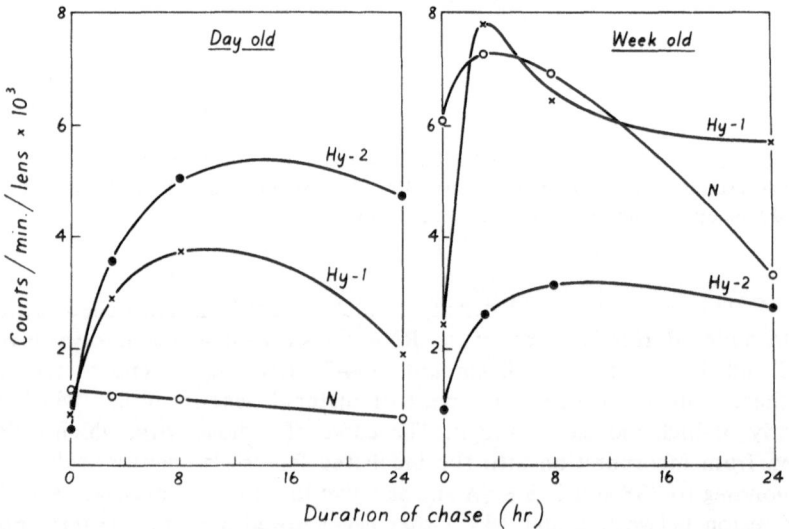

Fig. 6. Time course of incorporation into 6-14S RNA following labelling for 1 hr with ^{3}H-uridine.

22

The results of chase incubation following 1 hr pulse labelling with respect to incorporation into 6-14S RNA are shown in Fig. 6. The time curves of these fractions are quite different from those of other RNA fractions. In all strains and at both ages there is evidence of turnover of RNA during the 24 hr period. In the day old chick the lenses of N birds show a rapid initial incorporation and a slight but steady decline in radioactivity during the chase period. The lenses of strain Hy-1 birds show rapid incorporation up to 8 hrs, but thereafter there is a loss of radioactivity indicating a relatively
pid turnover of this fraction of RNA. Strain Hy-2 lenses show a most marked incorporation up to 8 hr after the pulse, and a slight decline up to 24 hr.

When lenses from one week old birds were examined, strain Hy-2 showed only a slight diminution in initial incorporation and, again, slight turnover after 8 hr. The N birds, however, showed a very rapid initial incorporation up to 8 hr, but considerable turnover after this time, while strain Hy-1 showed a high rate of incorporation up to 3 hr and less turnover in the one week old birds than in the day old birds.

Effect of incubation

The results described above have all been based on consideration of a 1 hr pulse labelling with ^{3}H-uridine followed by chase incubations in unlabelled

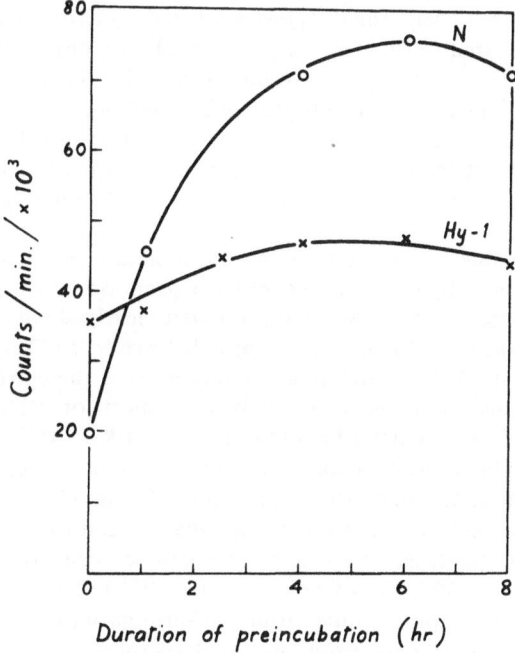

Fig. 7. Effect of preincubation for various times on incorporation of ^{3}H-uridine into total RNA of day-old chick lenses during a period of 1 hr.

medium. Interpretation of the data requires consideration of the effect of incubation itself. This has been investigated to some extent by measuring the incorporation into total RNA over a one hr period following various periods of preincubation. Strains Hy-1 and N were examined over a period of up to 8 hr and the results are shown in Fig. 7. As in the previous experiments the initial incorporation without preincubation was less in N than in Hy-1 lenses, but after one hr preincubation the incorporation rate of N lenses had risen to above that in Hy-1 and after about 6 hr the rate of incorporation in N lenses was about 150 per cent of that in Hy-1. Thus it appears that the incubation conditions had a stimulating effect on N lenses, while Hy-1 lenses were apparently little affected by the conditions of incubation.

DISCUSSION

Whenever attempts are made to estimate rates of synthesis of macromolecules by measuring the incorporation of a radioactive precursor the interpretation must always consider the possibility of differential dilution of the labelled precursor by endogenous molecules within the cell. In the case of the data presented in this paper it might be argued that the high rate of uridine incorporation in lenses of strain Hy-1 compared with N is due to a relatively high concentration of endogenous uridine in the cells of the lenses of N birds. This possibility cannot be ruled out. However, when comparisons are made between classes of RNA, then so simple an explanation is not possible. For example, as we reported earlier, lenses of the hyperplastic strains show a relatively rapid transfer of radioactivity from nucleus to cytoplasm compared with N (CLAYTON et al., 1976a). If the differences between strains were merely the result of variation in pool sizes, then all classes of RNA (nuclear and cytoplasmic) would show the same kinetics, merely with the specific incorporation showing different values. When comparison is made between the different classes of RNA studied and the three strains of birds, then it appears that there are significant variations in RNA metabolism.

Another possible explanation of the differences in RNA metabolism between the strains might lie in the relative proportions of epithelial cells found in the lenses. Data previously presented clearly show that the hyperplastic strains have an abundance of epithelial material (CLAYTON, 1975; CLAYTON et al., 1976a) and it is established that the epithelial cells are sharply distinguished from fibre cells in respect of RNA metabolism (HANNA, 1965; PAPACONSTANTINOU & JULKU, 1968; REEDER & BELL, 1965). However, two lines of evidence support the belief that the strains differ in more than the proportion of epithelial material: firstly studies on clonal cultures have established that the individual epithelial cells of the hyperplastic lenses have a greater rate of cell division in culture (EGUCHI et al., 1975; CLAYTON et al., 1972). Secondly, and more directly, autoradiographic studies using ^{3}H-uridine have shown distinctive features of uridine incorporation in the hyperplastic lenses, rather than merely showing the presence of additional epithelium with features on incorporation similar to normal (CLAYTON et al., 1976a).

24

If, then, we can take the data on uridine incorporation at its face value then it appears that the lenses with hyperplastic epithelium show abnormal characteristics of incorporation into soluble RNA (which is presumably tRNA since this would be expected to form the bulk of the post ribosomal supernatant RNA), into ribosomal RNA, and into RNA of 6-14S size derived from polysomes. This latter class of RNA corresponds to the material which we have shown previously to have the ability to prime for crystallin synthesis in cell-free systems (10) and so can be regarded as containing at least some of the mRNA although it will not include mRNA of a higher molecular such as that for δ-crystallin (ZELENKA & PIATIGORSKY, 1974). This may possibly be associated with the tendency of much of the hyperplastic epithelium to become differentiated into fibre-like cells, whose mRNA might, by analogy with normal ontogenic studies, be more stable. On the other hand, epithelial cells of N are more readily stimulated into mitosis by FCS and the synthesis of enzymes on short lived messages may be stimulated by these conditions of culture. Studies of the turnover of this 6-14S RNA (Fig. 6) show that its kinetic properties are quite different from the other classes of RNA. In the day-old birds the hyperplastic strains show a high rate of incorporation into this RNA, which also shows a correspondingly high rate of turnover. In the week-old birds the Hy-1 and Hy-2 strains show that this class of RNA becomes more stable than it does in the N. Of course this class of RNA, in as much as it is messenger RNA, would also be expected to contain mRNA for non-crystallin proteins as well as crystallins. An attempt has been made, using actinomycin D, to estimate the stability of messengers for specific crystallins in the N, Hy-a and Hy-2 strains (CLAYTON et al., 1976b). More direct estimates using immunological fractionation methods (CLAYTON et al., 1972; 1974) have yet to be applied to these strains.

A further difference between the N and Hy-1 lenses which requires investigation and which can affect the interpretation of labelling experiments in organ culture is in the manner of response to incubation in the conditions used for these experiments (Fig. 7). The N strain lenses show an ability to respond to the conditions of culture by an increase in incorporation which is almost four-fold over six hours, while Hy-1 lenses show much less change. One consequence of this is that in experiments involving prolonged incorporation the relative activities of the different strains may appear to be much changed. Somewhat similar changes are also observed in amino acid incorporation into soluble proteins and membrane proteins in lenses of these strains (CLAYTON et al., 1976b).

These data indicate that the regulation of the rate of synthesis of each class of RNA is under genetic control.

ACKNOWLEDGEMENTS

We are grateful to Mr J. Hunter and the late A.I. Hannah for skilled technical assistance, Dr I. Thomson for helpful discussions and to E.D. Roberts for the diagrams.

We thank Sterling Poultry Products, Midlothian and the Poultry Research Centre, Edinburgh for the generous provision of day-old chicks.

Our work is supported by the M.R.C. and C.R.C.

REFERENCES

CLAYTON, R.M. Failure of growth regulation of the lens epithelium in strains of fast-growing chicks. *Genet. Res., Camb.* 25: *79-82* (1975).

CLAYTON, R.M., EGUCHI, G., TRUMAN, D.E.S., PERRY, M.M., JACOB, J. & FLINT, O.P. Abnormalities in the differentiation and cellular properties of hyperplastic lens epithelium from strains of chickens selected for high growth rate. *J. Embryol. exp. Morph.* 35: *1-23* (1976a).

CLAYTON, R.M., TRUMAN, D.E.S. & CAMPBELL, J.C. A method for direct assay of messenger RNA turnover for different crystallins in the chick lens. *Cell Diffn.* 1: *25-35* (1972)

CLAYTON, R.M., TRUMAN, D.E.S. & HANNAH, A.I. RNA turnover and translational regulation of specific crystallin synthesis. *Cell Diffn.* 3: *135-145* (1974).

CLAYTON, R.M., TRUMAN, D.E.S., HUNTER, J., ODEIGAH, P.G. & DE POMERAI, D. Protein synthesis and its regulation in the lenses of two strains of chicks (Hy-1 and Hy-2) with hyperplastic lens epithelium. Docum. Ophthal. Proc. Ser. 8: *27-37* (1976b).

EGUCHI, G., CLAYTON, R.M. & PERRY, M.M. Comparison of the growth and differentiation of epithelial cells from normal and hyperplastic lenses of the chick: studies of in vitro cell cultures. *Dev. Growth and Diffn.* 17: *395-413* (1975).

HANNA, C. Changes in DNA, RNA and protein synthesis in the developing lens. *Invest. Ophthalmol.* 4: *480-491* (1965).

PAPACONSTANTINOU, J. & JULKU, E.M. The regulation of ribosomal RNA synthesis and ribosomal assembly in the vertebrate lens. *J. Cell Physiol.* 72: Suppl. 1: *161-180* (1968).

REEDER, R. & BELL, E. Short- and long-lived messenger RNA in embryonic chick lens. *Science* 150: *71-72* (1965).

WILLIAMSON, R., CLAYTON, R.M. & TRUMAN, D.E.S. Isolation and identification of chick lens crystallin messenger RNA. *Biochem. Biophys. Res. Commun.* 46: *1936-1943* (1972).

WILLIAMSON, R., MORRISON, M., LANYON, G., EASON, R. & PAUL, J. Properties of mouse globin messenger ribonucleic acid and its preparation in milligram quantities. *Biochemistry* 10: *3014-3021* (1971).

ZELENKA, P. & PIATIGORSKY, J. Isolation and *in vitro* translation of δ-crystallin mRNA from embryonic chick lens fibers. *Proc. Natn. Acad. Sci.* 71: *1896-1900* (1974).

Keywords:

Lens
Chick
Epithelium
RNA
Hyperplasia
Genetics

Authors' address:

Institute of Animal Genetics
University of Edinburgh
West Mains Road
Edinburgh EH9 3JN, U.K.

PROTEIN SYNTHESIS AND ITS REGULATION IN THE LENSES OF NORMAL CHICKS AND IN TWO STRAINS OF CHICKS WITH HYPERPLASIA OF THE LENS EPITHELIUM

R.M. CLAYTON, D.E.S. TRUMAN, J. HUNTER, P.G. ODEIGAH &
D.I. DE POMERAI

(Edinburgh, U.K.)

ABSTRACT

Comparisons have been made of the regulation of the synthesis of crystallins and membrane proteins in the lenses of normal chicks (N) and two strains (Hy-1 and Hy-2) showing hyperplasia of the lens epithelium. Quantitative differences were found in the rate of crystallin synthesis and qualitative changes in membrane composition. Genetic differences between the strains were found in the response to preincubation, stability of synthesis to Actinomycin D and sensitivity to Daunomycin.

INTRODUCTION

Two strains of chick have been described with epithelial hyperplasia (Hy-1 and H-2) (CLAYTON, 1975) which show folding and multiple layering of the epithelium, with a tendency to differentiate into fibre-like cells within the layers. A comparison of epithelium from Hy-1 and a normal strain (N) has shown abnormalities in cellular properties which include mitotic rate, cell behaviour, and propensity for differentiation, which are intrinsic properties of the cells (CLAYTON et al., 1976; EGUCHI et al., 1975). The ontogeny of specific crystallin synthesis is modified from normal in Hy-1 and Hy-2 (McDEVITT & CLAYTON, 1965) and effects on protein synthesis (CLAYTON et al., 1976; EGUCHI et al., 1975) nucleic acid synthesis (TRUMAN et al., 1976) and the pattern of response to different culture conditions (CLAYTON et al., in press) have also been found. This paper reports on further investigations into the synthesis of proteins in these lenses.

MATERIALS AND METHODS

Chicks

Day-old chicks of the two hyperplastic strains (Hy-1 and Hy-2) and the morphologically normal control strain (N) were obtained from the Poultry Research Centre, Edinburgh and Sterling Poultry Products, Midlothian.

Culture of Lenses

Lenses were explanted into medium 199 + 10% foetal calf serum (F.C.S.) (Flow Laboratories) as described previously (CLAYTON et al., 1976)

27

except that $10\,\mu g/ml$ Actinomycin-D (AmD) was added where indicated. Proteins were labelled by transferring lenses after incubation in medium (with or without AmD) to the same medium containing $25\,\mu Ci/ml$ of ^{14}C-mixed amino acids for 2 or 3 hrs as indicated. DNA was labelled in medium containing ^{3}H-thymidine at $50\,\mu Ci/ml$ for 1 hr and RNA by incubation with ^{14}C-uridine at $10\,\mu Ci/ml$ for 1 hr. Incorporation of proline into membrane fractions was obtained by culturing lenses for 3 hrs in medium containing $76\,\mu Ci/ml$ of ^{3}H-proline.

Where indicated, some lenses were cultured in medium 199 alone without the addition of F.C.S.

In all experiments, material after labelling was washed repeatedly in cold Hank's solution or cold buffered saline at 4 °C and stored in liquid nitrogen until analyzed.

Preparation of soluble proteins

These were prepared as described previously (TRUMAN et al., 1972). Before isoelectric focussing an equal volume of 11 M urea containing 200 mM β-mercaptoethanol and 20% sucrose was added.

Preparation of membrane fractions

The membrane fraction was prepared according to ALCALA, et al. (1975). For analysis in gels it was then sonicated in the solubilising solution of MINER & HESTON (1972) for 15-20 min, centrifuged at 30 000 g for 30 mins at 4 °C, and the supernatant used for analysis.

Isoelectric focussing in polyacrylamide gels in dissociating conditions

Gels were prepared according to WRIGLEY (1968) but modified to contain 8 M urea, 10 mM β-mercaptoethanol and a mixture of equal amounts of ampholine in the pH ranges 3.5-10, 4-6, 6-8 (BURNS, 1975). Gels were stained in Coomassie Blue (CRAMBACH et al., 1967), scanned in a Kipp and Zonen or a Joyce-Loebl densitometer, sliced in a Gilson Automatic Dispenser in 1 mm or in 2 mm slices, solubilised with 0.5 ml of 10 vols H_2O_2 overnight, and counted after the addition of PPO-POPOP-Triton scintillant, as described elsewhere (TRUMAN et al., 1976).

Estimation of radioactivity in aliquots

All labelled aliquots were processed as described in CLAYTON et al. (1976) and TRUMAN et al. (1976).

RESULTS

The accumulation of proteins in the lenses of N, Hy-1 and Hy-2 lenses are shown in the densitometer traces in Fig. 1. The profile is very similar for all three stains. The incorporation of ^{14}C-amino acids is also represented in Fig. 1, and it may be seen that the pattern of incorporation is broadly similar but not quantitatively identical between strains.

Differences in the rates of synthesis between strains may be observed in the components of a high pI (which include some β-crystallins but may also contain non-crystallins) and in αA2 and the β-crystallins of lowest pI, all of which are more actively synthesised in N than in Hy-1 and H-2, in αB$_2$, which is synthesised at a lower rate in Hy-2 than in N and Hy-1, and in the relative distribution of activity in two peaks in the major δ zone, where Hy-2 differs from N and Hy-1. The β-crystallin which is poorly separated from the δ of intermediate pI behaves differently in all three strains.

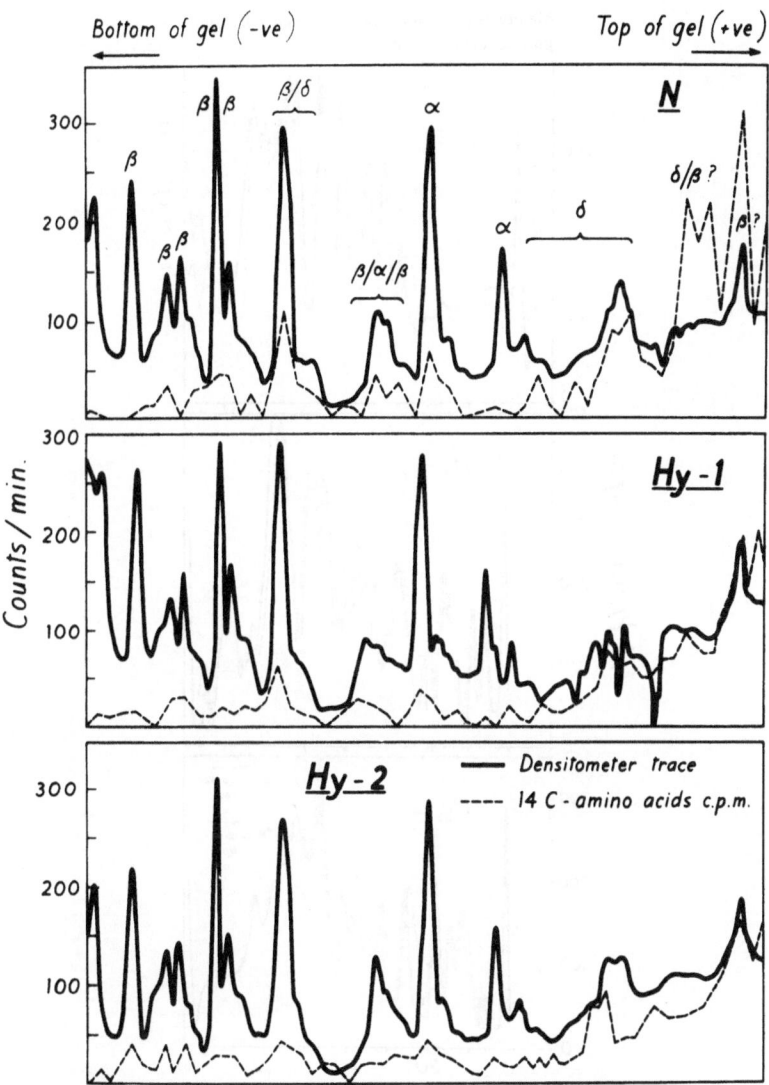

Fig. 1 Incorporation of ¹⁴C-amino acids into soluble proteins of lenses of three strains fractionated by isoelectric focussing on polyacrylamide gels.

It is particularly noticeable that the rate of labelling is apparently un-related to the quantity of protein already accumulated in the lens.

Fig. 2 shows the pattern of accumulation of polypeptides and the rate of synthesis of the membrane proteins. In marked contrast to the soluble proteins, the densitometer profile is quite distinct for each of the three strains, but the rates of synthesis closely follow the densitometer trace, showing a direct relationship between the rate of synthesis and the quantity present for each component.

The level of protein synthesis overall between 2 and 4 hrs of incubation is shown for each strain in Table 1. The effect of AmD on ^{3}H-uridine

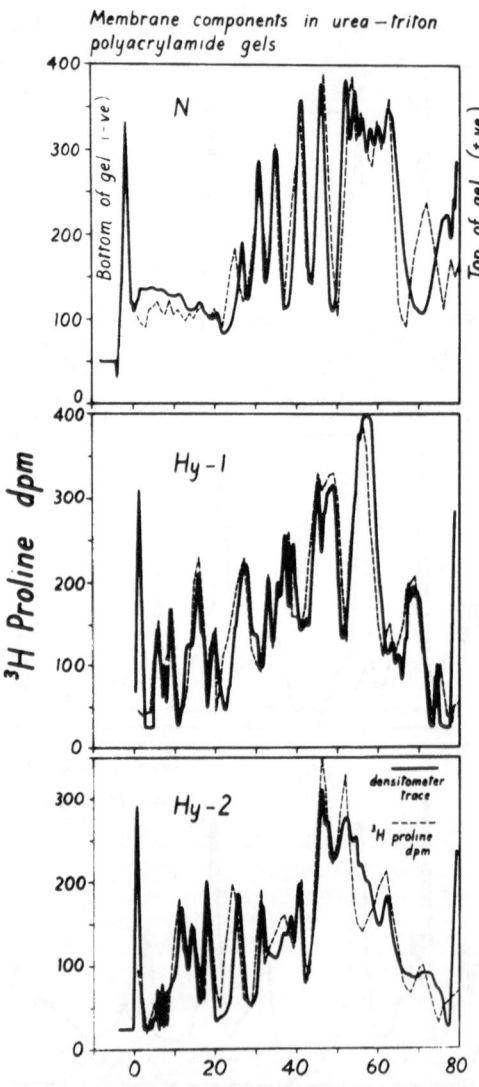

Membrane components in urea – triton polyacrylamide gels

Fig. 2. Incorporation of ^{3}H-proline into membrane proteins of lenses of three strains fractionated by isoelectric focussing on polyacrylamide gels.

Table I. Amino acid incorporation into total proteins and the effect of Actinomycin D.
Lenses were incubated ± AmD for 2 hr then labelled for 2 hr with 14 C-amino acids (2 μCi/ml) ± AmD.

Strain	Counts/min/lens x 10^3 ± S.D. (N = 20)		
	N	Hy-1	Hy-2
Amino acid incorporation in control	1.13 ± .119	2.66 ± .077	2.36 ± .053
Amino acid incorporation after AmD treatment	1.11 ± .068	2.38 ± .525	2.06 ± .075
$\dfrac{\text{AmD}}{\text{Control}}$ x 100	98.2	89.4	87.3

incorporation is to reduce it to less than 9% within an hour and to very low levels (0.8%-2.14%) thereafter. The effect on ^{14}C-amino acid incorporation after two hours of incubation in AmD-containing medium followed by 2 hrs of incubation in medium with AmD and ^{14}C-amino acids is shown in Table 1 and it is evident that the larger part of protein synthesis is rather stable to the effect of AmD in all three strains, Hy-1 and Hy-2 being slightly more affected than N. The synthesis of proteins and their stability to AmD subsumes the properties of soluble and membrane proteins. Table 2 shows this over a total period of 4 hrs in culture. In all three strains the rate of synthesis of membrane proteins is about 5% of that of the soluble proteins. The soluble and the membrane proteins are both rather stable to the effect of AmD in N, but behave differently from each other in Hy-1 and Hy-2, the synthesis of the membranes being less stable, while incorporation into the soluble proteins is stimulated.

Table II. Amino acid incorporation into soluble and membrane proteins and the effect of Actinomycin D.
Lenses were incubated ± AmD for 1 hr, then labelled for 3 hr with 14 C-amino acids (2.5 μCi/ml) ± AmD.

	Strain	Counts/min/lens x 10^3		
		N	Hy-1	Hy-2
Amino acid incorporation in control	Soluble proteins	13.2	12.2	11.2
	Membrane proteins	0.668	0.713	0.631
$\dfrac{\text{AmD}}{\text{Control}}$ x 100	Soluble proteins	91	107	102
	Membrane proteins	96	72	79

During the course of our observations in Hy-1 and Hy-2, in which various periods and conditions of incubation were employed, we observed certain inconsistencies in the comparative rates of synthesis and the effect of incubation in AmD, which appears to result in slight stimulation of protein synthesis in some experiments and various degrees of inhibition in others. In order to elucidate the cause of the apparent inconsistencies we have studied the effect on the pattern of synthesis with various times of preincubation before labelling and assay. Fig. 3 shows the time course of incorporation of label into soluble and membrane proteins from N and Hy-1 respectively.

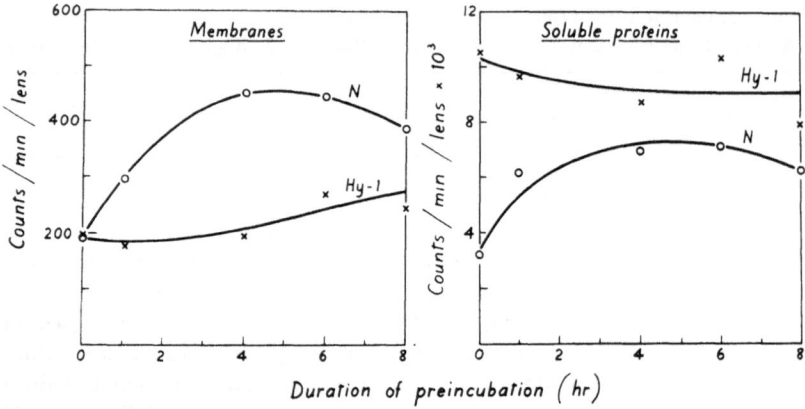

Fig. 3. Incorporation of ^{14}C-amino acids into soluble and membrane proteins during a period of 1 hr. following preincubation for various times of lenses of strains N and Hy-1.

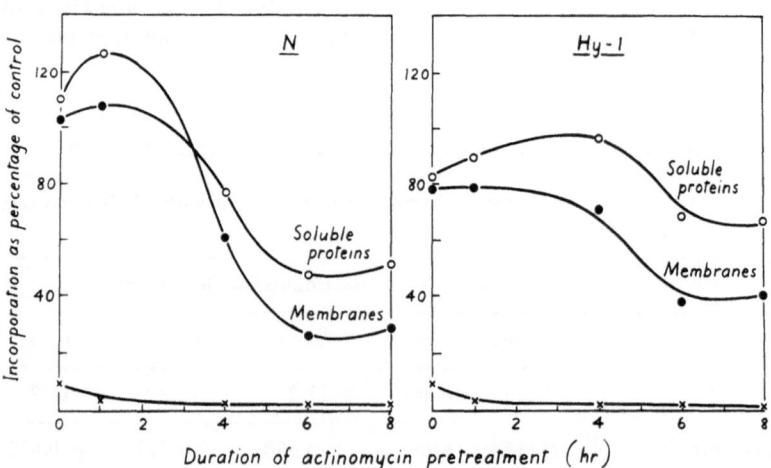

Fig. 4. Effect of preincubation with AmD on amino acid incorporation into soluble and membrane proteins of lenses of strains N and Hy-1. The lenses were preincubated for various times, then labelled for 1 hr. Values are expressed as a percentage of controls preincubated in the absence of AmD.

The level of synthesis is clearly affected by the duration of the pre-incubation and this time course of effect distinguishes the soluble and membrane fractions from each other and is quite different between strains. In particular, N is most responsive to a 4-6 hr pre-incubation, but Hy-1 responds very little and more slowly to these conditions. Thus comparisons between strains will show a degree of distinction from each other which depends on the duration of the experiment. Fig. 4 shows the effect of different periods of pre-incubation on the response to AmD of N and Hy-1. In both strains the soluble proteins and membranes show a biphasic response indicating an unstable and a stable component of protein synthesis. However, the strains differ in that an initial decline in Hy-1 is followed by a transitory rise to control values at about 4 hrs, while in N the immediate response is an apparent stimulation of synthesis in both classes of protein at 1 hr. At 3 hrs both classes appear to be unaffected compared to controls but by 4 hrs marked inhibition of synthesis is observed in both classes of protein. In both strains, the AmD-unstable component appears to have declined and a stable response at a lower level than controls is observed from 6 hrs.

The importance of the period of pre-incubation is probably due to changes leading to the cycle of cell divisions stimulated by culture conditions. The incorporation of ^{3}-H-thymidine into the DNA and ^{14}C-uridine into the RNA is shown for Hy-2 over a 70 hr period in Fig. 5. Although we have not followed the other two strains for a comparable period it seems likely that they do not have the same phasing, as indicated in part by Figs. 3 and 4 and also by the differences between these strains, both in DNA synthesis and in response to the stimulatory effect of F.C.S., as shown in Table 3.

We found previously that after 3 hrs incubation in the presence of F.C.S. the rate of thymidine incorporation in Hy-1 is close to 150% of that in N

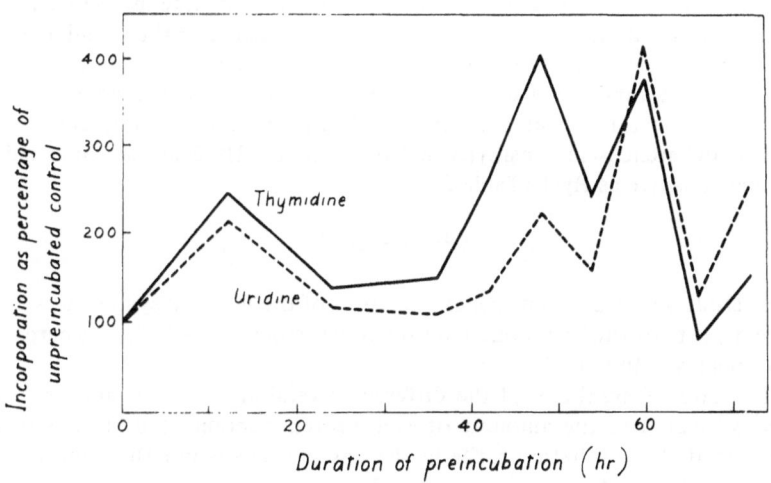

Fig. 5. Effect of preincubation on thymidine and uridine incorporation into lenses of strain Hy-2. Labelling was for 1 hr after preincubation for the times indicated. Values are expressed as a percentage of the control which was not preincubated.

Table III. Thymidine incorporation into lenses and the effect of culture conditions. Lenses were incubated for 21 hr under the various culture conditions then labelled for 3 hr with ^{3}H-thymidine (50 μCi/ml).

	Disintegrations/min x 10^3		
	N	Hy-1	Hy-2
Medium 199	356	434	382
Medium 199 + 10% FCS	904	533	1244
Medium 199 + 10% FCS + 4 mM Daunomycin	729	501	583
Effect of FCS ($\frac{\text{FCS medium}}{\text{control}} \times 100$)	239	123	324
Effect of Daunomycin in presence of FCS ($\frac{\text{Daunomycin + FCS}}{\text{FCS}} \times 100$)	81	93	47
Residual FCS-induced effect after Daunomycin as % of incorporation in Medium 199	20	33	80

and of Hy-2 close to 300% of that in N (CLAYTON et al., 1976). Table 3 shows that after 24 hrs in the presence of F.C.S., thymidine incorporation in Hy-1 is now 60% of that of N, and Hy-2 about 130% of that in N. This difference between the strains at the 3 hr and the 24 hr point is due to their responses to F.C.S., since in its absence, the ^{3}H-thymidine incorporation is low compared to that in the presence of F.C.S. and is rather similar in all three strains. (Hy-1 is 118% of N, and Hy-2 is essentially the same as N). The level of Daunomycin used is not sufficient to produce complete inhibition in this material over a 24 hr period, and permits the observation of marked differences in sensitivity between strains, Hy-2 in particular being twice as sensitive as Hy-1 (Table 3).

DISCUSSION

These studies indicate some general features of the lens cell system as well as some aspects of the metabolic modifications associated with the hyperplasia in strains Hy-1 and Hy-2.

The rate of synthesis of the different crystallins does not appear to be directly related to the amounts of each protein accumulated. This is to be expected if the synthetic profile in the day-old lens is not the same as that in earlier stages of development, which is in general agreement with data from many developmental studies (CLAYTON, 1970; 1974). It is not possible from the present data to distinguish between the possibilities that crystallins showing no amino acid incorporation in the day old lens are post-translational products or that they are metabolically stable proteins synthesised only at an earlier stage of development.

In spite of the quantitative disparities in the rates of synthesis of particular crystallins when strains are compared, the profile of accumulated proteins is essentially similar. Although there appear to be some alterations of the normal ontogenic sequence of some crystallins in the first few days of development *in ovo* (McDEVITT & CLAYTON, 1965) the morphological abnormalities in epithelial organisation are not found before 16 days of incubation (McDEVITT & CLAYTON, in preparation), so that the day-old lens has an abnormal epithelium on a fibre mass which is usually morphologically normal (CLAYTON, 1975) (except for that small proportion of lenses with vacuolated cells in the youngest cortical fibres.) The similar gross compositions found may therefore reflect the normality of the major part of the fibre mass.

In contrast to the crystallins and other cytoplasmic proteins the membrane proteins demonstrate a synthetic profile which follows exactly the profile of accumulated protein. Either there are no significant ontogenic changes in the composition and synthesis of membrane components or, in contrast to the crystallins, there is turnover throughout the lens during development. In support of this latter suggestion is an unpublished observation that the half-life of soluble proteins in the Hy-2 lens is 48 hr but is only 11 hrs for the insoluble proteins, which include the membrane components. A rapid turnover of membrane components has been found especially for non-dividing cells, and has been discussed by WARREN (1969), although it is unlikely that this could apply to the membranes in the lens nucleus. The synthesis of membrane proteins is more sensitive than that of soluble proteins to AmD, but both fractions show a biphasic response indicating that there are two classes of messenger RNAs, one unstable, the other relatively stable, associated with both groups of proteins. The sensitivity to AmD of the messenger RNAs for both soluble proteins and membranes is strongly modified by the genotype. A stimulation of the incorporation of label after actinomycin D treatment may be observed but it is obviously transitory suggesting that it is not due to an increased rate of synthesis but probably to initially diminished competition from proteins synthesised on messengers with a very short half life. A relationship between the cell cycle and the biosynthesis of enzymes and other components of the cell has been reported by several authors as has the change in availability of several cell surface markers such as the B and H antigens, the H-2 antigen and lectin-agglutinable sites. These topics have been reviewed by LENGEROVA (1972) and by RAPIN & BURGER (1974).

The time course of response to culture conditions, both for crystallins and for membrane proteins, is strain specific. In addition a comparison of the data presented in this paper with previous findings suggest to us that the differentials between the strains in levels of DNA, RNA and protein synthesis increase or decrease according to the time elapsed after explantation. These two observations are consistent with one another and would be explained if the levels of synthesis are related to the stage of the cell cycle and if the strains differ in the periodicity of the cycle and its sensitivity to modification. We have previously shown that epithelial cells of Hy-1 have a higher intrinsic mitotic rate than those of N. However, the growth conditions must also affect the mitotic cycle, although differently for each strain. The rate of DNA synthesis is most similar for all strains in unsupplemented medium 199 which does not facilitate mitosis, but shows a strain specific response both to F.C.S., which promotes mitosis (HARDING et al., 1971) and to a partially inhibitory level of Daunomycin, an inhibitor of DNA synthesis (THEOLOGIDES et al., 1967).

The effect of F.C.S. on protein synthesis in the short term is most marked in N, and it may be significant that this is the strain with the lowest intrinsic mitotic rate. However at the 21 hour point Hy-2 has the highest rate of DNA synthesis in the presence of F.C.S.

Differences in mitotic phase may account for the fluctuation of the values obtained when comparing the strains at any particular time interval. The extent of the divergence from normal in parameters such as rates of syntheses of different macromolecules appears to be greater than can be accounted for by differences in mitotic phase alone, but is a strain-specific characteristic.

Similarly the striking differences in membrane composition between the strains is a feature of the whole lens and therefore cannot be explained wholly in terms of the mitotic phase of the cells in the epithelium.

We have shown previously (CLAYTON et al., in press) that conditions affecting mitosis and contact between epithelial cells and fibres and conditions affecting metabolism are among the signals which affect the quantitative profile of crystallin synthesis and that Hy-1 and Hy-2 have a response to these signals which differs from normal. Furthermore the turnover of the 6-14S fraction, which includes some of the mRNA, differs between these strains (TRUMAN et al., 1976). The effect of AmD reported here suggests that mRNA stability is among the genetically different properties of these strains and this might be expected to be responsive to changes in the duration of the cell cycle, in turn affecting protein synthesis.

The nature of the relationship between the cell surface properties of these cells, including their cell behaviour, their membrane composition and their mitotic periodicity, and of the relationship between these properties and the parameters of protein synthesis requires further investigation.

ACKNOWLEDGEMENTS

We are grateful to Mr. R.N. Roy for cooperation in the experiment shown in Fig. 5 and to A.G. Gillies, the late A.I. Hannah and H.J. MacKenzie for excellent technical assistance. We are grateful to the Poultry Research Centre, Edinburgh and Sterling Poultry Products, Midlothian for day-old chicks. Our work is supported by the C.R.C. and the M.R.C.

REFERENCES

ALCALÁ, J., LIESKA, N. & MAISEL, H. Protein composition of bovine lens cortical fiber cell membranes. *Expl. Eye Res.* 21: *581-595* (1975).

BURNS, A.T.H. RNA and protein synthesis in the differentiation of the lens. Ph.D. Thesis. Edinburgh (1975).

CLAYTON, R.M. Problems of differentiation in the vertebrate lens. *Current Top. Devl. Biol.* 5: *115-180* (1970).

CLAYTON, R.M. Comparative aspects of lens proteins. *The Eye* 5: *400-494* Ed.H. Davson & L.T. Graham (Academic Press, London 1974).

CLAYTON, R.M. Failure of growth regulation of the lens epithelium in strains of fast-growing chicks. *Genet. Res.*, Camb. 25: *79-82* (1975).

CLAYTON, R.M., EGUCHI, G., TRUMAN, D.E.S., PERRY, M.M., JACOB, J. & FLINT, O.P. Abnormalities in the differentiation and cellular properties of hyperplastic lens epithelium from strains of chickens selected for high growth rate. *J. Embryol. exp. Morph.* 35. *1-23* (1976).

CLAYTON, R.M., ODEIGAH, P.G., DE POMERAI, D.I., PRITCHARD, D.J., THOMSON, I. & TRUMAN, D.E.S. Experimental modifications of the quantitative pattern of crystallin synthesis in normal and hyperplastic lens epithelia. In 'Biology of the Epithelial Lens Cells in Relation to Development, Ageing and Cataract' Ed. by Courtois, Y. and Regnault. F. (Les Colloques de l'I.N.S.E.R.M., Paris, 1976). (in press)

CRAMBACH, A., REISFELD, R.A., WYCHOFF, M. & ZACCAR, J. A procedure for rapid and sensitive staining of protein fractionated by polyacrylamide gel electrophoresis. *Anal. Biochem.* 20: *150-154* (1967).

EGUCHI, G., CLAYTON, R.M. & PERRY, M.M. Comparison of the growth and differentiation of epithelial cells from normal and hyperplastic lenses of the chick: studies of in vitro cell cultures *Dev. Growth and Diffn.* 17: *395-413* (1975).

HARDING, C.V., REDDAN, J.R., UNAKAR, N.J. & BAGCHI, M. The control of cell division in the ocular lens. *Int. Rev. Cytol.* 31: *215-300* (1971).

LENGEROVA, A. The expression of normal histocompatibility antigens in tumour cells. *Adv. Cancer Res.* 16: *235-271* (1972).

McDEVITT, D.S. & CLAYTON, R.M. Ontogeny and localization of α, β and δ crystallins in the Hy-1 chick lens. *J Cell Biol.* 67: *2732* (1965).

MINER, G.D. & HESTON, L.L. Methods for acrylamide gel isoelectric focussing of insoluble brain proteins. *Anal. Biochem.* 50: *313-316* (1972).

RAPIN, A.M.C. & BURGER, M.M. Tumor cell surfaces: general alterations detected by agglutinins. *Adv. Cancer Res.* 20. *1-91* (1974).

THEOLOGIDES, A., YARBRO, J.W. & KENNEDY, B.J. Daunomycin inhibition of DNA and RNA synthesis in normal and malignant tissues. *Proc. Amer. Assoc. Cancer Res.* 8: *67* (1967).

TRUMAN, D.E.S., BROWN, A.G. & CAMPBELL, J.C. The relationship between the ontogeny of antigens and of the polypeptide chains of the crystallins during chick lens development. *Expl Eye Res.* 13: *58-69* (1972).

TRUMAN, D.E.S., CLAYTON, R.M., GILLIES, A.G. & MACKENZIE, H.J. RNA synthesis in the lenses of normal chicks and in two strains of chicks with hyperplasia of the lens epithelium. *Docum. Ophthal. Proc. Ser.* 8: *17-26* (1976).

WARREN, L. The biological significance of turnover of the surface membrane of animal cells. *Current Topics in Dev. Biol.* 4: *197-222* (1969).

WRIGLEY, C.M. Gel electrofocussing. A technique for analysing multiple protein samples by isoelectric focussing. *Science Tools* 15: *17-23* (1968).

Keywords:

Lens
Epithelium
Hyperplasia
Genetic
Mitosis

Membrane
Crystallin
Synthesis
Regulation

Authors' address:

Institute of Animal Genetics
University of Edinburgh
West Mains Road
Edinburg EH9 3JN, U.K.

EPITHELIUM OF THE ADULT LENS IN TISSUE CULTURE*

J. FRANÇOIS & V. VICTORIA-TRONCOSO

(Ghent, Belgium)

There are two types of lens cultures:
1. The organotypical culture, where the lens is cultivated in toto in order to study the metabolism and the transparence of the organ.
2. The histotypical culture, which has been made by several authors, following upon the initial work of KIRBY (1926), and which makes research possible at the cellular level. The development of the cells, their metabolism and their biosynthesis can so be studied.

The importance of tissue culture in the study of the lens metabolism has been stressed by NORDMANN (1954, 1962), PIRIE & VAN HEYNINGEN (1956), VAN HEYNINGEN (1962) and LUCAS (1965).

The histochemical and lysosomal study has not, up to the present time, been carried out. Therefore we thought it worthwhile to undertake it.

MATERIAL AND METHODS

We made cultures of the lens epithelium of the rabbit, using adult albino Flanders Giants weighing between 2 and 3 kg. After enucleation, the eyes were placed in two successive baths of penicillin (10.000 I.U. per ml) for 20 minutes. These eyes were then dissected in a sterile chamber with laminate airstream, bacterial filters and UV lamp.

After having removed the cornea and the iris, the lens was detached at the same time as the vitreous, the latter being separated from the lens with the aid of a spatula.

A square of capsule and epithelium of about 1 cm² was removed at the level of the anterior surface of the lens, in order to avoid any contamination by other cells. This specimen, which was divided into quarters, was then placed in a Petri dish with a drop of culture medium. We used the plasma clot technique. The pieces of the specimen were transplanted in Leighton tubes with glass lamina in order to obtain monocellular layers, in T flasks and in Petri dishes 3 cm in diameter. They were orientated in such a fashion that the epithelium was on top and the capsule underneath.

A drop of chicken embryo extract was added to each specimen, which had been incubated for 2 hours before the culture medium was added.

---

* This paper has been written in honour of Prof. J. Nordmann at the occasion of his eightieth anniversary.

We used two culture media:

Solution A:	T 199 (Difco)	40%
	Hanks (B.S.S.)	40%
	El 100 Chick Embryo extract (Difco)	7.5%
	Homologous serum	12.5%
Solution B:	L-proline	4.8 mg
	L-hydroxyproline	1.2 mg
	Glycin	6 mg
	Glucose	0.5 mg
	Solution A	100 ml

Solution B was filtered on bougie.

For the study of the lysosomes we used the technique already described (FRANÇOIS et coll., 1976).

The histochemical techniques are summarised in Tables I and II.

Table I

Method	Granules	Cytoplasmic matrix	Nucleus
PAS 5′ oxidation	·	+	−
PAS 15′ oxidation	−	++	−
Alcian blue pH 1	+ for the fine granules in the cell pseudopodia	−	−
Alcian blue pH 2,5	+ for the fine granules in the cell pseudopodia	−	−
Wilder's reaction (reticulin)	·	++	−
Colloidal iron	++ in many cyto-plasmic granules	−	+
Toluidine blue pH 6,5	achromasia	β-metachro-masia	α-metachro-masia
Acridine orange (nucleic acids)	·	RNA orange fluorescence	DNA green fluorescence
Hemotoxyline-eosine	−	eosinophilia	basophilia

Table II

Method	Lysosomes	Mitochondria
G-6-PD	–	++
Lacto-dehydrogenase	–	++
Acid phosphatase (Takeuchi-Tanoue)	++	–
Acid phosphatase (Standard cupling azo-dye method)	++	–
Incubation in a medium containing Acridine orange (vital staining)	Red to orange fluorescence	green fluorescence

RESULTS

I. Development of the cultures

The cells began to migrate already during the first 24 hours (Figs. 1 and 2). They formed a 'fibrillar pattern' (Fig. 2).

After 48 to 72 hours, they increased in size by augmenting their cytoplasm (Fig. 3) and formed rounded shapes (Fig. 4).

Subsequently they tended to form an irregular mosaic (Fig. 5) which showed nevertheless a growth front, at the level of which they were more elongated.

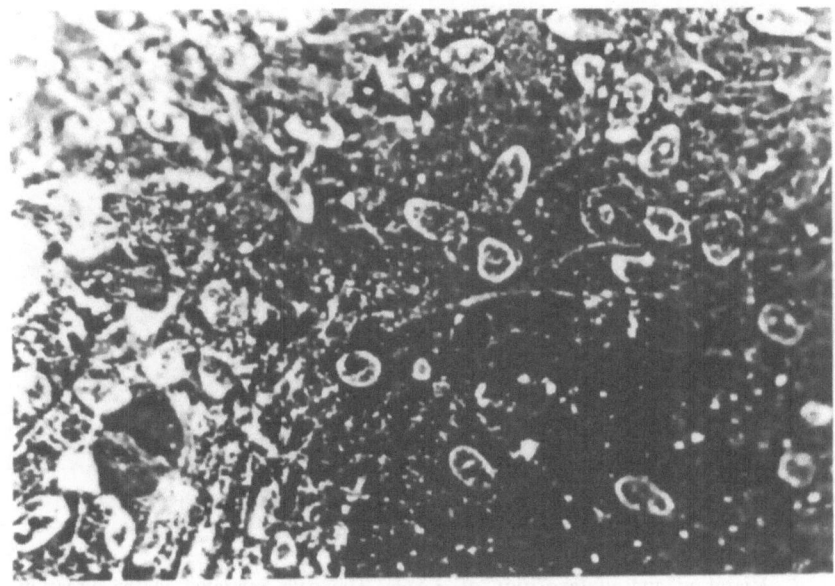

Fig. 1. Migration of cells on the specimen. Phase contrast microscope (obj. x 20).

The development of the cultures of the lens epithelium is very rapid. The cells, which continue to increase from the specimen, tend always to take on an elongated shape and the appearance of a fibre (Fig. 6). Subsequently there are rounded shapes and more peripherically they form a mosaic. The growth centre remains the co   ny of cells located on the lens capsule (Figs. 1 and 2).

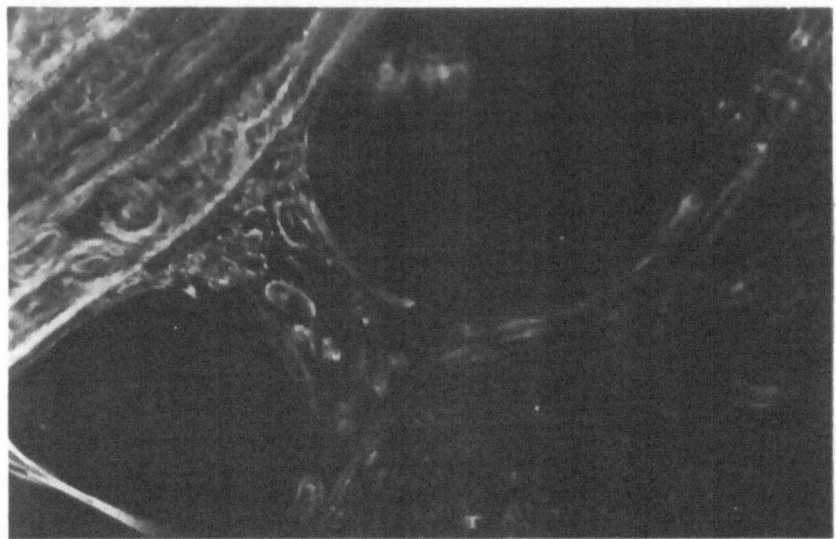

Fig. 2. Growth of cells from the lens capsule (above at the left). Phase contrast microscope (obj. x 20).

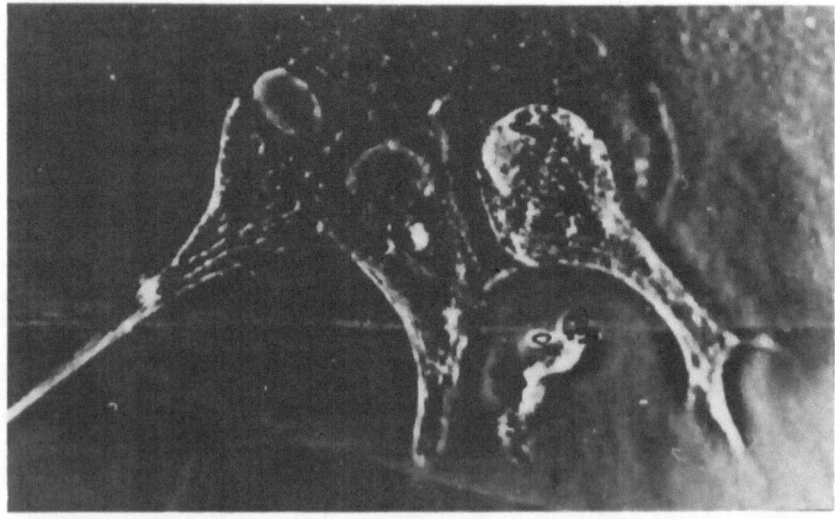

Fig. 3. Migration and juxtaposition of 3 cells. The cells migrated in the direction indicated by the arrows. Phase contrast microscope (obj. x 20).

II. The fresh cultures under the phase-contrast microscope

There are two kinds of cells: (1) elongated cells of fibrillar shape and (2) cells with abundant cytoplasm.

1. *The elongated cells of fibrillar shape* have lengths between 60 and 100 μ (Fig. 6).

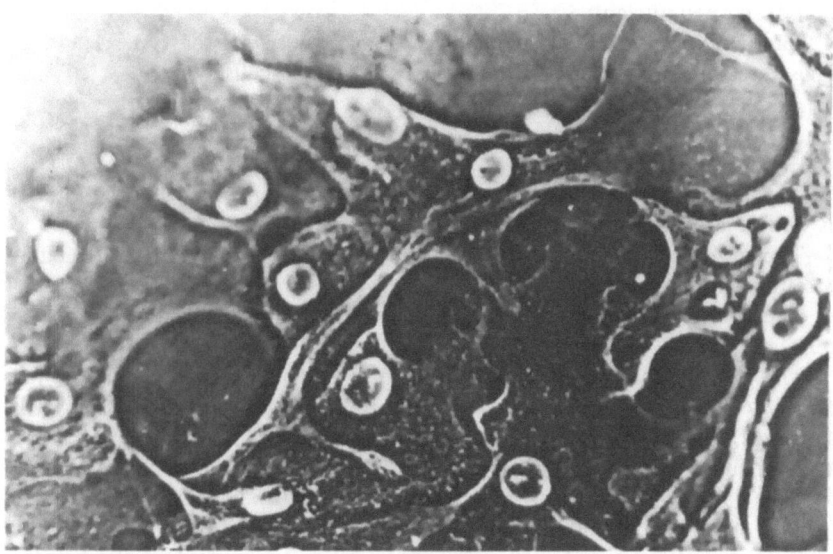

Fig. 4. Cells disposed in round figures. The cytoplasm contains many round or rod-like granules. Phase contrast microscope (obj. x 20).

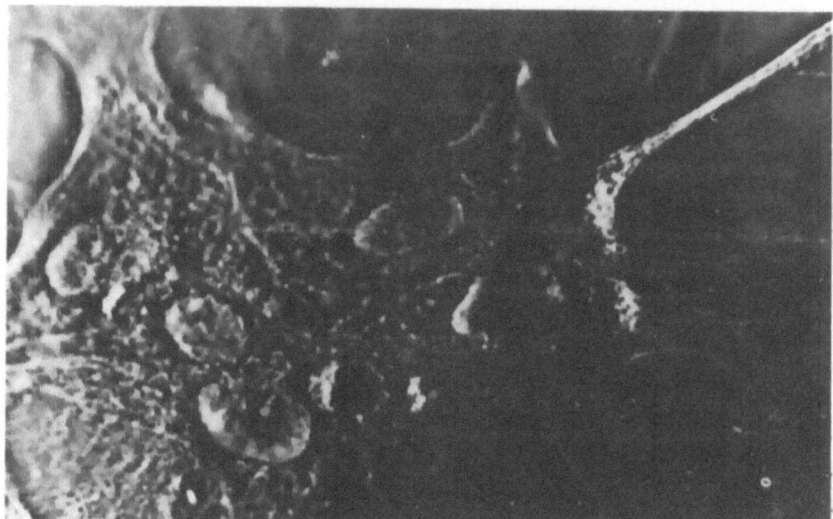

Fig. 5. Cells disposed in mosaic. Dark granules of various sizes are visible in the cytoplasm. Phase contrast microscope (obj. x 50).

They have a more or less central nucleus. They generally cluster together in groups of 2 or 3 (Fig. 3). The cytoplasm contains uniformly distributed dark granulations and mitochondria which show the shape of rods.

2. *The cells with abundant cytoplasm* (Figs. 2 and 3) are polygonal or star-shaped. They have diameters between 30 and 50 μ. They contain numerous granulations and mitochondria regularly distributed throughout the cytoplasmic matrix. The nuclei are oval or rounded and contain 1 to 3 very well developed nucleoli.

There are some cells of shapes intermediate between the types 1 and 2. These are spindle-shaped or more or less star-shaped cells.

III. Histochemical study (Tables I and II)

It is curious to observe that the colloidal iron colours positively the nuclei, as well as a certain number of cytoplasmic granules.

The cytoplasmic matrix is PAS positive. Wilder's reaction for reticulin colours it homogeneously.

The very fine granulations, which are identified in the extensions of the cells, are positive for alcian blue pH 1 and pH 2,5.

The cytoplasmic granules are lysosomes, because they are positive for acid phosphatase and display a red fluorescence after vital staining with acridine orange (FRANÇOIS et al., 1976), whereas the mitochondria display a green fluorescence. The distribution of the lysosomes is homogeneous in the two cell types. The lysosomes are abundant both in the cells which grow on the capsule and also in the cells which develop on the glass lamina. Their distribution is different from that which is observed in the keratocytes, the hyalocytes or the goniocytes.

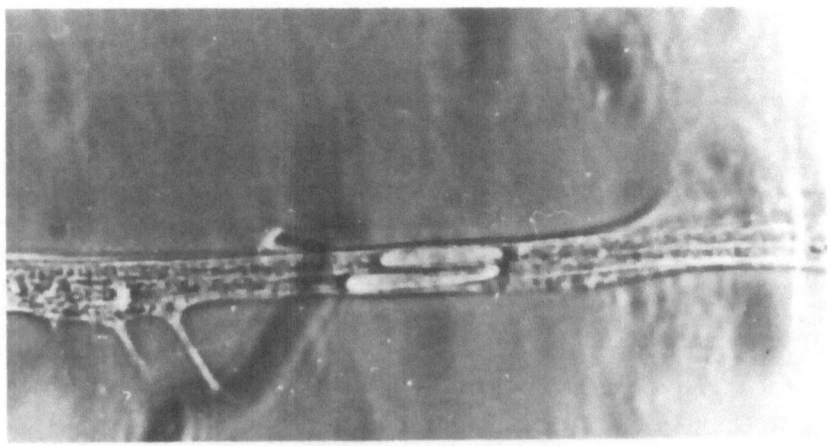

Fig. 6. Cells resembling lens fibres. Very fine pseudo-podia are visible. Phase contrast microscope (obj. x 50).

CONCLUSIONS

The study of the cultures of the lens epithelium is very rewarding. The cells which develop close to the capsule have an appearance which resembles that of the lens fibres, both as regards their elongated shape and also as regards the disposition of the nucleus (Fig. 6). However, as the distance from the specimen increases, the cells appear to become dedifferentiated.

APPELMANS et al. (1968) drew attention to the possible role of the lysosomes in the genesis of cataract. Moreover, we were able to demonstrate a particularly well developed lysosomal system. That fact justifies a number of hypotheses:

1. Certain congenital cataracts might be due to a storage through lack of a lysosomal enzyme.
2. The activation of the lysosomes in traumatic cataracts might give rise to areas of lens necrosis and consequently cause the progression of the opacification.
3. The accumulation, in the course of aging, of 'dense bodies', which constitute the terminal stage of the intralysosomal digestion, might produce a deterioration of the lens cells and cause senile opacification.

The mitochondria are positive for two enzymes: (1) glucose-6-phosphate-dehydrogenase (G-6-PD), which plays a part in anaerobic glycolysis, and (2) lacto-dehydrogenase, which plays a part in aerobic glycolysis. The two respiratory types are therefore possible.

There are small granulations positive for alcian blue pH 1 and pH 2.5. They are probably glycoproteins.

Because the cytoplasmic matrix is positive for PAS and for reticulin, it very probably contains glycoproteins.

The tests for the nucleic acids show that the cells of the lens epithelium can very rapidly display a very great activity of biosynthesis.

SUMMARY

The lens epithelium develops very rapidly in tissue culture. The cells become dedifferentiated as the distance from the specimen increases. They have a very important lysosomal system, which might play a part in the genesis of congenital, traumatic and senile cataracts. The lens uses two respiratory modes, aerobic and anaerobic. The cytoplasmic matrix contains glycoproteins.

REFERENCES

APPELMANS, M., MICHIELS, J. & MISSOTTEN, L. L'autolyse du cristallin: Y a-t-il des lysosomes dans la lentille. In: Biochemistry of the Eye, Ed. by M.V. Dardenne & J. Nordmann, S. Karger, Basel, pp. *344-347* (1968).

KIRBY, D.B. A study of the nutrition of the cristalline lens. The cultivation of the lens epithelium. *Trans. Amer. Acad. Ophthal. Otolaryng.* 31: *137-142* (1926).

LUCAS, D.R. Special cytology of the eye. In: Cells and Tissues in Culture. Methods, Biology and Physiology, Ed. E.N. Willmer, vol. II, Academic Press, London, N.Y. (1965).

NORDMANN, J. Biologie du cristallin. Masson, Paris (1954).

NORDMANN, J. Acquisitions récentes dans le domaine de la biologie du cristallin. *Adv. Ophthal.*, Karger, Basel, 59: *1-47* (1962).

PIRIE, A. & VAN HEYNINGEN, R. Biochemistry of the Eye. Blackwell, Oxford (1956).

VAN HEYNINGEN, R. The lens. In: The Eye, vol. I. Vegetative Physiology and Biochemistry (Ed. H. Davson), Academic Press, N.Y. (1962).

Authors' address:
University Eye Clinic
de Pintelaan 135
Ghent
Belgium

46

ON THE STABILITY OF THE DIFFERENTIATED STATE
– REACTIVATION OF LENS FIBER CELLS TO MITOTIC GROWTH –*

M. IWIG & D. GLÄSSER

(Halle, G.D.R.)

ABSTRACT

Differentiated nuclei containing fiber cells from adult bovine eye lenses are reactivated to mitotic growth in vitro. This process was linked with a transformation of the fiber cells into motile epithelium like cells. These dedifferentiated fiber cells were morpho-logically indistinguishable from cultured lens epithelial cells.

INTRODUCTION

The differentiation of lens epithelial cells into fiber cells is linked with characteristic morphological and biochemical changes (PAPACONSTANTI-NOU, 1967; GLÄSSER, 1971; IWIG & GLÄSSER, 1972; PIATIGORSKY, 1974; PIATIGORSKY et al., 1972; RAFFERTY & ESSON, 1974). One major characteristic of the differentiation process is, that DNA replication and mitosis become less frequent and finally cease in the prospective fiber cells as they differentiate into definitive fibers (MODAK et al., 1968) where-as protein synthesis continues (PAPACONSTANTINOU, 1967; PIATI-GORSKY et al., 1972). During terminal lens cell differentiation fiber cell nuclei become pycnotic, accompanied by a progressive loss of DNA (MODAK et al., 1969). Therefore it was suggested, that in fiber cells the replicative activity is irreversibly inhibited (PAPACONSTANTINOU, 1967; IWIG & GLÄSSER, 1972/73). This proposition was favoured further by tissue culture experiments. Since the early studies of KIRBY (1926) it was suggested that in culture the only cells which survive and multiply are those of the subcapsular epithelium, whereas lens fibers dissolve in the medium within the first 2 to 3 days (MANN, 1948). Here we show, that nuclei containing fiber cells in culture dedifferentiate to replicating epithelium-like cells.

MATERIALS AND METHODS

Tissue culture medium according to Eagle (MEM); phosphate buffered salt solution (PBS) (Staatliches Institut für Immumpräparate und Nährmedien,

---

* Dedicated to Prof. Dr. J. Nordmann on his 80th birthday.
Abbreviations:
MEM: Minimal Essential Medium according to Eagle
PBS: Phosphate Buffered Salt solution

Berlin-GDR). Trypsin cryst. (Spofa, Prague-CSSR). Calf serum, abattoir collected, inactivated.

Cultivation and subcultivation of lens epithelial cells as described previously (IWIG & GLÄSSER, 1975).

Cultivation of lens fiber cells: The lenses were removed from the eyes of

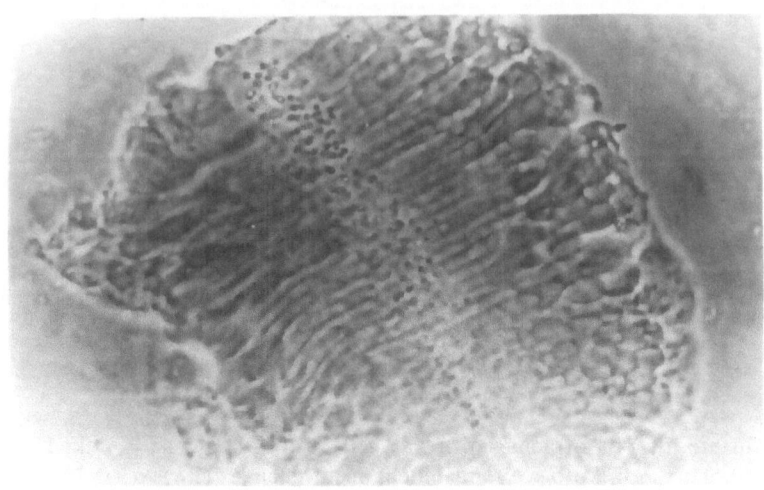

Fig. 1. Bundle of fiber cells dissected from the equator of the lens: The microphotograph shows nuclei containing fiber cells 1 hour after explantation. The ends of the fiber cells are swollen and rounded up. Phase contrast; 100 x

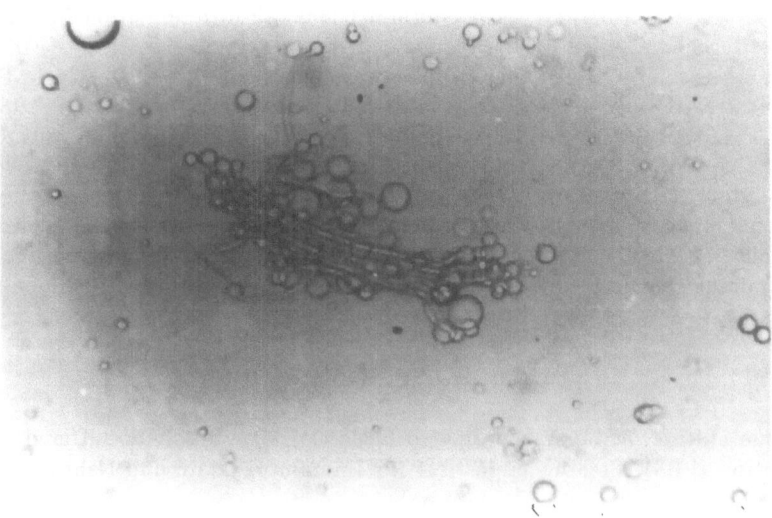

Fig. 2. Bundle of fiber cells after trypsinization: Trypsinized fiber cells $2\frac{1}{2}$ hours after explantation. The ends of the fiber cells are swollen and rounded up. Some fiber cells are subdivided into globules. Microphotograph 50 x

1 to 2 years old animals 2 to 3 hours after sacrificing. The lens capsule was incised and pulled off. Thereafter pieces of the superficial layer of fiber cells were cut along the equator of the lens and transferred to Petri dishes or culture bottles. In some experiments large bundles of fiber cells were trypsinized (0.1% (w/v) trypsin in MEM) for 5 to 20 min and/or mechanically

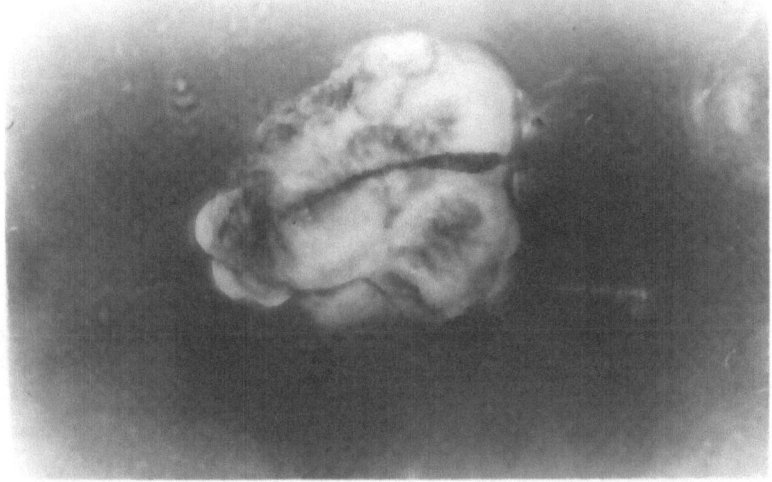

Fig. 3. Fiber cell aggregate: 2 days after explantation of fiber cells a small aggregate adhere to the bottom of the culture vessel. Phase contrast: 100 x

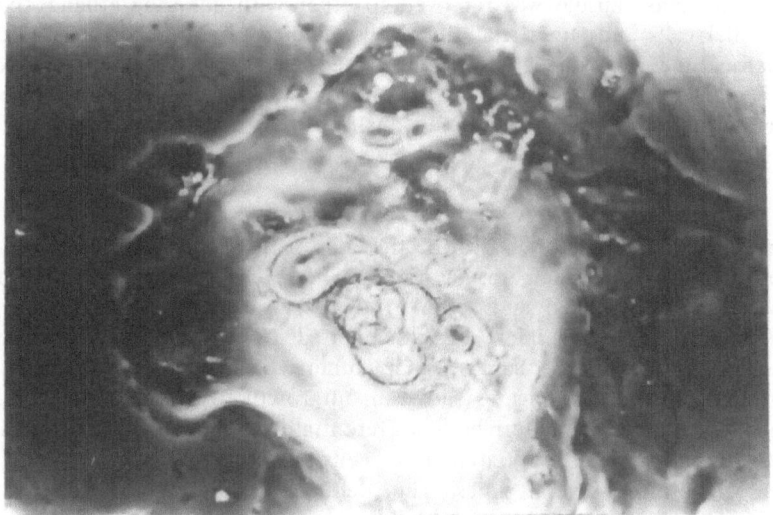

Fig. 4. Fiber cell aggregate with outgrowth of 'dedifferentiated' fiber cells: The fiber cell preparation was made after a 30 sec. ethanol treatment of the intact lens. The outgrowth of epithelium like fiber cells was observed 9 days after explantation. Phase contrast: 100 x

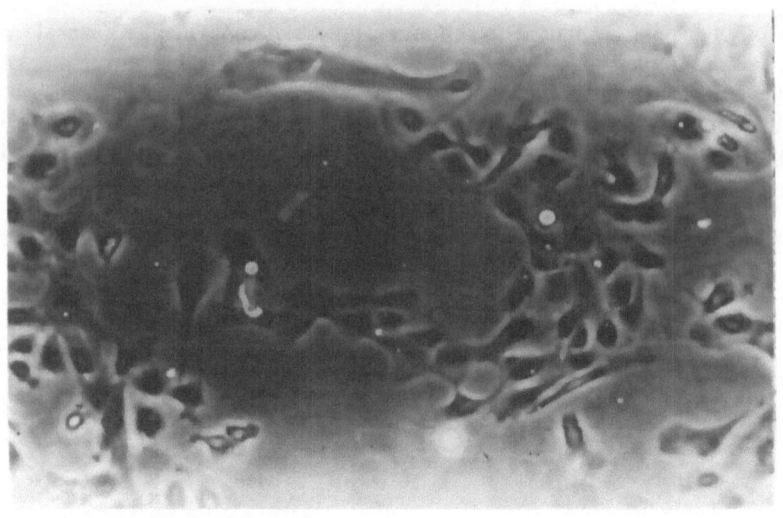

Fig. 5. Subcultured 'dedifferentiated' fiber cells: The fiber cell preparation was taken from a lens immersed in ethanol for 30 sec. The microphotograph shows cells of the sixth subculture. Phase contrast; 100 x

separated. The culture medium was MEM supplemented with 10% calf serum. Fiber cell preparations without being contaminated with epithelial cells were obtained in the following way: Intact lenses were immersed in ethanol (70%; v/v) during 10 to 60 sec. and rinsed with MEM for 20 sec. Then the lens capsule was removed together with adhering ethanol-fixed epithelial cells and superficial fiber cells. Thereafter the fiber cells of the equator zone were dissected and cultivated as described above. For reference epithelial cells of the central zone of the same ethanol-treated lens were cultured under identical conditions.

RESULTS

During the first hours of cultivation the ends of the fiber cells round up and swell to many times their normal volume (Fig. 1). After trypsinization this process is strengthened and some of the fiber cells are subdivided into several globules (Fig. 2). Many of these bloated structures undergo autolysis; others go to form dense aggregates and adhere to the bottom of the culture vial (Fig. 3). These aggregates show an outgrowth of epithelium-like cells (Fig. 4), in the following termed 'dedifferentiated' fiber cells. During further cultivation the 'dedifferentiated' fiber cells show mitotic growth and have been subcultured several times. The 'dedifferentiated' fiber cells (Fig. 5) were morphologically indistinguishable from subcultured epithelial cells (Fig. 6) as judged by light microscopy. Among normal-shaped 'dedifferentiated' fiber cells sometimes we found very large, flattened fiber cells (Fig. 7). Some of them were observed over a period of 3 months, but we never found any mitosis.

By reason of the morphological identity between 'dedifferentiated' fiber cells and cultured epithelial cells a contamination of fiber cell preparations by epithelial cells has to be excluded. Therefore the epithelial cells were fixed with ethanol before making fiber cell preparations as described in methods. Table I demonstrates the effect of ethanol treatment on the viabil-

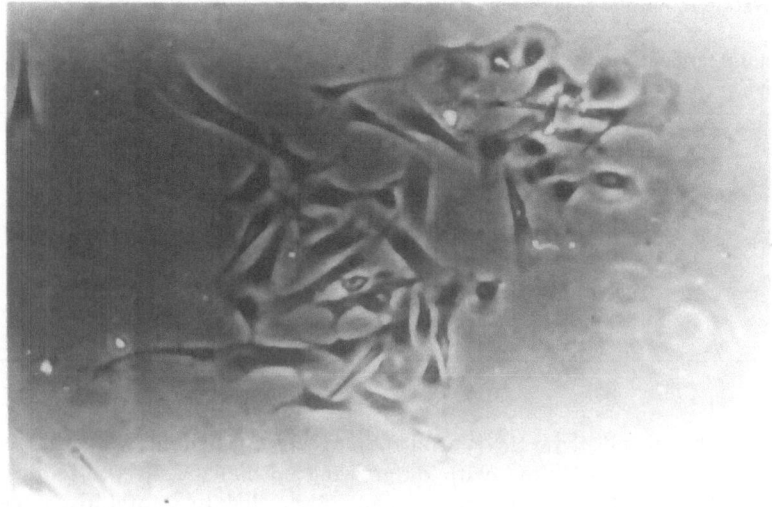

Fig. 6. Subcultured epithelial cells from bovine eye lenses: The microphotograph shows epithelial cells of the 29th subculture. Phase contrast: 100 x

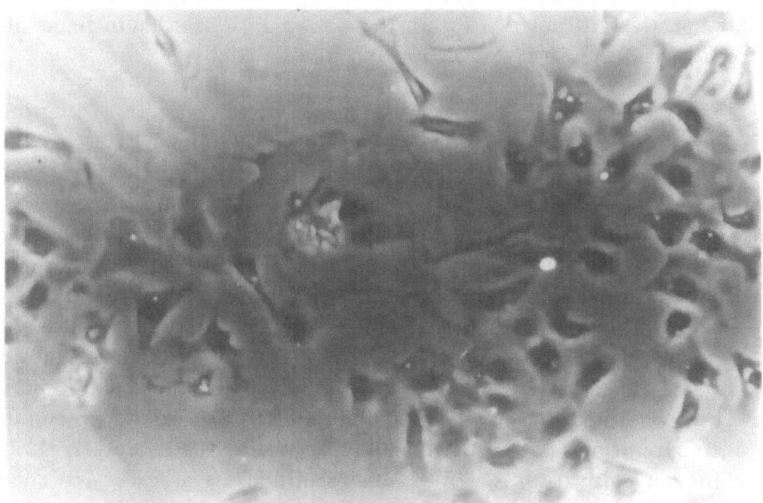

Fig. 7. Large, flattened 'fiber' cell: The fiber cell preparation was made after a 30 sec. ethanol treatment of the lens. The microphotograph was taken from the first subculture and shows a very large flattened 'fiber' cell in the midst of normal shaped epithelium like, 'dedifferentiated' fiber cells. Phase contrast: 100 x

Table I. Effect of ethanol-treatment of intact bovine eye lenses on mitotic growth of epithelial cells and fiber cells.

Intact lenses were immersed in ethanol (70%; v/v) for the time indicated. Then epithelial cells and fiber cells were cultured as described. The cultures were observed for mitotic growth over a period of 3 weeks. The quotient gives numbers of preparations with reactivation to mitotic growth per total numbers of preparations.

Ethanol-treatment Seconds	Epithelial cell preparation	Fiber cell preparation
0	14/14	6/7
10	5/5	
15	0/1	1/1
20	2/5	
25	0/5	
30	0/25	10/19
40	0/8	2/6
60	0/3	0/3

ity of epithelial cells from the central zone of lens epithelium. Above 10 sec. the number of preparations with outgrowing epithelial cells was reduced. Ethanol treatment lasting for more than 25 sec. led to a total loss in cell viability. Cell sheets of fixed epithelial cells swam in the culture medium without any ability to aggregate or to adhere to the substratum. Although ethanol treatment of 25, 30, and 40 sec. respectively led to a total loss in viability of epithelial cells, mitotic growth was found with 10 from 19 and 2 from 6 fiber cell preparations cultured after an ethanol treatment of 30 or 40 sec. respectively (Table I). Within these preparations ethanol fixed fiber cells from the superficial layers were often found.

DISCUSSION

Contrary to the statements of KIRBY (1926) and MANN (1948) our results demonstrate that lens fiber cells can be reactivated to mitotic growth in vitro. During cultivation lens fiber cells undergo essential morphological changes. First of all the ends of the fiber cells round up and swell to many times their normal volume. These pherical structures may be identical with the so-called Morgagnian globules, which appear in the cleft after lens injury in vivo and are considered to be breakdown products of the lens fibers (RAFFERTY & GOOSSENS, 1975). Studying wound repair in needle injured organ cultured lenses, these bubble like entities were also seen, but related to alterations of the epithelial cells (WEINSIEDER et al., 1970). During further cultivation the fiber cells form dense aggregates and adhere to the bottom of the culture vessel. Thereafter an outgrowth of epithelium-like cells was observed, morphologically indistinguishable from epithelial cells.

Mitotic growth was only found after transformation of fiber cells into motile epithelium-like cells. It is worth stressing that this phenomenon of dedifferentiation was not a matter of 'overgrowth' of fiber cells by a small number of contaminating epithelial cells. Contamination of the fiber cell preparations was excluded by the ethanol-fixation procedure, as described above. Therefore we suppose, that the process of dedifferentiation is a precondition for the reactivation of fiber cell nuclei. Similar observations were made with other differentiated cells. In vitro liberated chondroblasts (HOLTZER & ABBOTT, 1968; SCHILTZ et al., 1973) and cells from a myogenic clone transform into motile cells that are morphologically indistinguishable from authentic fibroblasts.

Our results on the reactivation of lens fiber cell nuclei are also in accordance with the reactivation of nuclei from other fully differentiated cells, e.g. chick erythrocytes (EGE et al., 1975).

Regarding lens fiber cells one must suggest that only cells of earlier differentiation stages can be reactivated to mitotic growth since during terminal differentiation the cell nuclei become pycnotic and lose their DNA.

The large flattened cell shown in Fig. 7 may represent a fiber cell population which has still retained the ability to adhere to and to flatten on the substratum but has already lost the ability to become reactivated to motile mitotically growing epithelium-like cells.

The relation between the regulation of growth and cell differentiation is of general importance. There are diverse factors effective in stimulating mitotic dormant epithelial cells of organ cultured eye lenses to mitosis (activation of $G_0 \rightarrow G_1$ transition) such as mechanical injury (BITO & HARDING, 1965; WEINSIEDER et al., 1970), calf serum (HARDING et al., 1968; BAGCHI et al., 1971) and insulin (REDDAN et al., 1972). Moreover reactivation to mitosis is observed after explantation of lens epithelial cells into a suitable culture medium (FRIEDRICH & GLÄSSER, 1971; SHAPIRO, et al., 1969) as well as after transplantation of epithelial cell nuclei into parthenogenetically activated eggs (MUGGLETON-HARRIS & PEZZELLA, 1972). On the other hand we have shown (GLÄSSER et al., 1975; GLÄSSER & IWIG, 1975) that cell adherence, cell flattening, and protein synthesis of primarily cultured lens epithelial cells can be specifically inhibited by low concentrations of C_6-substituted purines. This in turn leads to a delay in the reactivation of mitotic growth (retardation of $G_0 \rightarrow G_1$ transition). In further investigations it has to be shown whether C_6-substituted purines are also effective in retarding the reactivation of lens fiber cells.

ACKNOWLEDGEMENT

The skilful technical assistance of Mrs. Barbara Michel is gratefully acknowledged.

REFERENCES

ABBOTT, J., J. SCHILTZ, S. DIENSTMAN & H. HOLTZER. The phenotypic complexity of myogenic clones. *Proc. Natl. Acad. Sci. USA* 71: *1506-1510* (1974).

BAGCHI, M., C. HARDING, N. UNAKAR & J. REDDAN. Experimental modification of the temporal aspects of the serum-induced cell cycle in the cultured adult rabbit lens. *Ophthal.Res.* 2: *133-142* (1971).

BITO, L.Z. & C.V. HARDING. Patterns of cellular organization and cell division in the epithelium of the cultured lens. *Exp. Eye Res.* 4: *146-161* (1965).

EGE, T., J. ZEUTHEN & N.R. RINGERTZ. Reactivation of chick erythrocyte nuclei after fusion with enucleated cells. *Somat. Cell Genet.* 1: *65-80* (1975).

FRIEDRICH, E. & D. GLAESSER. Zum Wachstum der Epithelzellen von Rinderaugenlinsen in der Primärkultur. *Acta biol. med. germ.* 27: *41-53* (1971).

GLAESSER, D. Enzymologische und enzymimmunologische Untersuchungen zur Zelldifferenzierung in Augenlinsen. Nova Acta Leopoldina, Neue Folge, No. 197, Vol. 36. Barth, Leipzig 1971.

GLÄSSER, D., M. IWIG & E. WEBER. Zur Regulation altersabhängiger Phänomene: Einfluss C_6-substituierter Purine auf Zellaggregation und Zellemigration in der Primärkultur von Linsenepithelzellen. *Z. Alternsforsch.* 30: *359-370* (1975).

GLÄSSER, D. & M. IWIG. Low concentrations of C_6-substituted purines retard the G_0 → G_1 transition of bovine lens epithelium cells. *FEBS Letters* 60: *205-209* (1975).

HARDING, C.V., W.L. WILSON, J.R. WILSON, J.R. REDDAN & V.N. REDDY. Triggering of the cell cycle in an organized tissue in vitro. *J. Cell Physiol.* 72: *213-220* (1968).

HOLTZER, H. & J. ABBOTT. Oscillations of the chondrogenic phenotype in vitro. In: The stability of the differentiated state. Ed. H. Ursprung. pp. 1-16. Springer, Berlin 1968.

IWIG, M. & D. GLAESSER. Investigations on mitotic activity, cell density, and enzyme activities in the bovine eye lens during cell differentiation. *Ophthal. Res.* 4: *328-342* (1972/73).

IWIG, M. & D. GLAESSER. DNS- und Protein-Synthese in kultivierten Linsenepithelzellen. I. Testsystem. *Acta biol. med. germ.* 34: *987-996* (1975).

KIRBY, D.B. Trans. Amer. Acad. Ophthal. Otolaryng. p. 137 (1926). cit. by Mann (1948).

MANN, I. Tissue cultures of mouse lens epithelium. *Brit. J. Ophthal.* 32: *591-596* (1948).

MODAK, S.P., G. MORRIS & T. YAMADA. DNA synthesis and mitotic activity during early development of chick lens. *Develop. Biol.* 17: *544-561* (1968).

MODAK, S.P., R.C. VON BORSTEL & F.J. BOLLUM. Terminal lens cell differentiation. II Template activity of DNA during nuclear degeneration. *Exptl. Cell Res.* 56: *105-113* (1969).

MUGGLETON-HARRIS, A.L. & K. PEZZELLA. The ability of the lens cell nucleus to promote complete embryonic development through to metamorphosis and its applications to ophthalmic gerontology. *Exp. Geront.* 7: *427-431* (1972).

PIATIGORSKY, J. Differentiation of lens fiber cells: a brief review of recent developments. *Develop Biol.* 40: *f21-f23* (1974).

PIATIGORSKY, J., H.E. DE WEBSTER & S.P. CRAIG. Protein synthesis and ultrastructure during the formation of embryonic chick lens fibers in vivo and in vitro. *Develop. Biol.* 27: *176-189* (1972).

PAPACONSTANTINOU, J. Molecular aspects of lens cell differentiation. *Science* 156: *338-346* (1967).

RAFFERTY, N.S. & E.A. ESSON. An electron-microscope study of adult mouse lens: some ultrastructural specializations. *J. Ultrastr. Res.* 46: *239-253* (1974).

RAFFERTY, N.S. & W. GOOSSENS. Ultrastructural studies of traumatic cataractogenesis Observations of a repair process in mouse lens. *Amer. J. Anat.* 142: *177-200* (1975).

REDDAN, J.R., C.V. HARDING, H. ROTHSTEIN, M.W. CROTTY, P. LEE & N. FREEMAN. Stimulation of mitosis in the vertebrate lens in the presence of insulin. *Ophthal. Res.* 3 *65-82* (1972).

SCHILTZ, J.R., R. MAYNE & H. HOLTZER. The synthesis of collagen and glycosaminoglycans by dedifferentiated chondroblasts in culture. *Differentiation* 1: *97-108* (1973).

SHAPIRO, A.L., I.M. SIEGEL, M.D. SCHARFF & E. ROBBINS. Characteristics of cultured lens epithelium. *Invest. Ophthal.* 8: *393-400* (1969).

WEINSIEDER, A., H. ROTHSTEIN & J. GIERTHY. A comparison of wound repair in cultured lenses with that occurring in the lenses of living animals. *Ophthal. Res.* 1: *279-291* (1970).

Keywords:

Lens fiber cells
Tissue cultivation
Dedifferentiation
Mitotic growth
Regulation of mitosis

Authors' address:

Physiologisch-chemisches Institut
Martin-Luther-Universität Halle-Wittenberg
402 HALLE (Saale)
Hollystr. 1
G.D.R.

ON THE CHROMOSOMAL PROTEINS OF LENS EPITHELIUM

ROBERT C. BRIGGS, NORMAN WAINWRIGHT & HOWARD ROTHSTEIN

(Burlington, Vermont)

ABSTRACT

Chromosomal proteins of lens epithelium from bullfrogs, leopard frogs, and rabbits have been isolated and compared. Gels of frog lens histones contain one more band than those of rabbits. Qualitatively, the NHCPs of the two amphibians are nearly identical. Coupling between histone and DNA synthesis in the rabbit lens was demonstrated by use of cytosine arabinoside. The block was reversed with deoxycytidine.

INTRODUCTION

There are two general types of chromosomal protein in eukaryotic organisms, the basic histones and the basic and acidic nonhistone chromosomal proteins (NHCPs). Histones are thought to be nonspecific repressors of gene transcription and are involved in the organization of DNA in the chromosomes (BONNER & GARRARD, 1974; ELGIN & WEINTRAUB, 1975). The specific control of gene transcription is believed by some to reside in the NHCPs (STEIN et al., 1974; ELGIN & WEINTRAUB, 1975; STEIN et al., 1975). The most definitive evidence for this separation of function between the two groups of chromosomal proteins comes from mixing-reconstitution experiments (see reviews by STEIN et al., 1974 and STEIN et al., 1975). Different experimental approaches indicate that some of the NHCPs are probably also involved in the organization of chromosomes and in the general mechanism of gene transcription and RNA processing (ELGIN & WEINTRAUB, 1975). Changes in NHCPs reportedly occur together with variations in gene transcription (such as during the cell cycle) (STEIN & BASERGA, 1970; STEIN & BORUN, 1972; GERNER & HUMPHREY, 1973; JOHNSON et al., 1974; KARN et al., 1974; BASERGA, 1975).

The suitability of the lens for work in these areas is well recognized (see reviews by PAPACONSTANTINOU, 1967; ROTHSTEIN, 1968; HARDING et al., 1971). However, the small amount of material available has limited the biochemical analysis of chromosomal proteins in these studies. Recently, a procedure has been developed for electrophoretic analysis of histones and NHCPs from rabbit lens epithelium. The initial application was an analysis of chromosomal protein changes associated with the cell cycle of lens epithelial cells maintained in organ culture (BRIGGS et al., 1976a). The findings were similar to those made in other *in vitro* systems (BHORJEE & PEDERSON, 1972; STEIN & BORUN, 1972; KARN et al., 1974). Since then, chromosomal proteins have been examined while the cells were traversing the cycle *in vivo* (BRIGGS et al., 1976b). Histone labeling was confined to the DNA synthetic phase in both cases with varying levels of NHCP labeling during all cycle phases.

The chromatin isolation procedure has also been adapted for use with amphibian lenses. In this report we will present a comparison of these proteins from the lenses of a number of species in addition to those originating from the frog erythrocyte.

In a previous account we reported the presence of an electrophoretic band with migration characteristics like the tissue-specific histone H5 (f2c)* (JOHNSON & ROTHSTEIN, 1970). Since the publication of that report, the embryonic chick lens was found not to contain this histone (TENG et al., 1974). The presence of the molecule was sought in rabbit lens and once again in the bullfrog. The problem of coupling histone and DNA synthesis was also reexamined.

MATERIALS AND METHODS

Lenses were obtained from either adult frogs (*Rana catesbeiana* and *Rana pipiens berlandieri*) or New Zealand white rabbits (2.0-2.6 Kg). The lenses were isolated by the posterior approach as previously described for frog (ROTHSTEIN, 1968) and rabbit (WILSON et al., 1967).

Rabbit lenses were cultured in 30 ml of medium 199 (Grand Island Biological Company, Grand Island, New York) with 20% rabbit serum (Pel Freez Biological Company, Rogers, Arkansas) (R20) in silicone-stoppered bottles at 34.8 °C with gentamicin (100 μg/ml). The inhibitors cytosine arabinoside (CA) (40 μg/ml) or fluorodeoxyuridine (FUdR) (10^{-5} M) were added initially and were also present during labeling. Labeling of chromosomal proteins was achieved by exposing lenses to Earle's balanced salt solution (Grand Island Biological Company), 2% fetal calf serum and ^{3}H-leucine (5 μCi/ml) (54 Ci/mM) with or without appropriate inhibitors. For the analysis of CA reversibility after 32 hr. of culture, the lenses were transferred to R20 containing deoxycytidine (80 μg/ml) and ^{3}H-Tdr (5 μCi/ml) (6.7 Ci/mM). Lenses were fixed in Carnoy's solution and prepared for autoradiography (ROTHSTEIN et al., 1966). The levels of inhibition achieved at 32 hr. in culture were determined by scintillation counting of lens epithelial whole mount preparations (ROTHSTEIN et al., 1966) after a 1 hr. exposure to ^{3}H-Tdr (1 μci/ml) (6.7 Ci/mM) for CA (40 μg/ml), or ^{3}H-Cdr (2 μCi/ml) (25 Ci/mM) for FUdR (10^{-5},M) in Earle's balanced salt solution.

Chromatin was isolated from lenses immediately after they were dissected free of the globe or after one hour of labeling (BRIGGS et al., 1976a). Ten rabbit lenses were used for the isolation. In the case of *Rana catesbeiana* and *Rana pipiens berlandieri*, 20 and 72 lenses were used respectively. Blood was obtained (5.0 ml) from a single *Rana catesbeiana* for the preparation of red blood cell chromatin. One-tenth volume of 0.15 trisodium citrate was added to prevent clotting and the cells were collected by centrifugation. The cells were then washed three times in SSC (0.14 M

---

* Ciba Symposium histone nomenclature H1, H2a, H2b, H3, H4, and H5.

sodium chloride, 0.01 M trisodium citrate) and chromatin was prepared as with the lens cells.

The chromosomal proteins were electrophoretically separated for analysis in the presence of DNA on sodium dodecyl sulfate (SDS), urea, 10% polyacrylamide gels (BRIGGS et al., 1976a). In some experiments histones were acid extracted (0.4 N H_2SO_4) from the chromatin and electrophoretically separated on the acid urea histone gels (PANYIM & CHALKLEY, 1969a).

RESULTS

The electrophoretic profile of the rabbit lens histones is very similar to that obtained from a commercial preparation of calf thymus histone (Fig. 1). Histones from bullfrog (*Rana catesbeiana*) lens epithelium have an extra band migrating between the H1 and H3 (Fig. 1) which may be H5 (EDWARDS & HNILICA, 1968; DICK & JOHNS, 1969). This band and the H1 were also selectively extracted from bullfrog lens chromatin with 5.0% perchloric acid. The H1 and H5 fractions are known to share this solubility property.

Bullfrog lens epithelial chromosomal proteins (NHCPs and histones) were electrophoretically separated on SDS, urea gels. The histone bands were identified by acid extraction and migration characteristics (Fig. 2A). Chromosomal proteins were also prepared from bullfrog erythrocytes (Fig. 2B). The major bands in the erythrocyte preparation correspond closely to the histones in the bullfrog lens chromatin. Histones have been found to be the major constituent of erythrocyte chromosomal proteins (HNILICA, 1972). The close similarity in electrophoretic profiles of *Rana pipiens berlandieri* (Fig. 2C) and *Rana catesbeiana* (Fig. 2A) NHCPs attests to the limited spe-

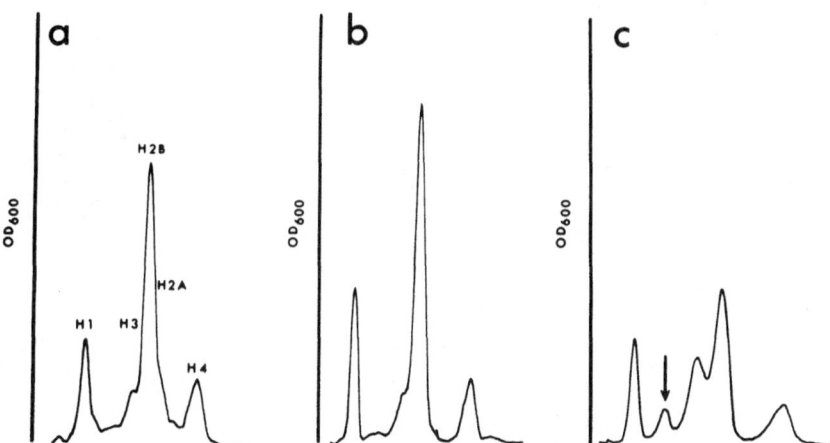

Fig. 1. Densitometric tracing of acid, urea, histone polyacrylamide gel electrophoresis. Histones obtained from (a) calf thymus (commercially acquired), (b) rabbit lens, (c) bullfrog lens. Note additional band migrating between H1 and H3 in the bullfrog lens preparation.

59

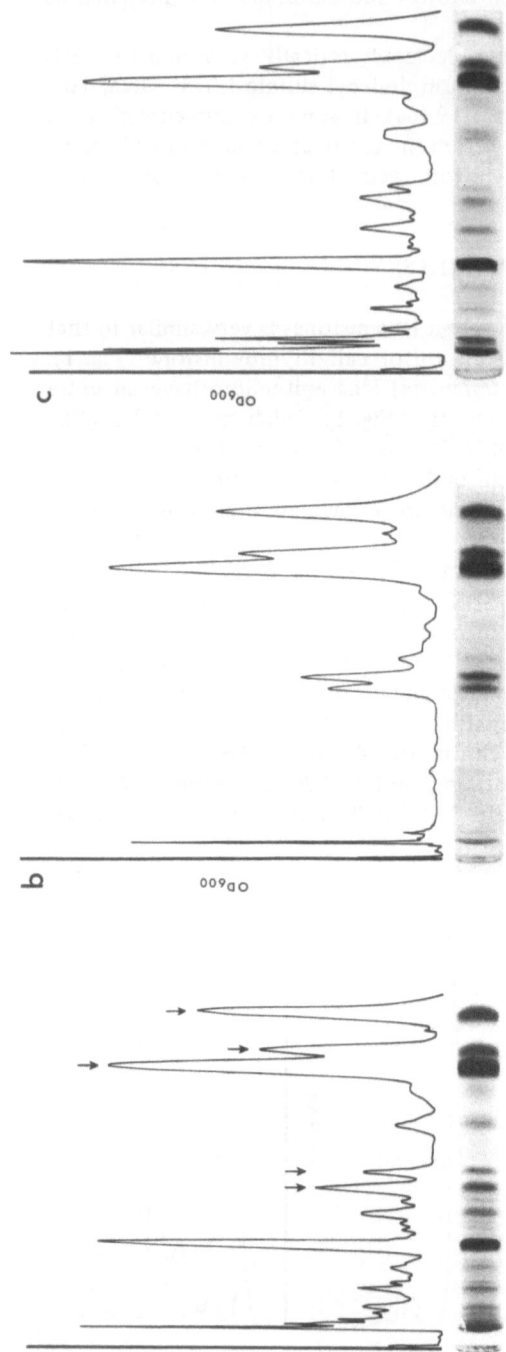

Fig. 2. Polyacrylamide, sodium dodecyl sulfate, urea, electrophoretic gels, and densitometric tracings of chromosomal proteins obtained from (a) *Rana catesbeiana* lens (histone bands indicated), (b) *Rana catesbeiana* erythrocytes, (c) *Rana pipiens berlandieri* lens.

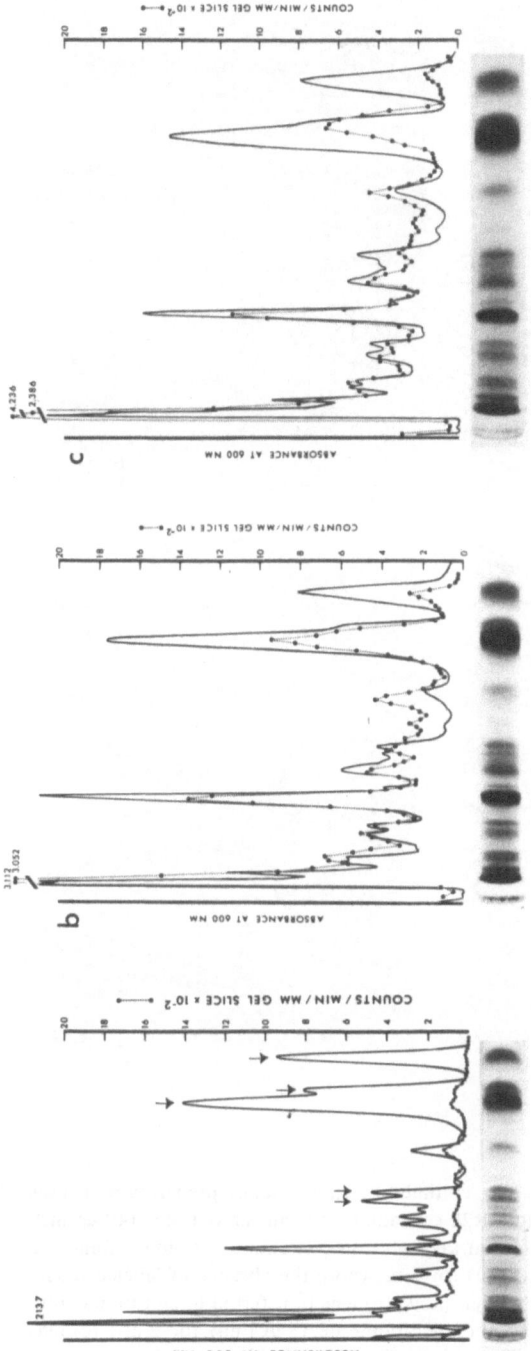

Fig. 3. Polyacrylamide, sodium dodecyl sulfate, urea, electrophoretic gels and densitometric tracings of chromosomal proteins. Lenses were exposed to ^{3}H-leucine (5 μCi/ml) with or without appropriate inhibitors for one hour prior to chromatin isolation. Incorporation was detected by gel slicing and scintillation counting. (a) Rabbit lens epithelium cultured in R20 (medium 199 with 20% rabbit serum) with cytosine arabinoside (40 μg/ml) for 32 hr. (histone bands indicated), (b) rabbit lens epithelium cultured in R20 for 32 hr. without inhibitors, (c) rabbit lens epithelium cultured in R20 with 10^{-5} M FUdR for 32 hr.

61

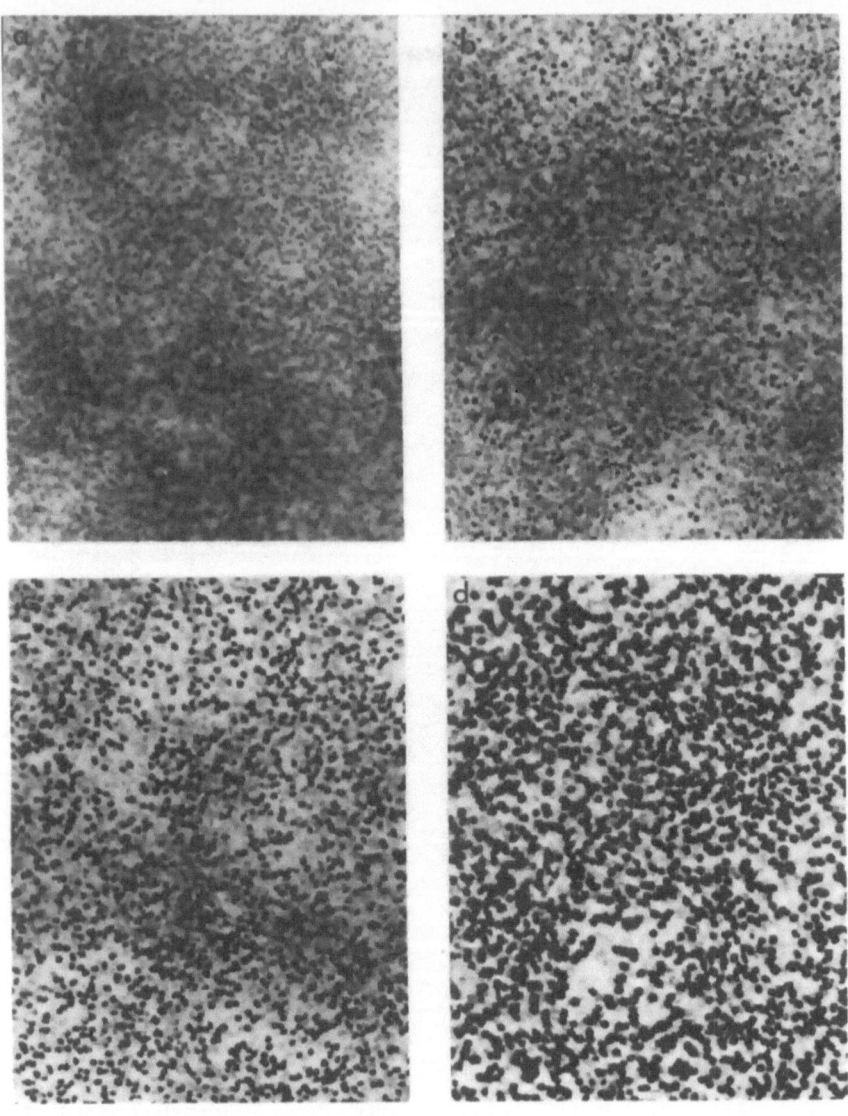

Fig. 4. Autoradiograms of rabbit lens epithelium whole mount preparation. Lenses cultured for 32 hr. in culture medium R20 containing cytosine arabinoside (40 μg/ml). (a) Lens transferred to Earle's balanced salt solution containing cytosine arabinoside (40 μg/ml) and ^{3}H-thymidine (5 μCi/ml) for 1 hr. (note the absence of labeled nuclei demonstrating the inhibition of DNA synthesis, (b) lens transferred to culture medium R20 with deoxycytidine (80 μg/ml) and ^{3}H-thymidine (5 μCi/ml) for 2 hr., (c) lens transferred to the same media described in (b) for 5.5 hr., (d) lens transferred to same media described in (b) for 20 hr. [Note increasing number of labeled nuclei with later times after cytosine arabinoside removal and addition of deoxycytine, (b) to (d)].

cies specificity of these proteins as detected by this analytical technique. Differences are more apparent between NHCPs of rabbit lenses (Fig. 3) and those of the amphibian lenses (Fig. 2A and 2C).

The rabbit chromosomal proteins in Figure 3A were obtained from lenses cultured for 32 hr. (DNA synthetic period) in serum containing media in the presence of CA, a DNA synthetic inhibitor. Note the low level of ^{3}H-leucine incorporation into the histone bands. After 32 hr. in serum culture without inhibitor, histone labeling was high (Fig. 3B). This labeling was not diminished by inhibiting DNA synthesis with 10^{-5} M FUdR (Fig. 3C). The inhibition of DNA synthesis in this case is about 60% as determined by ^{3}H-Cdr incorporation. The level of NHCP and histone labeling is the same as found after 32 hr. of serum culture without FUdR (Fig. 3B). The DNA synthesis inhibition with CA was greater than 90% as determined by ^{3}H-Tdr incorporation. Under these conditions, histone labeling is depressed as is that of NHCPs (but to a lesser degree). The ratio of NHCPs to histones in the chromatin isolated from CA-treated lenses is 1.14 as determined from the respective areas under the absorbance curve in Figure 3A. This ratio is noticeably lower than that in the culture without inhibitor (1.40) (Fig. 3B) and in the presence of 10^{-5} M FUdR (1.30) (Fig. 3C). After CA removal and addition of deoxycytidine, the block of DNA synthesis was released as shown by incorporation of ^{3}H-Tdr (Fig. 4).

DISCUSSION

We have reported the presence of a histone in the bullfrog lens with electrophoretic migration characteristics similar to that of H5 (JOHNSON & ROTHSTEIN, 1970). This histone was not found in the embryonic chick lens (TENG et al., 1974) or in that of the adult chicken (JOHNSON, A.W., personal communication). In this report we show it is absent in the adult rabbit lens. Its presence in bullfrog lens has been corroborated. A histone band with similar characteristics was detected in a number of nondividing tissues (PANYIM & CHALKLEY, 1969b). The functional significance of H5 is unknown (ELGIN & WEINTRAUB, 1975). The electrophoretic and solubility characteristics of the histone found in the bullfrog lenses indicate a probable relationship to H5. Amino acid analysis of the lens histone has not, however, been performed. Its presence in bullfrog and absence in rabbit and chicken lenses does not help in assigning a physiological role. Lens epithelial cells in all of these species are active in transcription and some are undergoing division in the germinative zone of all these tissues. The time of appearance of the crystallins during development in the frog lens does not appear to be different from other species (MCDEVITT et al., 1969). Although the classes of crystallins are similar in the frog to other species, the quantities are different (MCDEVITT, 1967). Changes in crystallins were observed in the post-metamorphic frog (POLANSKY & BENNETT, 1973). Whether the unique frog lens histone is related to these changes in crystallins has not been determined.

The functional separation of histones and NHCPs is supported by the comparison of bullfrog lens and erythrocyte total chromosomal proteins (Fig. 2). The paucity of NHCPs obtained from the erythrocyte is notable, while the histone bands of the two tissues correspond closely. The total lens chromosomal protein fractions of the two amphibian species are clearly identical. The difference between frog and rabbit NHCPs is more significant indicating the existence of limited species specificity.

The employment of CA has allowed the demonstration of a coupling mechanism between histone and DNA synthesis. FUdR probably does not prevent histone synthesis in lenses because it does not prevent that of DNA sufficiently. CA almost obliterates DNA synthesis and was observed to stop incorporation of tritiated leucine into histones. The present studies also confirm the independence of NHCP synthesis from that of DNA. When DNA synthesis is disrupted during S phase, the NHCP labeling remains at S phase levels (STEIN & BORUN, 1972; STEIN & THRALL, 1973; KRAUSE et al., 1975). However, when cells are prevented from beginning DNA synthesis, as in our lens experiments, the NHCP labeling levels are not characteristic of S (compare Fig. 3A with Fig. 3B) but of Gl (GERNER & HUMPHREY, 1973; BRIGGS et al., 1976a). The inhibitor may exert non-specific influences but the effects observed cannot be due to cell death as shown by their reversibility. The reversal of the CA block has been observed by IWIG & GLASSER (1975) to require an extended period of time. Those authors advised against the use of CA for synchronizing lens cells. Our results support this caveat and also show that the delay noted may be due, in part, to nonsynchronous release of the cells from the block.

This work was supported by USPHS grant EY00281-11 from the National Eye Institute.

REFERENCES

BASERGA, R. Non-histone chromosomal proteins in normal and abnormal growth. *Life Sci.* 15: *1057-1071* (1975).

BHORJEE, J.S. & PEDERSON, T. Nonhistone chromosomal proteins in synchronized HeLa cells. *Proc. Nat. Acad. Sci. USA* 69: *3345-3349* (1972).

BONNER, J. GARRARD, W.T. Biology of the histones. *Life Sci.* 14: *209-221* (1974).

BRIGGS, R.C., ROTHSTEIN, H. & WAINWRIGHT, N. Cell cycle variations in chromosomal proteins of the lens epithelium. *Exptl. Cell Res.* 99: *95-105* (1976a).

BRIGGS, R.C., WAINWRIGHT, N. & ROTHSTEIN, H. Biochemical events associated with healing of a chemical injury in the rabbit lens. (in preparation) (1976b).

DICK, C. & JOHNS, E.W. A quantitative comparison of histones from immature and mature erythroid cells of the duck. *Biochim. Biophys. Acta* 175: *414-418* (1969).

EDWARDS, L.J. & HNILICA, L.S. The specificity of histones in nucleated erythrocytes. *Experientia* 24: *228-229* (1968).

ELGIN, S.C.R. & WEINTRAUB, H. Chromosomal proteins and chromatin structure. *Ann. Rev. Biochem.* 44: *725-773* (1975).

GERNER, E.W. & HUMPHREY, R.M. The cell-cycle phase synthesis of nonhistone proteins in mammalian cells. *Biochim. Biophys. Acta* 331: *117-127* (1973).

HARDING, C.V., REDDAN, J.R., UNAKAR, N.J. & BAGCHI, M. The control of cell division in the ocular lens. *Int. Rev. Cytol.* 31: *215-300* (1971).

HNILICA, L.S. The structure and biological functions of histones, first edition. Cleveland: CRC Press 1972.

IWIG, M. & GLÄSSER, D. DNA- und Protein-Synthesis in kultivierten Linsenepithelzellen II. Einfluss synthetischer Effektoren. *Acta biol. med. germ.* 34: *997-1005* (1975).

JOHNSON, A. & ROTHSTEIN, H. Amphibian lens histones and their relation to the cell cycle. *J. Gen. Physiol.* 55: *688-702* (1970).

JOHNSON, E.M., KARN, J. & ALLFREY, V.G. Early nuclear events in the induction of lymphocyte proliferation by mitogens. *J. Biol. Chem.* 249: *4990-4999* (1974).

KARN, J., JOHNSON, E.M., VIDALI, G. & ALLFREY, V.G. Differential phosphorylation and turnover of nuclear acidic proteins during the cell cycle of synchronized HeLa cells. *J. Biol. Chem.* 249: *667-677* (1974).

KRAUSE, M.O., KLEINSMITH, L.J. & STEIN, G.S. Properties of genome in normal and SV40 transformed Wl38 human diploid fibroblasts. I. Composition and metabolism of nonhistone chromosomal proteins. *Exptl. Cell Res.* 92: *164-174* (1975).

MCDEVITT, D.S. Separation and characterization of the lens proteins of the amphibian, *Rana pipiens. J. Exp. Zool.* 164: *21-30* (1967).

MCDEVITT, D.S., MEZA, I. & YAMADA, T. Immunofluorescence localization of the crystallins in amphibian lens development with special reference to the γ-crystallins. *Develop. Biol.* 19: *581-607* (1969).

PANYIM, S. & CHALKLEY, R. High resolution acrylamide gel electrophoresis of histones. *Arch. Biochem. Biophys.* 130: *337-346* (1969a).

PANYIM, S. & CHALKLEY, R. A new histone found only in mammalian tissues with little cell division. *Biochem. Biophys. Res. Commun.* 37: *1042-1049* (1969b).

PAPACONSTANTINOU, J. Molecular aspects of lens cell differentiation. *Science* 156: *338-346* (1967).

POLANSKY, J.R. & BENNETT, T.P. Alterations in physical parameters and proteins of lens from *Rana catesbeiana* during development. *Develop. Biol.* 33: *380-408* (1973).

ROTHSTEIN, H. Experimental techniques for investigation of the amphibian lens epithelium. In: Methods in cell physiology, vol. 3, Prescott, D.M., ed. New York: Academic Press 45-74 (1968).

ROTHSTEIN, H., FORTIN, J. & YOUNGERMAN, M.L. Synthesis of macromolecules in epithelial cells of the cultured amphibian lens. I. DNA and RNA. *Exptl. Cell Res.* 44: *303-311* (1966).

STEIN, G.S. & BASERGA, R. The synthesis of acidic nuclear proteins in the prereplicative phase of the isoproterenol-stimulated salivary gland. *J. Biol. Chem.* 245: *6097-6105* (1970).

STEIN, G.S. & BORUN, T.W. The synthesis of acidic chromosomal proteins during the cell cycle of the HeLa S-3 cells. *J. Cell Biol.* 52: *292-307* (1972).

STEIN, G.S., SPELSBERG, T.C. & KLEINSMITH, L.J. Nonhistone chromosomal proteins and gene regulation. *Science* 183: *817-824* (1974).

STEIN, G.S., STEIN, J.S. & KLEINSMITH, L.J. Chromosomal proteins and gene regulation. *Sci. Am.* 232: *47-57* (1975)

STEIN, G.S. & THRALL, C.L. Uncoupling of nonhistone chromosomal protein synthesis and DNA replication in human diploid Wl-38 fibroblasts. *FEBS Letters* 34: *35-39* (1973).

TENG, N.N.H., PIATIGORSKY, J. & INGRAM, V.M. Histones of chick embryonic lens nuclei. *Develop. Biol.* 41: *72-76* (1974).

WILSON, W.L., HARDING, C.V. & WILSON, J.R. Quantitative studies on the stimulation of mitosis and DNA synthesis in the cultured rabbit ocular lens. *Exp. Eye Res.* 6: *343-350* (1967).

Authors' address:

Department of Zoology
Marsh Life Science Building
The University of Vermont
Burlington, Vermont 05401, USA

TRIGGERING OF MITOSIS IN THE CULTURED
MAMMALIAN LENS BY PROTEOLYTIC ENZYMES[1,2]

JOHN R. REDDAN, NALIN J. UNAKAR,
EVAMARIE KRASICKY & DOROTHY WILSON

(Rochester, Michigan)

ABSTRACT

Rabbit lenses were cultured in medium KEI-4 or in KEI-4 containing trypsin, thrombin, or soybean trypsin inhibitor. Lenses were exposed to soybean trypsin inhibitor and/or trypsin (5 μg/ml) for the initial 30 minutes of culture and were subsequently maintained in medium KEI-4 alone for a total of 52 hrs of culture. Whole-mounts of the epithelium were analyzed for mitosis and cell migration.

A brief exposure of the isolated lens to trypsin, in a completely defined serum-free medium, is sufficient provocation to induce cell division and migration throughout the normally quiescent central lens epithelium. If soybean trypsin inhibitor is present, the proliferative and migratory response normally induced by tripsin fails to materialize. If thrombin (5 μg/ml) is continuously present throughout the entire 52 hr culture period a central mitotic stimulation ensues which is not accompanied by extensive cell migration. The possible role of proteolytic enzymes in the induction of cell division and tissue repair in the injured lens *in vivo* is discussed.

INTRODUCTION

Environmental factor(s) are known to modulate the entrance of cells into the cell cycle (HARDING et al., 1971). One aim of our investigations is to gain a better understanding of the factor(s) that control cell division and wound healing in the ocular lens. The lens is avascular, lacks innervation and is enclosed within a basement membrane, i.e., the lens capsule. It is therefore possible to extricate the lens from its surrounding tissue without interruption of either a blood or nerve supply and to study the effect of various agents on an isolated organ that retains an overall level of organization similar to that found *in vivo*.

Cell division in the adult mammalian lens is primarily confined to the peripheral region of the epithelium, i.e., the germinative zone (REDDAN, 1974). Although the cells throughout the central lens epithelium are normally amitotic, they can be programmed to divide as a result of mechanical (HARDING & SRINIVASAN, 1961) or chemical insult (WEINSIEDER et al., 1975) *in vivo*, or by exposure of the isolated lens to whole serum (REDDAN et al., 1970), to aqueous humor obtained subsequent to ocular injury (WEINSIEDER, REDDAN & WILSON, 1976), or to crystalline insulin (REDDAN et al., 1972, 1975). As a result of mechanical or chemical

[1] Dedicated to Professor Jean Nordmann
[2] This work was supported by grant EY-00362 from the National Eye Institute

injury to the lens, the protein content of the aqueous increases and numerous blood cells with their accompanying hydrolytic enzymes are found in the anterior chamber (UNAKAR et al., 1973). As a case in point, acid phosphatase has been detected at extracellular sites following mechanical injury to the lens (UNAKAR et al., 1975). In many instances a fibrin clot has been detected in the anterior chamber following mechanical trauma, implying the presence of the various factors involved in the blood clotting mechanism.

In view of the known mitogenic effect of proteolytic enzymes on various mammalian cells maintained in tissue culture (BURGER, 1970; SEFTON & RUBIN, 1970) and in view of the known insulin-like activity of some of the proteolytic enzymes (KONO & BARHAM, 1971), the effect of specific proteases on the epithelium of the cultured lens was investigated. Our results show that a brief exposure of the isolated lens to trypsin or continuous exposure to thrombin, triggers a pronounced mitotic response throughout the central lens epithelium. Of added importance is the finding that the mitotic activation induced by the proteolytic enzymes occurs in the absence of whole serum and can be obtained in a culture medium that is of known composition.

MATERIALS AND METHODS

New Zealand white rabbits 8-12 weeks of age were killed by an air embolism. The eyes were enucleated and lenses isolated as previously described (REDDAN et at., 1975). Lenses were cultured in medium KEI-4 (see REDDAN et al., 1975 for formulation) or in medium KEI-4 containing: (1) trypsin [type III 2x crystallized from bovine pancreas]; (2) trypsin plus soybean trypsin inhibitor [type I-S at a concentration of $10\,\mu g/ml$]; (3) thrombin [grade 1]; (4) whole rabbit serum; or (5) secondary aqueous humor, [2°AH]. The proteolytic enzymes and the soybean trypsin inhibitor (STI) were obtained from Sigma Chemical Co., St. Louis, MO. Whole-serum and aqueous humor collected 15 minutes after initial paracentesis, i.e. 2°AH, was obtained as in prior experiments (WEINSIEDER, REDDAN & WILSON, 1976). The protein content of the aqueous humor or whole-serum was determined colorimetrically with rabbit serum albumin serving as a standard as previously described (WEINSIEDER et al., 1976). Trypsin, thrombin, 2°AH and whole-serum were used at a concentration of $5\,\mu g/ml$ for the initial 30 minutes of culture. Following the 30 minute exposure, lenses were cultured in medium KEI-4 alone for 51.5 hrs with 3 additional media changes. Some lenses were exposed to thrombin ($5\,\mu g/ml$) for the entire culture period. Lenses were fixed in Carnoy's fluid and whole mounts (HOWARD, 1952) of the epithelium were assayed for cellular migration and mitosis.

RESULTS

Lenses cultured in medium KEI-4 alone for 52 hrs exhibited mitosis in that region of the epithelium thought to correspond to the germinative zone under *in vivo* conditions. The cells throughout the central region of the epithelium remained amitotic. Lenses exposed to 5 µg/ml trypsin for 30 minutes and subsequently cultured for a total of 52 hr in a serum-free medium for the remainder of the culture period exhibited cellular migration and mitosis throughout the entire epithelial layer (Fig. 1). If the culture medium contained both trypsin and soybean trypsin inhibitor at a ratio of 1: 2, the pronounced migratory response normally brought about by trypsin alone was completely suppressed (Fig. 2). Moreover, no central mitotic response was found in whole-mount preparations of lenses exposed simultaneously to trypsin and STI but dividing cells were noted in region of the germinative zone. Clearly, certain of the epithelial cells can divide in the presence of soybean trypsin inhibitor. The appearance of whole-mount preparations obtained from lenses treated with trypsin and STI is ostensibly similar to those observed in lenses cultured for 52 hrs in medium KEI-4 alone.

In the majority of cases, an initial 30 minute exposure of the cultured lens to thrombin did not induce mitosis or migration after 52 hrs of culture. However, if the cultured lens was continuously exposed to 5 µg/ml thrombin throughout the culture period, a central mitotic response was realized (Fig. 3). As is evident in Fig. 3, the hyperplastic response elicited by thrombin was not accompanied by the extensive cellular disorganization which characterized the trypsin-induced mitotic response (Fig. 1).

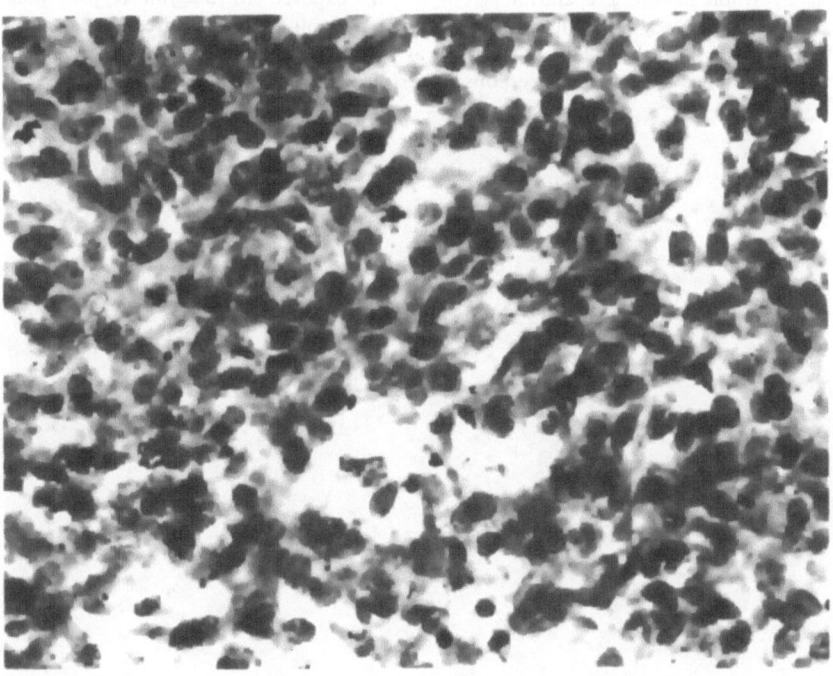

Fig. 1. Whole-mount preparation from a lens exposed to 5 µg/ml trypsin for the initial 30 minutes of culture. The lens was then cultured in medium KEI-4 and fixed at 52 hrs. Note pronounced cellular disorganization and numerous mitotic figures. Harris hematoxylin (x 650)

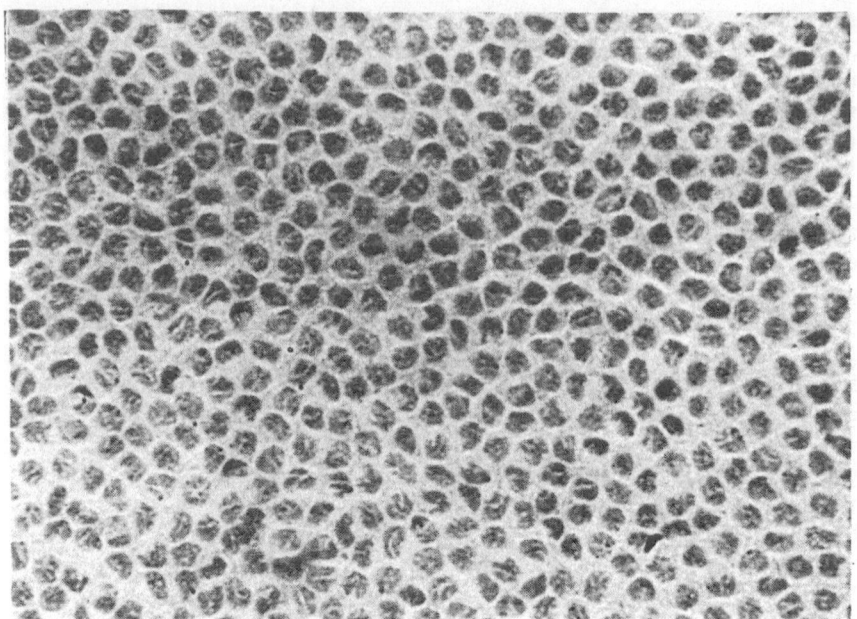

Fig. 2. Whole-mount preparation from a lens exposed to 5 µg/ml trypsin plus 10 µg/ml trypsin soybean inhibitor for the initial 30 minutes of culture. The lens was then cultured in medium KEI-4 and fixed at 52 hrs. Note lack of cellular disorganization and absence of the mitotic response. Harris hematoxylin (x 650)

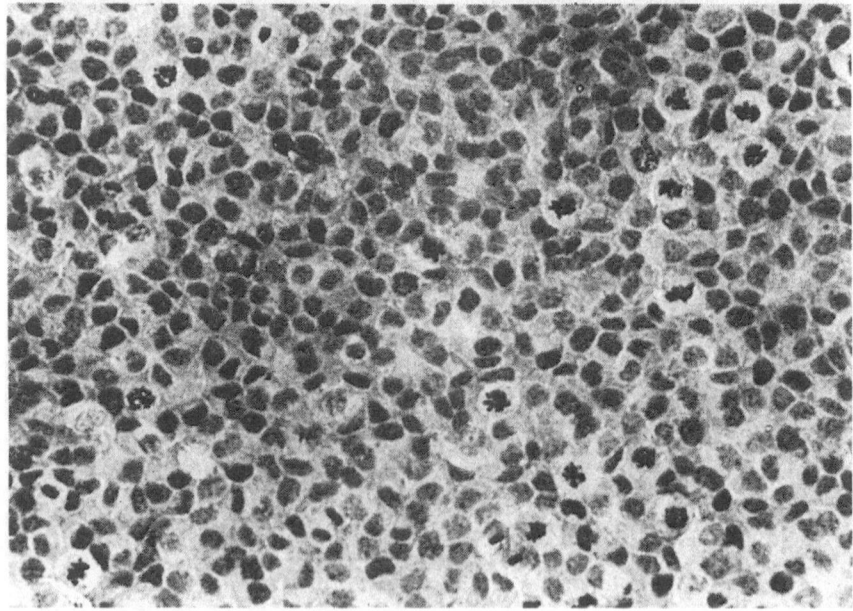

Fig. 3. Whole-mount preparation from a lens fixed after 52 hrs of culture. The lens was exposed to thrombin (5 µg/ml) throughout the culture period. Note dividing cells and absence of pronounced cellular disorganization. Harris hematoxylin (x 650)

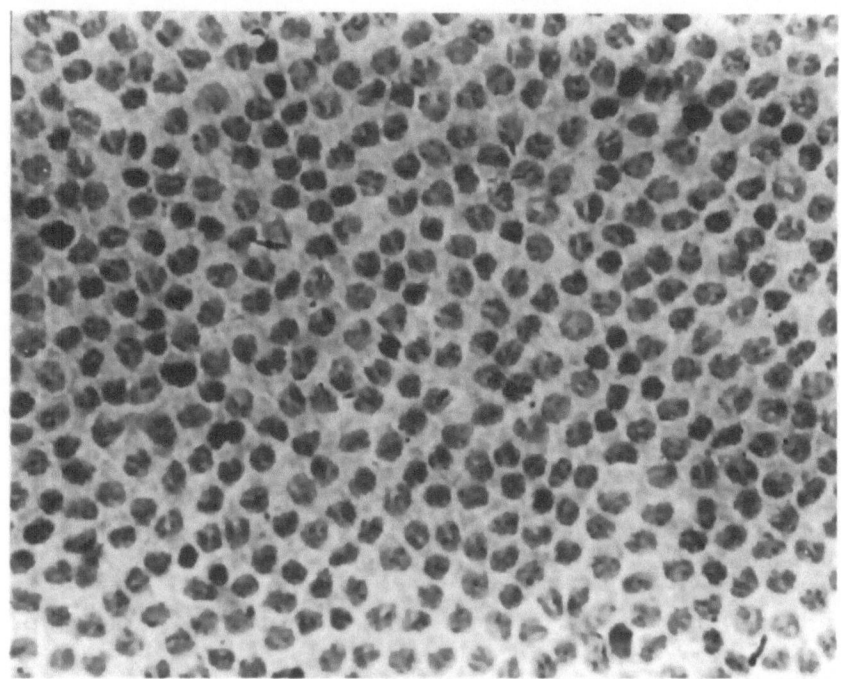

Fig. 4. Whole-mount preparation from a lens exposed to secondary aqueous humor containing 5 μg/ml protein for the initial 30 minutes of culture. The lens was then cultured in KEI-4 alone and fixed following 52 hrs of culture. Note the orderly arrangement of the epithelium and dearth of mitotic figures. Harris hematoxylin (x 650)

The presence of a proteolytic enzyme in the medium represents, in effect, the addition of a certain amount of protein to the environment of the cultured lens. In order to exclude the possibility that the mitogenic response was due solely to the quantity of protein, lenses were exposed to whole-rabbit serum and to secondary aqueous humor at a protein concentration and time interval equivalent to that in the above noted trypsin experiments. Exposure of the lens to whole-rabbit serum or to secondary aqueous humor at a concentration of 5 μg/ml for the initial 30 minutes of culture did not initiate cell division or cellular migration in the lens epithelium after 52 hrs of culture. Indeed, the morphology of the epithelium and the distribution of mitotic figures in lenses briefly exposed to either serum or secondary aqueous humor was similar to that detected in lenses cultured in trypsin-STI or in medium KEI-4 alone for a period of 52 hrs.

DISCUSSION

The data reported herein clearly indicate that trypsin and thrombin exert a potent mitogenic effect on the cultured mammalian lens epithelium. The mitogenic response occurs in the absence of whole-serum and can be obtained in a completely defined medium. The migratory response engendered by trypsin is comparable to that obtained in lenses in which the epithelium has been prompted to undergo mitosis by continuous exposure to whole rabbit serum (REDDAN et al., 1970). The present results indicate that both trypsin and thrombin can effectively substitute the entire spectrum of serum factors that are normally required for the induction of cell division in the cultured mammalian lens (HARDING et al., 1971). Although a brief exposure to trypsin is sufficient to stimulate mitosis, we have not excluded the possibility that the enzyme may remain bound to the tissue at intervals beyond 30 minutes. It has been suggested that proteolytic enzymes remain bound to the cell surface and retain their activity for intervals as long as 24 hrs (POSTE, 1971). Thrombin, which is an important enzyme in the blood clotting mechanism, brings about a mitotic activation in the lens and has been shown to stimulate mitosis in cultured chicken fibroblast cells (CHEN & BUCHANAN, 1975). Other mitogens, i.e. whole rabbit serum and secondary aqueous humor, when used at concentrations and intervals equivalent to that of trypsin, do not engender mitosis. This data coupled with the repression of the tripsin induced response brought about by soybean trypsin inhibitor suggests that the mitogenicity of the enzymes is attributable to their proteolytic activity. Additional studies will be needed to verify this possibility.

Insulin triggers a central mitotic stimulation in the cultured lens (REDDAN et al., 1972, 1975). It is of interest that trypsin mimics the action of insulin in certain cell types, and is thought to interact with insulin receptor sites (KONO & BARHAM, 1971). Irrespective of whether the proteases interact with insulin receptors or not, they are known to alter the physiological properties of the cell surface (BLUMBERG & ROBBINS, 1975; BURGER, 1970; HOLLEY, 1975). The exact mechanism(s) by which proteolytic enzymes or polypeptide hormones initiate cell growth to be elucidated.

In our previous studies we have suggested that acid hydrolases play a role in initiating the hyperplasia resultant to mechanical injury in the lens *in vivo* (UNAKAR et al., 1973, 1975). In addition to these enzymes, aggregates of fibrin have been detected at the wound locus in the mechanically injured lens. Thus the microenvironment of the lens in the immediate area of trauma comes to contain proteolytic enzymes. If such proteolytic enzymes are not inactivated by various serum proteins at the site of the wound or if they remain bound to the cell surface or to fibrin in an active form then these enzymes may be responsible for the triggering of mitosis and cell migration which are essential prerequisites for wound healing. The results of the current study support, but do not prove, such an hypothesis.

Studies beyond this preliminary inquiry will be needed in order to define the role of proteolytic enzymes in those events associated with the restoration of tissue transparency in the injured or cataractous lens.

REFERENCES

BLUMBERG, P.M. & ROBBINS, P.W. Effect of proteases on activation of resting chick embryo fibroblasts and on cell surface proteins. *Cell* 6: *137-147* (1975).
BURGER, M.M. Proteolytic enzymes initiating cell division and escape from contact inhibition of growth. *Nature* 227: *170-171* (1970).

CHEN, L.B. & BUCHANAN, J.M. Mitogenic activity of blood components. I. Thrombin and prothrombin. *Proc. Nat. Acad. Sci.* 72: *131-135* (1975).

HARDING, C.V., REDDAN. J.R., UNAKAR, N.J. & BAGCHI, M. The control of cell division in the ocular lens. *Int. Rev. Cytol.* 31: *215-300* (1971).

HARDING, C.V. & SRINIVASAN, B.B. A propagated stimulation of DNA synthesis and cell division. *Exptl. Cell Res.* 25: *326-340* (1961).

HOLLEY, R.W. Control of growth of mammalian cells in cell culture. *Nature* 258: *487-490* (1975).

HOWARD, A. Whole-mounts of rabbit lens epithelium for cytological study. *Stain Technol.* 27: *313-315* (1952).

KONO, T. & BARHAM, F.W. The relationship between the insulin-binding capacity of fat cells and the cellular response to insulin. *J. Biol. Chem.* 216: *6210-6216* (1971).

POSTE, G. Tissue dissociation with proteolytic enzymes. Adsorption and activity of enzymes at the cell surface. *Exptl. Cell Res.* 65: *359-367* (1971).

REDDAN, J.R. Development and structure of the lens. In: Cataract and Abnormalities of the Lens. J. Bellows (ed.) Grune & Stratton, Inc., N.Y. p. 29-42 (1974).

REDDAN, J.R., CROTTY, M.W. & HARDING, C.V. Characterization of macromolecular synthesis in the epithelium of cultured rabbit lenses. *Exp. Eye Res.* 9: *165-174* (1970a).

REDDAN, J.R., HARDING, C.V., ROTHSTEIN, H., CROTTY, M.W., LEE, P. & FREEMAN, N. Stimulation of mitosis in the vertebrate lens in the presence of insulin. *Ophthal. Res.* 3: *65-82* (1972).

REDDAN, J.R., UNAKAR, N.J., HARDING, C.V., BAGCHI, M. & SALDAÑA, G. Induction of mitosis in the cultured rabbit lens initiated by the addition of insulin to medium KEI-4. *Exp. Eye Res.* 20: *45-61* (1975).

SEFTON, B.M. & RUBIN, H. Release from density dependent growth inhibition by proteolytic enzymes. *Nature* 227. *843-845* (1970).

UNAKAR, N.J., BINDER, L.I., REDDAN, J.R. & HARDING, C.V. Histochemical localization of acid phosphatase in the injured rabbit lens. *Ophthal. Res.* 7: *158-169* (1975).

WEINSIEDER, A., BRIGGS, R., REDDAN, J., ROTHSTEIN, H., WILSON, D. & HARDING, C.V. Induction of mitosis in ocular tissue by chemotoxic agents. *Exp. Eye Res.* 20: *33-44* (1975).

WEINSIEDER, A., REDDAN, J. & WILSON, D. Aqueous humor in lens repair and cell proliferation. *Exp. Eye Res.* In press, (1976).

Keywords:

Lens epithelium
Organ culture
Mitosis
Cell migration
Proteolytic enzymes
Trypsin
Thrombin
Wound healing

Authors' address:

Department of Biological Sciences
Oakland University
Rochester, Michigan 48063, USA

ISOELECTRIC FOCUSING OF CRYSTALLINS FROM DIFFERENT PARTS OF THE BOVINE AND DOG LENS IN DEPENDENCE ON AGE*

J. BOURS, KARIN DOEPFMER & O. HOCKWIN

(Bonn, B.R.D.)

ABSTRACT

The crystallin composition of various parts of the bovine and dog lens is determined by thin-layer isoelectric focusing in dependence on age. In the equator and the anterior and posterior cortex there is in both species a distinct decrease in concentration of γ-crystallin and its components and a considerable increase of β-crystallin and its components in dependence on age. The per cent of α-crystallin shows especially for bovine a decrease in all parts, but an increase in absolute amounts in the equator, a slight increase in the anterior and posterior cortex, and a distinct decrease in absolute amounts in the lens nucleus in dependence on age.

In the bovine and the dog lens a disappearance of specific β- and γ-crystallin components is observed in dependence on age, e.g. in the lens nucleus a certain β-crystallin component, and in the lens equator and anterior cortex a low molecular weight β-crystallin. Specific γ-crystallin .components are absent in the bovine and dog lens equator and anterior and posterior cortex with progressed age of the lens.

INTRODUCTION

In the mammalian lens considerable changes in crystallin composition occur during the aging process. Generally, when crystallins of the bovine whole lens are analysed, a slight decrease after an initial increase of α-crystallin is observed, along with an increase in β-crystallins and a sharp decrease in γ-crystallin concentration (HOCKWIN, NEUMANN & KLEIFELD, 1958; BOURS, WEBER & HOCKWIN, 1976a, b). But particularly it is of interest to analyze the composition of the crystallin components in the different lens parts in dependence on age, like the equator (the growth zone containing always the youngest, just synthesized proteins), the anterior and posterior cortex (the fiber cell regions) and the nucleus (the former embryonic part and therefore being the oldest region of an individual lens).

Since longer time it is known that marked differences in crystallin composition exist between the lens cortex and the nucleus. The β crystallins are dominating in the equator and the cortex of the lens, because the amount of γ-crystallin is very low (HOCKWIN et al., 1958; MÜLLER et al., 1958; VAN KAMP & HOENDERS, 1973; BOURS & BRAHMA, 1973) and disappears even in very old age. One of the low molecular weight β-crystallins, the $β_s$-crystallin (VAN DAM, 1966) is synthesized and accumulated in increasing amounts in the adult bovine lens (CROFT, 1973; SLINGSBY & CROFT, 1973). The γ-crystallins have a different nature and distribution in

* Research supported by the 'Deutsche Forschungsgemeinschaft' (Ho 249/8).

the lens equator and in the nucleus: the γ-crystallins present in the nucleus have a fetal character (FRANÇOIS & RABAEY, 1956; FUCHS & KLEIFELD, 1956; PAPACONSTANTINOU, 1965; RABAEY & LAGASSE, 1971; KABASAWA & KINOSHITA, 1974), and are differing from the γ-crystallins present in the adult lens cortex (PAPACONSTANTINOU, 1965; BOURS, 1973b). Also the amount of 'cortical' γ crystallins in the equator of the lens is much lower than in its nucleus (MÜLLER et al., 1958; BJÖRK, 1961; NEWSOM & HOCKWIN, 1967; CRISTINI & NEGRONI, 1968; VAN KAMP & HOFNDERS, 1973; BOURS, 1973b, 1974; YU & EAST, 1975).

Finally, the γ-crystallins from the bovine lens nucleus and cortex differ in molecular weight (KABASAWA & KINOSHITA, 1974).

In addition, though the general appearance of the α-, β- and γ-crystallin distribution in the mammalian lens parts may be the same, considerable differences in composition of the crystallins of the various species in detail may exist, which is strongly expressed as a species-specificity (WEBER, BOURS & HOCKWIN, 1976; BOURS & HOCKWIN, 1976).

Purpose of this study is to demonstrate by thin-layer isoelectric focusing the qualitative and quantitative differences in distribution of α-, β- and γ-crystallins and their components in the various lens parts in dependence on age, of the two mammalian species: bovine and beagle-dog.

MATERIALS AND METHODS

Preparation of crystallins from lens tissues

Calf and adult bovine eyes of various age were transported from the slaughter house under ice, and the lenses were removed immediately and dissected

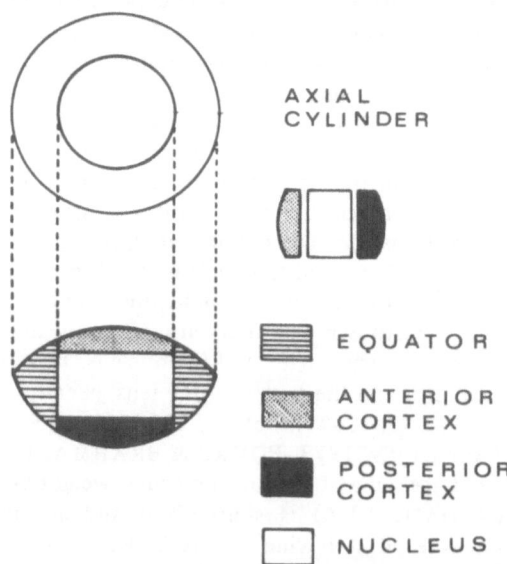

Fig. 1. The division of the lens into equator, anterior and posterior cortex, and nucleus. The diameter of the remaining nucleus is 80% from that of the lens.

76

Table I. Determination of the amount of protein extract in the different parts of the bovine lens in dependence on age

Fig 2:	AGE (years)	LENS PORTION	FW (g)	WS (mg)	WI (mg)	WS/WI (Ratio)
a.	0.16	EQ	–	102	2	46
e.	12.2	EQ	–	163	9	18
j.	18.7	EQ	–	179	14	13
b.	0.16	AC	–	37	3	14
f.	12.2	AC	–	122	12	10
k.	18.7	AC	–	110	21	5
c.	0.16	PC	–	39	1	39
g.	12.2	PC	–	86	19	4
l.	18.7	PC	–	67	14	5
d.	0.16	N	–	91	3	31
h.	12.2	N	–	260	35	7
m.	18.7	N	–	298	55	5
a-d	0.16	WL	1.125	269	9	30
e-h	12.2	WL	2.686	631	75	8
j-n	18.7	WL	2.819	654	105	6

Table II. Determination of the fresh weight and the amount of protein extract in the different parts of the dog lens in dependence on age

Fig 3:	AGE (years)	LENS PORTION	FWP (mg)	DW (mg)	WS (mg)	WI (mg)	WS/WI (Ratio)
a.	1.34	EQ	211	63	43	10	4
e.	7.8	EQ	261	78	64	8	8
j.	9.8	EQ	278	90	71	10	7
b.	1.34	AC	84	32	15	2	9
f.	7.8	AC	101	38	26	8	3
k.	9.8	AC	73	28	19	6	3
c.	1.34	PC	94	46	17	9	2
g.	7.8	PC	124	50	29	11	3
l.	9.8	PC	147	62	36	19	2
d.	1.34	N	156	62	34	3	12
h.	7.8	N	186	95	43	37	1.2
m.	9.8	N	188	96	40	47	0.8
a-d	1.34	WL	595	203	109	24	4
e-h	7.8	WL	696	261	162	64	2.5
j-n	9.8	WL	716	276	166	82	2.0

Legend:
FW = fresh weight lens
FWP = fresh weight lens portion
DW = dry weight lens portion
WS = water-soluble proteins: crystallins
WI = water-insoluble proteins: albuminoid
– = not determined

EQ = lens equator
AC = anterior cortex
PC = posterior cortex
N = lens nucleus
WL = whole lens

free from surrounding tissues. The dog lenses (beagle) of different age were prepared from the enucleated eyes immediately after killing of the animals. The intact lenses were frozen at $-20\ °C$ and the equatorial part was cut out using a trepane of 80% of the lens equatorial diameter. Then the inner cylinder was cut into the anterior and posterior part and the remaining nucleus (Fig. 1) (HOCKWIN & KLEIFELD, 1965). These lens parts were homogenized at $4\ °C$ in c. 5 ml distilled water, or dried first and then homogenized, centrifuged at 38,000 g for 1 hr at $4\ °C$ and the supernatants were lyophilized. The residues were washed two times with distilled water to extract most of the soluble materials. The fresh weights of whole lenses (bovine, dog) and of the different lens portions (dog), and the mg amounts of protein extract in the lens parts were determined by weight in dependence on age (Table 1, Table 2).

Thin-layer isoelectric focusing

Isoelectric focusing experiments were carried out essentially as described earlier (BOURS, 1971). Useful indications and alterations when using the Multiphor electrophoresis equipment (LKB 2117) were published later (BOURS, 1975). The photographs of the stained isofocused crystallin components (Fig. 2, 3) were scanned with a Chromoscan recording reflectance densitometer (Joyce & Loebl & Co, Ltd, London). The value or weight of each crystallin or crystallin component was calculated in per cent of total crystallin (Fig. 4, 6) or in absolute quantity of mg per lens part (Fig. 5, 7).

RESULTS

a. The amount of crystallin and albuminoid in different parts
of the bovine and dog lens in dependence on age

From the data of Tables 1 and 2 some general observations may be stated:
1. an increase is observed of crystallins and albuminoid in all lens parts with aging.
2. the lens equator always contains lowest amounts of crystallins and albuminoid.
3. the nucleus of the older lens shows a high and significant increase of the amount of albuminoid.

b. The different parts of the bovine lens

In the young bovine lens of 0.16 years the composition of the lens crystallins is determined by isoelectric focusing and calculated in per cent of total crystallin and in absolute amounts in mg per lens part. The composition of the anterior and posterior cortex is about the same, and to some extent this is also the case for the lens equator [Fig. 2(a-c); Fig. 4, 5]. The nucleus of the lens, which is the former embryonic part, contains a lower amount of α-crystallin (molecular weight 825,000 Daltons) than the equator. The nucleus contains a higher amount of γ-crystallins, whereas the amount of high-molecular weight β-crystallins (components Nr 1-8) is also higher in the

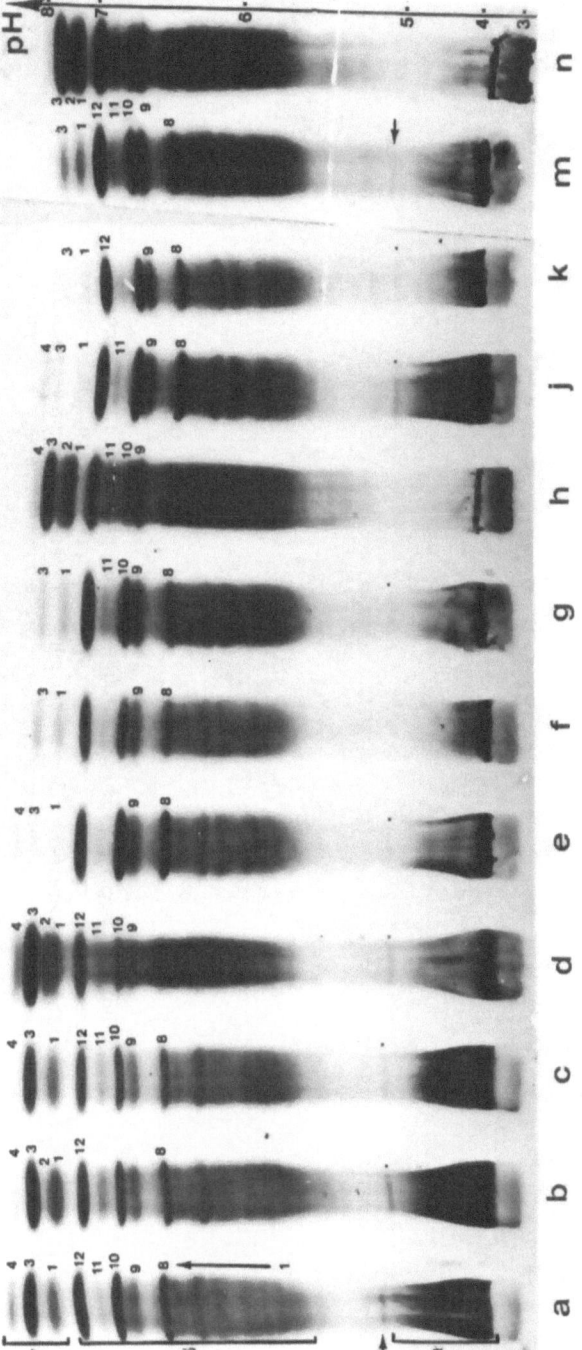

Fig. 2. Thin-layer isoelectric focusing patterns of different parts of the bovine lens in dependence on age. a, e, j = equator; b, f, k = posterior cortex; c, g, m = anterior cortex; d, h, n = nucleus. a-d = 0.16-year-old; e-h = 12.2-year-old; j-n = 18.7-year-old. The pH is measured at 4 °C. α = α-crystallin; arrow and squares = pre- α-crystallin; β₁-β₈ = β-crystallin components of high molecular weight; β₉-β₁₂ = β-crystallin components of low molecular weight; γ₁-γ₄ = γ-crystallin components.

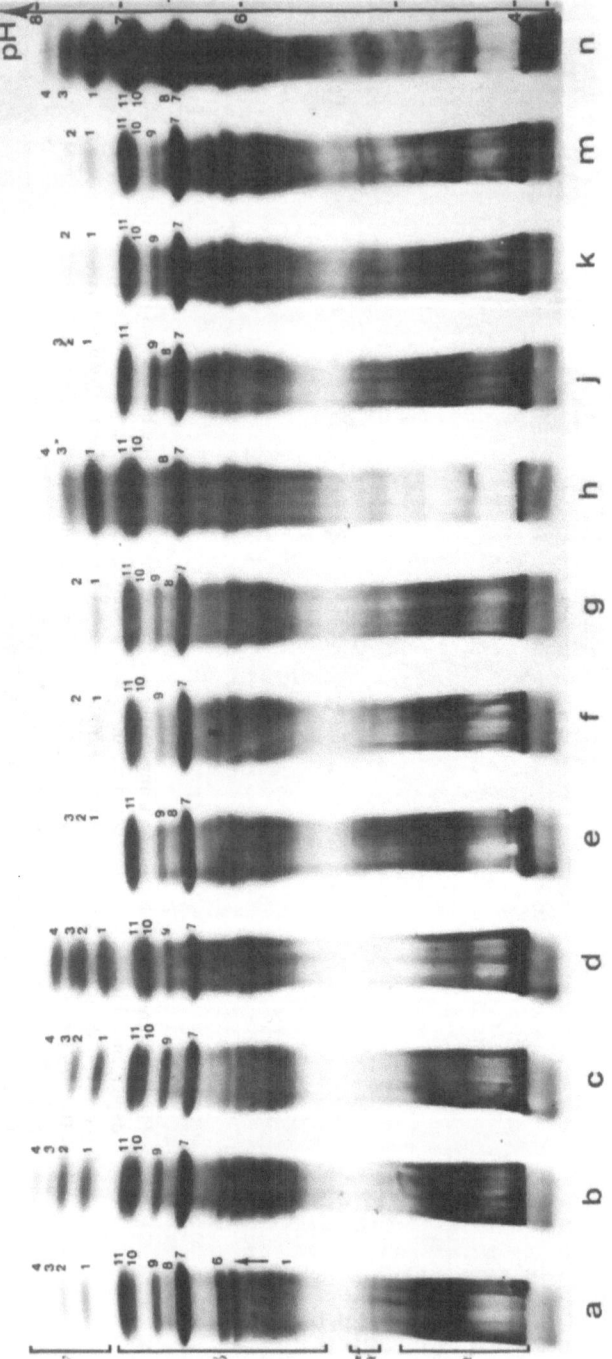

Fig. 3. Thin-layer isoelectric focusing patterns of different parts of the dog (beagle) lens in dependence on age. a, e, j = equator; b, f, k = posterior cortex; c, g, m = anterior cortex; d, h, n = nucleus. a–d = 1.34-year-old; e–h = 7.9-year-old; j–n = 9.8-year-old. The pH is measured at 4 °C. α = α-crystallin; pre-α = pre-α-crystallins; β_1-β_{11} = β-crystallin components; γ_1-γ_4 = γ-crystallin components.

nucleus. There is an increasing complexity in this β-crystallin region, and also there is a deterioration of sharpness of the isofocused bands. The pre-α-crystallin, which is in fact a low-molecular weight β-crystallin (BOURS & BRAHMA, 1973) (Fig. 2) appears as one single band. The low-molecular weight proteins like the β-crystallin components Nr 9-12, and the γ-crystallin components are sharply focused zones and are very prominent in all four parts of the young bovine lens [Fig. 2(a-d)]. The β_{12}-crystallin component is the β_s-crystallin and was first isolated in a pure form by VAN DAM (1966). The γ_3-crystallin component is the most prominent band of the γ-crystallins in the young bovine lens [Fig. 2(a-d)] and in the embryonic bovine lens (BOURS & BRAHMA, 1973).

In the old bovine lens of 12.2 and 18.7 years the composition of the equator, and both the anterior and posterior cortex shows also similarities [Fig. 2(e-g); 2(j-m); Fig. 4, 5]. The posterior cortex shows a lower amount of α-crystallin than the anterior part and the equator. In the older lens the

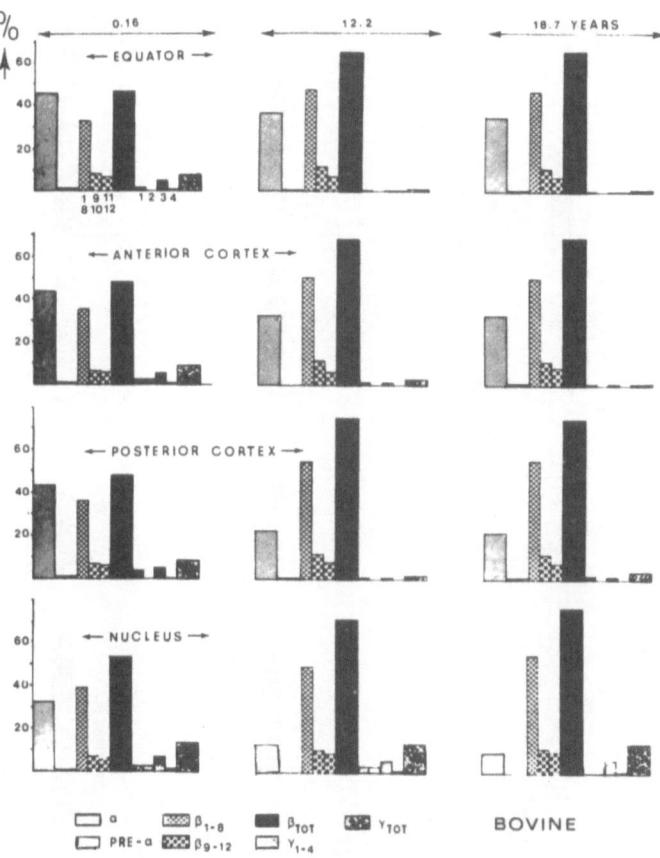

Fig. 4. The distribution (in per cent) of α-crystallin and of β- and γ-crystallin components in different parts of the bovine lens in dependence on age, evaluated by densitometry of thin-layer isoelectric focusing patterns.

γ-crystallin contents of the lens nucleus remains prominent compared to the other parts of the old bovine lens.

c. The bovine lens in dependence on age

When the amounts of crystallins of the various parts of the lens are determined in dependence on age, an increase of the β-crystallins in each lens part is observed [Fig. 4, 5]. However, the loss of the greater part of the amount of γ-crystallins in the equator and both the anterior and posterior cortex is very clear [Fig. 2(e-g); 2(j-m)]. This diminishment in concentration of γ-crystallin and its components is not seen in the nucleus, where the γ-crystallin content is almost constant [Fig. 2(d, h, n); Fig. 4, 5]. In the older lens nucleus of 12.2 and 18.7 years the pre- α-crystallin is absent [Fig. 2(h, n)]. Especially in the lens nucleus the α-crystallins of lower molecular weight decrease in per cent, but are rather constant in absolute

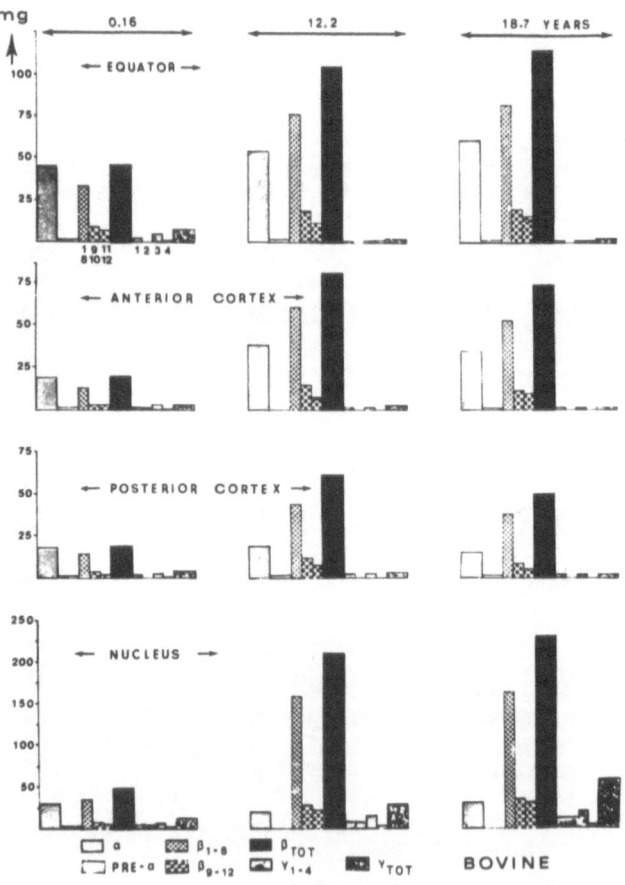

Fig. 5. The absolute amount of crystallin (in mg) in the different parts of the bovine lens in dependence on age. Values are obtained by evaluation of densitometer data after isoelectric focusing, with respect to the dry weight of the soluble crystallins.

82

amounts, while, on the other hand, there is a considerable increase of β-crystallins. In detail, the amount of high molecular weight β-crystallin components (β_1-β_6) increases markedly in the nucleus, and also the low molecular weight β-crystallins (β_9-β_{12}) increase and are rather constant in older age (12.2 and 18.7 years). There is a sharp decrease of the amount of γ-crystallin and its components in the equator and in the anterior and posterior cortex in dependence on age.

The protein composition of the *single* crystallin components in the various lens parts in dependence on age is different. In these parts occasionally a number of the components are entirely missing or have been reduced to low concentrations: 1. the pre- α-crystallin in the nucleus [Fig. 2(h, n)] and sometimes in the anterior cortex [Fig. 2(f)]; 2. the β_8 -crystallin in the nucleus [Fig. 2(d, h, n)], due to a deterioration of sharpness of the iso-focused zones; 3. the β_{11} -crystallin in the equator and the anterior cortex [Fig. 2(e, f); 2(k)]; 4. the γ_2 -crystallin in the equator, and in both the

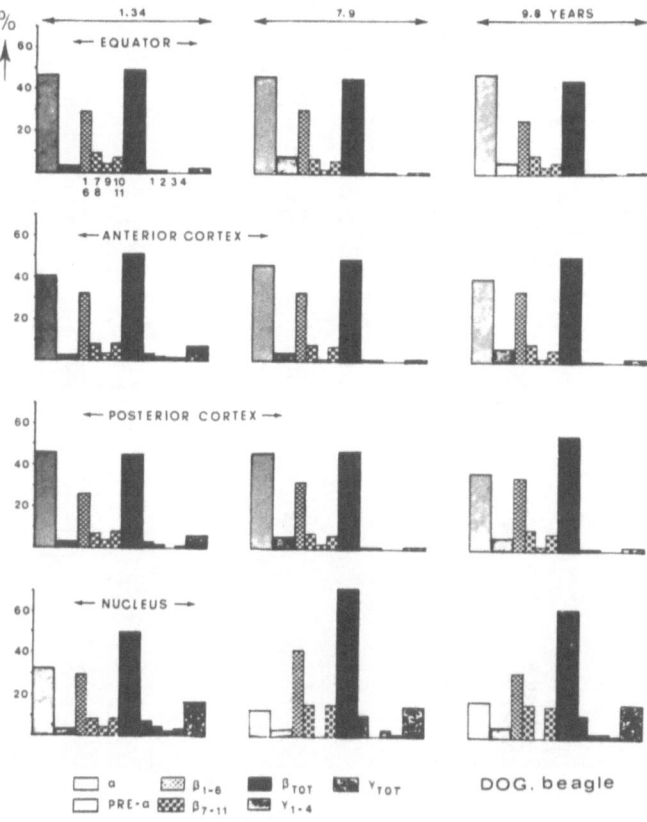

Fig. 6. The distribution (in per cent) of α-crystallin and of β- and γ-crystallin components in different parts of the dog (beagle) lens in dependence on age, evaluated by densitometry of thin-layer isoelectric focusing patterns.

83

anterior and posterior cortex of the lens [Fig. 2(c, e, f, g, j, k, m)]. In the nucleus the four γ-crystallin components are always detected.

d. The different parts of the dog lens

In the young dog lens (age 1.34 years) the composition of the soluble lens crystallins is about the same for the lens equator and the anterior and posterior cortex [Fig. 3(a-c); Fig. 6]. The lens nucleus has a lower per cent of α-crystallins and a higher amount of γ-crystallins compared to the other three parts of the lens, which is also demonstrated for the bovine lens [Fig. 2(d, h, n)]. In the dog lens the pre- α-crystallin consists of three iso-focused bands at isoelectric points ranging from pI 5.2 to 5.4, contrary to the same compound in the bovine lens, which is only one single band at pI = 5.25. The β-crystallin components (β_1-β_6) are sharply focused only in the young dog lens (age 1.34 years) and the β-crystallin components Nr 7-11 are

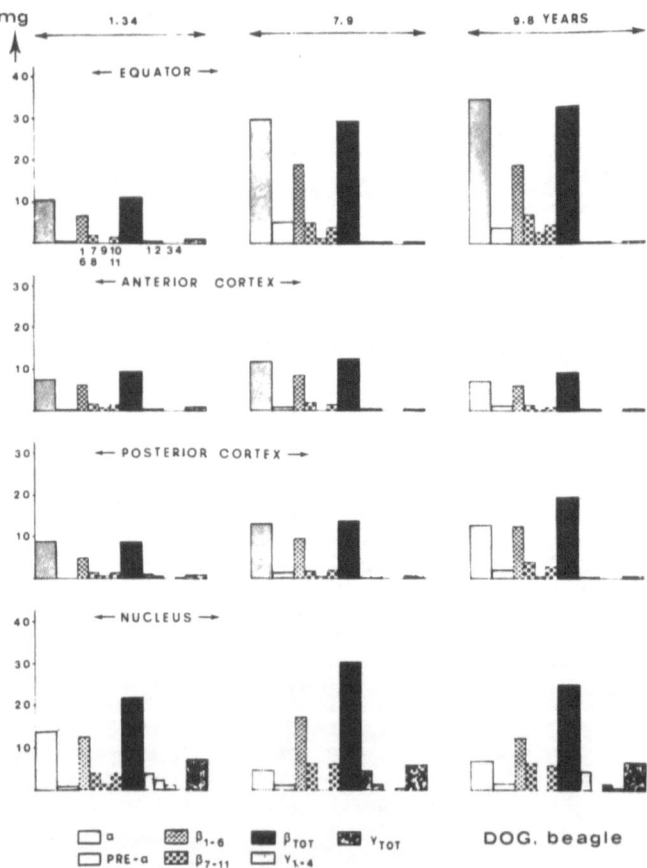

Fig. 7. The absolute amount of crystallins (in mg) in the different parts of the dog (beagle) lens in dependence on age. Values are obtained by evaluation of densitometer data after isoelectric focusing, with respect to the dry weight of the soluble crystallins.

84

quite prominent in the young lens [Fig. 3]. There are four γ-crystallin components, two of which are the most prominent ones in the equator and both the anterior and posterior cortex. Four γ-crystallin components are found in the young dog lens nucleus (age = 1.34 years) in relative high amounts.

e. The dog lens in dependence on age

The composition of the dog lens crystallins is also calculated in per cent of total crystallin [Fig. 6] and in absolute amounts of mg per lens part [Fig. 7]. In general, the per cent of α- and β-crystallins is fairly constant in the equator and both the anterior and posterior cortex in dependence on age. In absolute amounts, there is an increase of α- and β-crystallin concentration in the equator and in the posterior cortex. In the dog lens nucleus a decrease is observed of α-crystallin, and a slight increase in β-crystallin concentration is recorded in both per cent and in mg per lens [Fig. 6, 7].

However, the diminution in concentration of the γ-crystallins in dependence on age is very clear [Fig. 3(e-g); 3(j-m)]. Like in the bovine lens this diminishment in concentration of γ-crystallins and its components is not observed in the lens nucleus, where the γ-crystallin concentration is almost constant [Fig. 3(d, h, n); Fig. 6, 7]. Contrary to the observations in the bovine lens the pre- α-crystallins are uniformly present in the dog lens and its parts during aging, and are also of a different nature [Fig. 3].

Concerning the protein distribution of the crystallin components in the dog lens there are some β-crystallin components missing in older animals, e.g. the β_9-crystallin component in the lens nucleus [Fig. 3(h, n)] and the β_{10}-crystallin component in the lens equator [Fig. 3(e, j)]. The γ-crystallin components Nr 3 and 4 are absent or reduced to low concentrations in the older anterior and posterior cortex [Fig. 3(f, g, k, m)] and the 4th component also in the equator [Fig. 3(e, j)]. The γ-crystallin component Nr 2 is missing in the 7.9- and the 9.8-year-old dog lens.

Generally, the components isofocused are sharp, and the deterioration of sharpness is not observed in the young lens but is only seen later in the 9.8-year-old lens, and in a lower degree compared to the old bovine lens.

Generally spoken, the isoelectric focusing patterns in both bovine and dog lens show similarities, especially in the diminishment of the γ-crystallins in the equator and in the anterior and posterior cortex.

f. The species-specificity of crystallins

Although a gross resemblance of isofocused patterns is observed (Fig. 2, 3), these experiments have revealed a high species-specificity for the crystallins of the bovine and dog lens, due to an obvious difference in isoelectric points and in composition between the protein components of these two mammalian crystallins belonging to the same group, e.g. the β- and γ-crystallins [Fig. 2, 3]. Also a difference is observed in α-crystallin composition [Fig. 4, 6], and a difference in number and concentration of the single β- and γ-crystallin components. There is no concomittance in isoelectric points of the two α-crystallins and the β- and γ-crystallin components [Fig. 2, 3].

85

DISCUSSION

Compared to obsolete electrophoretical techniques like paper-, agar-, and cellulose-acetate electrophoresis, the thin-layer isoelectric focusing technique has a very good resolving power and a very good reproducibility. The crystallins are separated in a great number of isofocused components: for the bovine lens at least 12 and for the dog lens at least 11 β-crystallin components, and 4 γ-crystallin components both for the bovine and the dog lens. However, there are a few drawbacks when this method is used to analyze lens crystallins. Proteins with a low isoelectric point, like α-crystallin (pI = 4.85) and albumin (pI = 4.90) precipitate during isoelectric focusing due to a low solubility at their isoelectric point (BOURS 1973a, b, 1974). Also, it cannot be prevented that the α-crystallin of a molecular weight of 620,000 to 825,000 Daltons (BOURS & BRAHMA, 1973) appears after staining as a smear on the gel [Fig. 2, 3]. The aggregates of α-crystallin of high molecular weights (1-50 million Daltons) (SPECTOR, FREUND, LI & AUGUSTEYN, 1971) even do not enter into the pores of the 5% polyacrylamide gel and precipitate under the sample paper at the origin on the plate [Fig. 2, 3]. Due to this phenomenon, the thin-layer isoelectric focusing method is not suitable for quantification of the high molecular weight α-crystallins. It may be a better approach to analyze these aggregates by analytical isotachophoresis (KJELLIN, MOBERG & HAL-LANDER, 1975).

Regarding particularly the γ crystallin composition in dependence of their synthesis, the lens equator, anterior and posterior cortex show an entirely different feature compared to the lens nucleus, both in bovine [Fig. 2, 4, 5] and in dog lens [Fig. 3, 6, 7]. The γ-crystallins synthesized after birth are of a different nature compared to those which have been synthesized before birth which are as such situated in the nucleus, because specific γ-crystallin components fail in the lens equator [Fig. 2, 3].

The crystallin composition of the lens changes continuously during aging, which is caused by three different processes:

1. the post-translational aging in the nucleus. This is a conversion of units of lower molecular weight into large complexes, e.g. of α-crystallins. Most probably also β-crystallins in the nucleus are involved in this process because the amounts of high molecular β-crystallin components increase in dependence on age in the bovine lens [Fig. 2, 4, 5], and less pronounced also in the dog lens [Fig. 3, 6, 7].

2. Aging of the lens equator (and cortex), which is seen as loss of the ability to synthesize certain new crystallins. Regarding the γ-crystallin composition in dependence of their synthesis, the amount of γ-crystallins and its components decreases in the lens equator which is caused by the lack of synthesis in situ while the differentiation is still present [Table 1, 2].

3. Aging of the lens crystallins, where there is a post-translational loss or conversion of single crystallin components. In each of the lens parts there is a specific occasional loss of single crystallin components post synthesis in dependence on age, e.g. in the bovine lens the components pre-α, β_8, β_{12}, γ_2 and γ_4 [Fig. 2] and in the dog lens the components β_9, β_{10}, γ_3 and γ_4 [Fig. 3].

Species-specificity of the bovine and the dog lens is demonstrated in Figures 2 and 3. The clear difference observed in isoelectric points of the isofocused components and their concentrations is also seen in many other mammalian and avian species and in amphibia (BOURS, 1974; BRAHMA & McDEVITT, 1974; WEBER et al., 1976; BOURS & HOCKWIN, 1976, BOURS, 1976).

Since the results presented here are only dealing with evaluated data from three events in the growth curve, it is the future aim of current research to perform longitudinal studies on the aging processes in the eye lens and its parts.

ACKNOWLEDGEMENTS

We thank Dr W. Schnitzlein and Dr Astrid Fischer, Department of Toxicology, Knoll, A.G., Ludwigshafen for the supply with beagle dog lenses and Mr H.J. Müller for the preparation of this material.

It is a pleasure to thank Mrs Elke Oellers and Miss Barbara Polenz for the photographic illustrations.

REFERENCES

BJÖRK, I. Studies on γ-crystallin from calf lens. I. Isolation by gel filtration. *Exp. Eye Res.* 1: *145-154* (1961).

BOURS, J. Isoelectric focusing of lens crystallins in thin-layer polyacrylamide gels. A method for detection of soluble proteins in eye lens extract. *J. Chromatogr.* 60: *225-233* (1971).

BOURS, J. The presence of lens crystallins as well as albumin and other serum proteins in chick iris extracts. *Exp. Eye Res.* 15: *299-319* (1973a).

BOURS, J. Free isoelectric focusing of bovine lens γ-crystallins. *Exp. Eye Res.* 16: *501-515* (1973b).

BOURS, J. Isoelectric focusing and immunochemistry of lens crystallins. *Docum. Ophthal.* 37: *1-46* (1974).

BOURS, J. Isoelectric focusing of lens crystallins. In: Progress in isoelectric focusing and isotachophoresis. Ed. P.G. Righetti. North-Holland Publ. Cy., Amsterdam, pp. *235-256* (1975).

BOURS, J. The immunological aspects of the lens: on the organ- and species-specificity of crystallins. In: Scientific Foundations of Ophthalmology. Eds. E.S. Perkins & D.W. Hill. William Heinemann Medical Books, Ltd., London. (in press) (1976).

BOURS, J. & S.K. BRAHMA. Isoelectric focusing of embryonic cow lens crystallins. *Exp. Eye Res.* 16: *131-142* (1973).

BOURS, J. & O. HOCKWIN. Artunterschiede bei Linsenproteinen nach Trennung mit Isoelektrofokussierung auf Polyacrylamid-Dünnschichtplatten. *Berl. & Münch. Tierärztl. Wschr.* (in press) (1976).

BOURS, J., A. WEBER & O. HOCKWIN. The crystallin distribution of the bovine lens during aging. Abstract in: *Exp. Eye Res.* 22: *302* (1976) (16th AER-meeting, Leiden, The Netherlands).

BOURS, J., A. WEBER & O. HOCKWIN. The crystallin distribution of the bovine lens during aging. In: INSERM Symp. 'Biology of the epithelial lens cells in relation to development, aging and cataract. Eds. Y. COURTOIS & F. REGNAULT. INSERM, Paris. Vol. 34 (1976) (in press).

BRAHMA, S.K. & D.S. McDEVITT. Ontogeny and localization of γ-crystallins in *Rana temporaria, Ambystoma mexicanum* and *Pleurodeles walthii* normal lens development. *Exp. Eye Res.* 19: *379-387* (1974).

CRISTINI, G. & L. NEGRONI. Starch gel electrophoresis of lens proteins treated with urea. *Exp. Eye Res.* 7: *216-220* (1968).

CROFT, L.R, Low molecular weight proteins of the lens. In: The human lens in relation to cataract. CIBA Foundn. Symp., Elsevier – Exc. Med. – North-Holl. Ass. Sci. Publ. Amsterdam, Vol. 19, pp. *207-226* (1973).

DAM, A.F. VAN. Purification and composition studies of β_S-crystallin. *Exp. Eye Res.* 5: *255-266* (1966).

FRANÇOIS, J. & M. RABAEY. De l'existence d'une protéine cristallinienne embryonaire. *Ann. Oculist.* 189: *836-854* (1956).

FUCHS, R. & O. KLEIFELD. Über das Verhalten des wasserlöslichen Linseneiweißes junger und alter Tiere bei papierelektrophoretische Untersuchung. *Albr. v. Graefes Arch. Ophthal.* 158: *29-33* (1956).

HOCKWIN O. & O. KLEIFELD. Das Verhalten von Fermentaktivitäten in einzelnen Linsenteilen unterschiedlich alter Rinder und ihre Beziehung zur Zusammensetzung des wasserlöslichen Eiweisses. In: Die Struktur des Auges. II. Symposium. Hrg. J.W. ROHEN, F.K. Schattauer Verlag, Stuttgart, pp. *395-401* (1965).

HOCKWIN, O., H.G. NEUMANN & O. KLEIFELD. Das Verhalten der Linseneiweiße in Abhängigkeit vom Alter bei Meerschweinchen- und Rinderlinsen. *Albr. v. Graefes Arch. Ophthal.* 160: *8-19* (1958).

KABASAWA, I. & J.H. KINOSHITA. Aging effects on the bovine lens γ-crystallins. *Exp. Eye Res.* 18: *457-466* (1974).

KAMP, G.J. VAN & H.J. HOENDERS. The distribution of the soluble proteins in the calf lens. *Exp. Eye Res.* 17: *417-426* (1973).

KJELLIN, K.G., L. MOBERG & L. HALLANDER. Analytical isotachophoreis of cerebrospinal fluid proteins – a preliminary report. *Science Tools* 22: *3-7* (1975).

MÜLLER, H.K., P. DARDENNE, O. HOCKWIN, O. KLEIFELD & G. SCHAFHAUSEN. Altersbedingte Veränderungen im Stoffwechsel der Linse. XVIII Concilium Ophthal., Belgica, pp. *750-763* (1958).

NEWSOM, W.A. & O. HOCKWIN. Chromatographic separation of calf and ox lens proteins. *Albr. v. Graefes Arch. Ophthal.* 171: *318-323* (1967).

PAPACONSTANTINOU, J. Biochemistry of bovine lens proteins. II: The γ-crystallins of adult bovine, calf and embryonic lenses. *Biochim. Biophys. Acta* 107: *81-90* (1965).

RABAEY, M. & A. LAGASSE. Changes in the protein composition of the mammalian lens during embryonic development and aging, with special reference to the proteins of low molecular weight. In: Protides of the Biological Fluids, 18th Colloq., Bruges, 1970. Ed. H. PEETERS. Pergamon Press. Oxford, New York, pp. *117-120* (1971).

SLINGSBY, C. & L.R. CROFT. Developmental changes in the low molecular weight proteins of the bovine lens. *Exp. Eye Res.* 17: *369-376* (1973).

SPECTOR, A., T. FREUND, L.-K. LI & R.C. AUGUSSTEYN. Age dependent changes in the structure of α-crystallin. *Invest. Ophthal.* 10: *677-686* (1971).

WEBER, A., J. BOURS & O. HOCKWIN. The species-specificity of lens crystallins. Abstract in: *Exp. Eye Res.* 22: *302-303* (1976) (16th Meeting AER, Leiden, The Netherlands).

YU, N.-T. & F. FAST. Laser raman spectroscopic studies of ocular lens and its isolated protein fractions. *J. Biol. Chem.* 250: *2196-2202* (1975).

88

Keywords:

Lens equator
Anterior & posterior cortex
Nucleus
α-, β-, γ-crystallins
Pre- α-crystallin
Albuminoid
Aging
Isoelectric focusing
Bovine
Dog (beagle)

Authors' address:

Division of Biochemistry of the Eye
Clinical Institute for Experimental Ophthalmology
University of Bonn
D-5300 Bonn-Venusberg, B.R.D.

IMPROVED SEPARATION OF LM (LOW MOLECULAR WEIGHT) CRYSTALLINS

HANS BLOEMENDAL & ANNEKE ZWEERS

(Nijmegen, the Netherlands)

ABSTRACT

An improved separation procedure based on centrifugation and gel filtration for low molecular weight (LM) crystallins is described. The isolated fractions have been analyzed by various gel electrophoretic techniques.

INTRODUCTION

Since MÖRNER (1894) classified the water-soluble eye lens proteins as α, β and γ crystallin, extensive studies have been undertaken to characterize these highly specific proteins.

The properties of α crystallin have been investigated most intensively (BLOEMENDAL, 1972; HARDING & DILLEY, 1976), eventually resulting in the elucidation of the complete primary structure of both subunits αA_2 and αB_2 (VAN DER OUDERAA, DE JONG & BLOEMENDAL, 1973; VAN DER OUDERAA, DE JONG, HILDERINK & BLOEMENDAL, 1974) which are under direct genetic control (BLOEMENDAL, BERNS, VAN DER OUDERAA & DE JONG 1972a).

β Crystallin represents the most heterogeneous population among the water-soluble lens proteins. Both the structure as well as the possible interrelationship between different β polypeptides are far from being unraveled. Gel filtration on Sephadex G-200 of total calf lens water-soluble extract yields two β fractions designated as $\beta_{H(igh)}$ and $\beta_{L(ow)}$ (BLOEMENDAL & HERBRINK, 1974; HERBRINK & BLOEMENDAL, 1974) which correspond to fractions B and C obtained after gel filtration on Biogel 300 by TESTA, ARMAND & BALAZS (1965). In addition to these major β fractions a β crystallin of low molecular weight (approximately 28,000 D) has been described (VAN DAM, 1966). This protein has been named β_s. In gel filtration on Sephadex G-200 it coincides with the γ crystallin fraction.

As far as the latter class of crystallins is concerned, despite valuable sequence data which are available now (CROFT, 1972), various questions remain still to be answered. For example, why is this group of proteins not acetylated at the N-terminus, while all subunits of α and β crystallin are? Secondly, why does γ crystallin not form hybrids with either α or β chains upon dissociation and reaggregation at high protein concentration? (BLOEMENDAL, ZWEERS & WALTERS, 1975; BLOEMENDAL, ZWEERS, BENEDETTI & WALTERS, 1975). In the third place: Does there exist a similar interrelationship between the γ crystallins as, for instance, between

αA_2 and αA_1? (BLOEMENDAL et al. 1972a).

A primary condition for an experimental approach to answer these questions is the availability of adequate isolation procedures which would allow the preparation of well-characterized pure starting material. In view of this consideration we designed an improved method to optimally separate β_S from the γ components. In the procedure to be described in the present paper we found a minor β component (β_M) which emerges after β_L from the gel filtration column.

MATERIALS AND METHODS

Calf eyes were obtained fresh from the slaughterhouse and kept on ice no longer than 6 hours. The lenses were isolated and decapsulated. Portions of one hundred lenses were stirred overnight at $4°$ in a buffer containing 0.05 M Tris-HCl, pH 7.6, 0.05 M NaCl, and 0.001 M EDTA (TESTA et al., 1965). The same buffer was used for the equilibration and elution of the gel filtration columns.

For gel filtration two types of packing material were applied, namely Ultrogel AcA 34 (LKB, Sweden) and Sephadex G-75 (Pharmacia, Sweden). Columns of 100 x 2.5 cm and 100 x 3.0 cm were used for Ultrogel and Sephadex G-75, respectively. In both cases elution was performed at a flow rate of 30 ml/h.

SE Sephadex chromatography in columns of 40 x 1.5 cm was performed as described by BJÖRK (1964). Elution was carried out at a flow rate of 30 ml/h.

Gel electrophoresis was performed as reported earlier (BLOEMENDAL, 1963) with or without 6 M urea. 12 x 0.6 cm tubes containing 7.5% acrylamide at pH 8.9 were used. SDS gel electrophoresis was performed according to the procedure of LAEMMLI (1970).

RESULTS AND DISCUSSION

The crystallins have been separated into three general classes by electrophoretic mobility and size, and indicated by the Greek letters α, β and γ, respectively. One may ask whether this classification is still justified.

Firstly, it has been shown that the α fraction consists of a population of aggregates of various sizes (BLOEMENDAL, BERNS, ZWEERS, HOENDERS & BENEDETTI, 1972b). In older lenses a number of aggregates appear to have extremely high molecular weights (SPECTOR, FREUND, LI & AUGUSTEYN, 1971; VAN KLEEF & HOENDERS, 1973). However, despite minor differences in subunit composition due to several stages of degradation from the C-terminal end (DE JONG, VAN KLEEF & BLOEMENDAL, 1974; VAN KLEEF, DE JONG & HOENDERS, 1975), the polypeptides making up the architecture of all aggregates are virtually identical. For this reason the general classification α crystallin for all native aggregates which have as major components αA_1, αA_2, αB_1 and αB_2 chains is tenable.

As far as the β crystallins are concerned the situation is already more complicated. Upon gel filtration on a Sephadex G-200 column two β fractions can be obtained, indicated as β_H and β_L, respectively (BLOEMENDAL

& HERBRINK, 1974; HERBRINK & BLOEMENDAL, 1974). A marked difference between these two fractions is the occurrence of one acidic and two highly basic polypeptides in β_H which are lacking in β_L. Since we were able to show that both fractions share, in addition to a number of minor components, the predominant polypeptide βB_p (BLOEMENDAL & HERBRINK, 1974; HERBRINK & BLOEMENDAL, 1974), one may argue that the protein type designation 'β' is correct.

At least in the case of the γ fraction the general classification is misleading. Already VAN DAM (1966) observed that a M_r 28,000 β component ('β_s') coincided with γ crystallin on a Sephadex G-200 column. Therefore, we suggest – in accordance with the proposal of RABAEY, RIKKERS & DE METS (1972) for bird γ crystallin – to utilize the designation LM (low molecular weight) crystallin for the corresponding fraction in mammalian lenses.

For routine preparations Ultrogel AcA 34 may successfully be applied instead of Sephadex G-200. Comparison of two gel filtration experiments on columns of similar size, one packed with Sephadex, the other one with

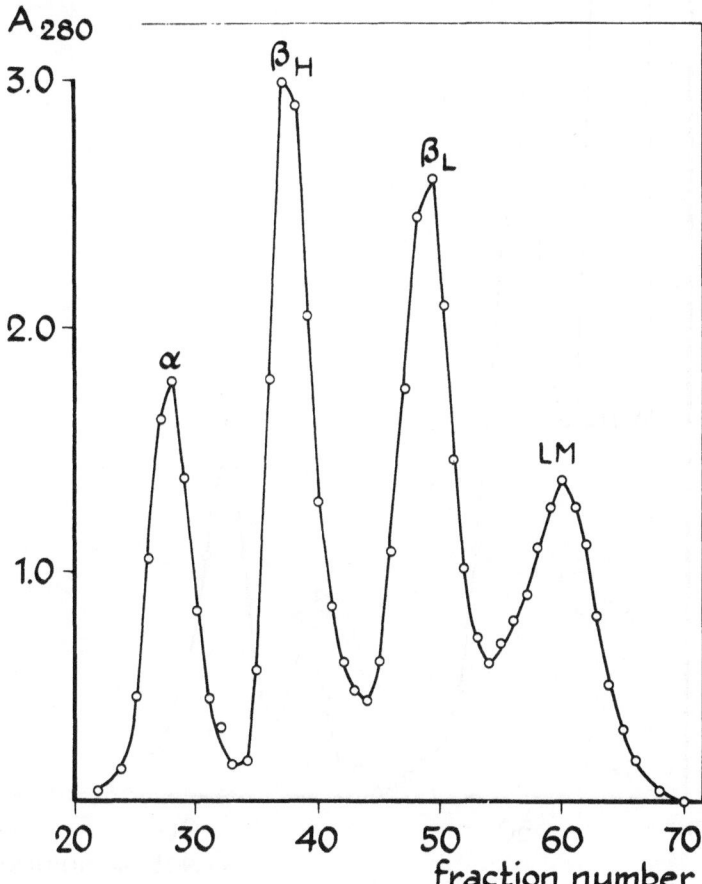

Fig. 1. Separation by gel filtration of the water-soluble lens proteins on an Ultrogel AcA 34 column, 300 OD units of protein have been applied.

Ultrogel, showed that the time needed for optimal separation can be reduced by a factor two when Ultrogel is used. The gel filtration experiment depicted in Fig. 1 required 20 h.

In contrast to α crystallin the LM crystallin obtained from these columns can be used for further fractionation only if lyophilization as intermediate

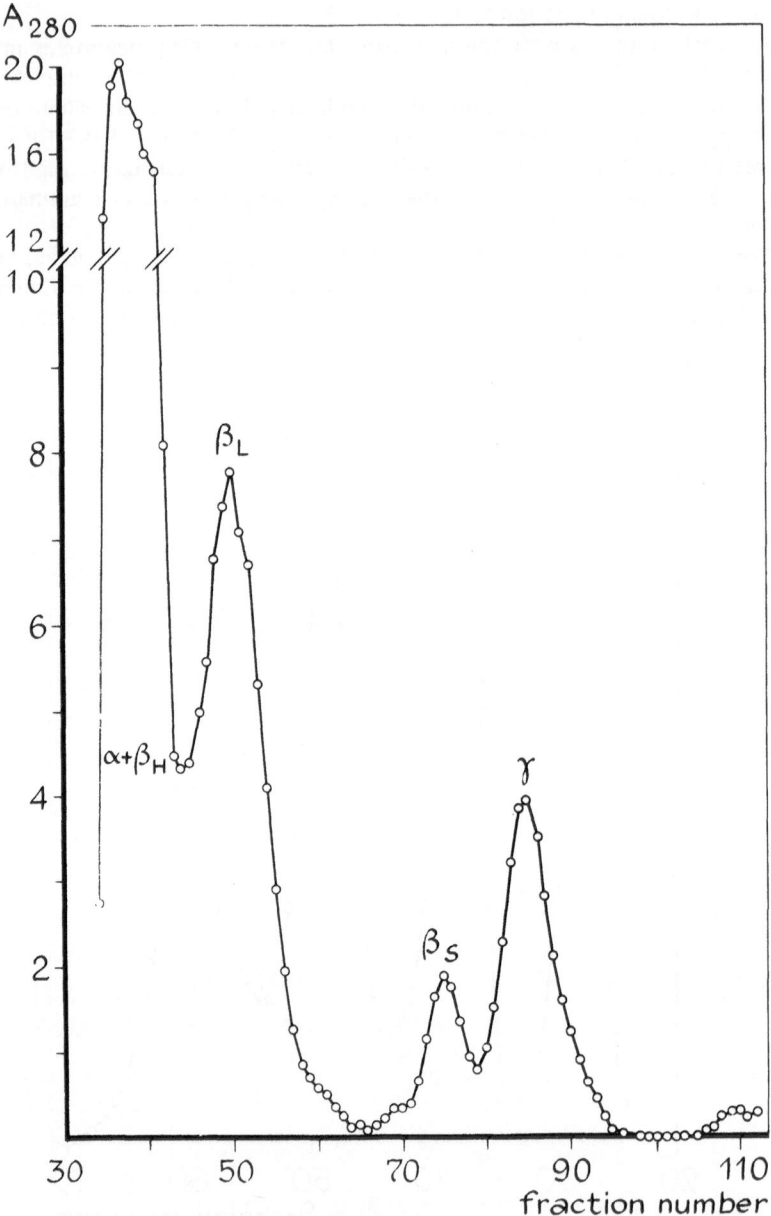

Fig. 2. Separation of the water-soluble lens proteins on a Sephadex G-75 column. Gel filtration was preceeded by centrifugation at 220,000 × g for 6 h. The upper two third of the supernatant fraction was used. 260 OD units of protein have been applied.

step can be avoided, since dialysis followed by lyophilization renders the proteins in the latter fraction completely insoluble.

BJÖRK (1961), VAN DAM (1966), and recently KABASAWA, KINO-SHITA & BARBER (1974) used Sephadex G-75 for the isolation of γ crystallin. We observed that on such columns α and β_H, although largely

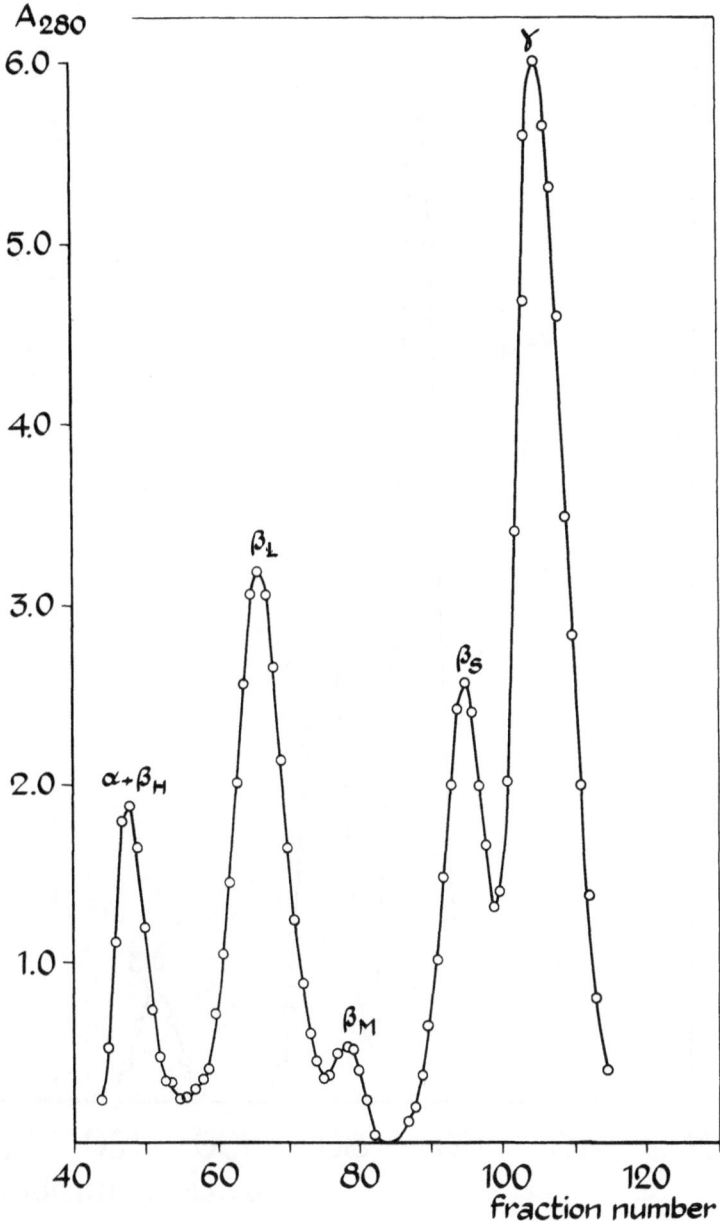

Fig. 3. Same experiment as described in the legend of Fig. 2, except that centrifugation was for 16 h instead of 6 h.

emerging with the void volume, interfere with optimal separation of the LM fraction. Therefore we introduced a centrifugation step prior to gel filtration of the total water-soluble lens protein mixture. Dependent on the time of centrifugation different profiles are obtained. After 6 h of centrifugation at 220,000 x g already a clear cut separation between β_s and γ crystallin is

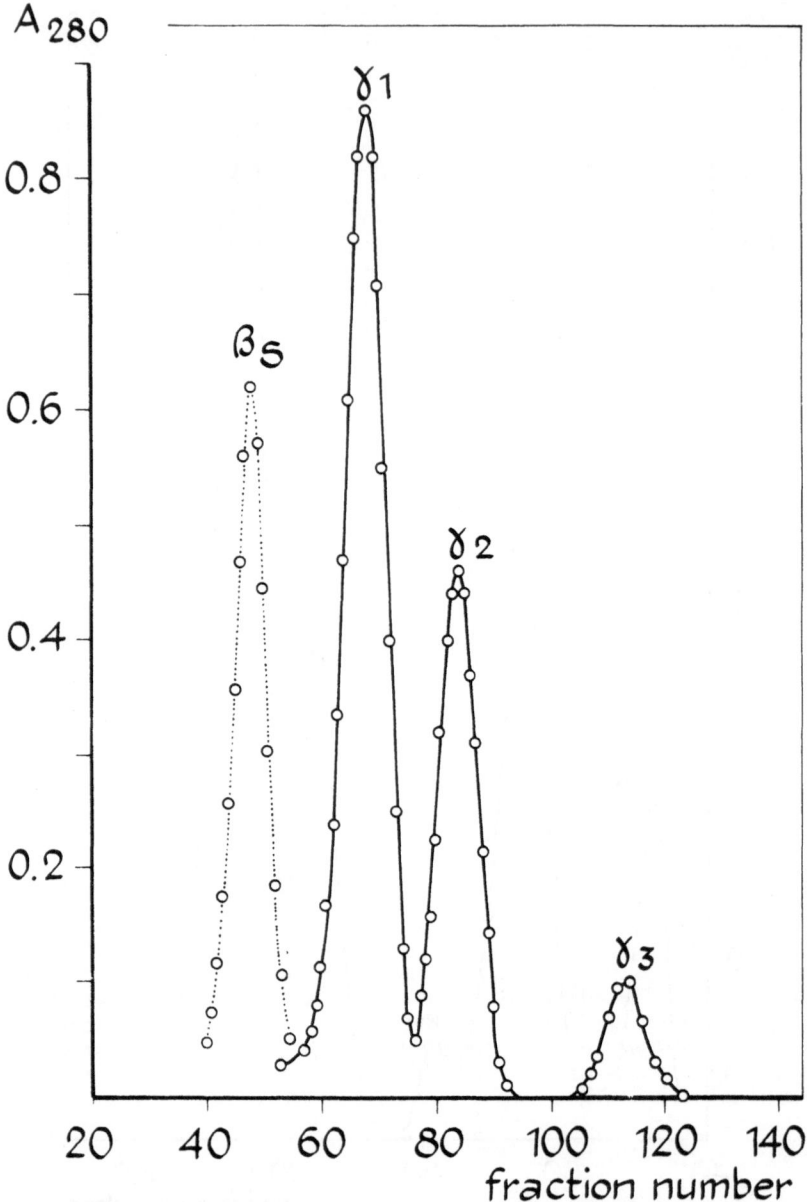

Fig. 4. SE Sephadex chromatography of the LM crystallin fraction. 100 OD units of protein have been applied. The peak fractions emerged at the following sodium acetate concentrations: β_s at 0.24 M; γ_1 at 0.28 M; γ_2 at 0.30 M; and γ_3 at 0.34 M.

96

obtained (Fig. 2). Obviously the separation is improved after a sedimentation time of 16 h (Fig. 3). The $\alpha + \beta_H$ mixture is considerably reduced, the β_L fraction emerges as a symmetrical component, and the relative amount of the separated β_s and γ crystallins is enhanced (compare Table I). The effect of centrifugation prior to gel filtration results in different ratio's $\beta_s : \gamma$ for cortex and nucleus. In the cortex this ratio is $1:3$ without any centrifu-

Table I. Percentages of crystallin fractions remaining after different centrifugation times

crystallin fraction	6h	16h
$\alpha + \beta_H$	50	10
β_L	22.5	26
β_s	4.5	16
γ	23	48

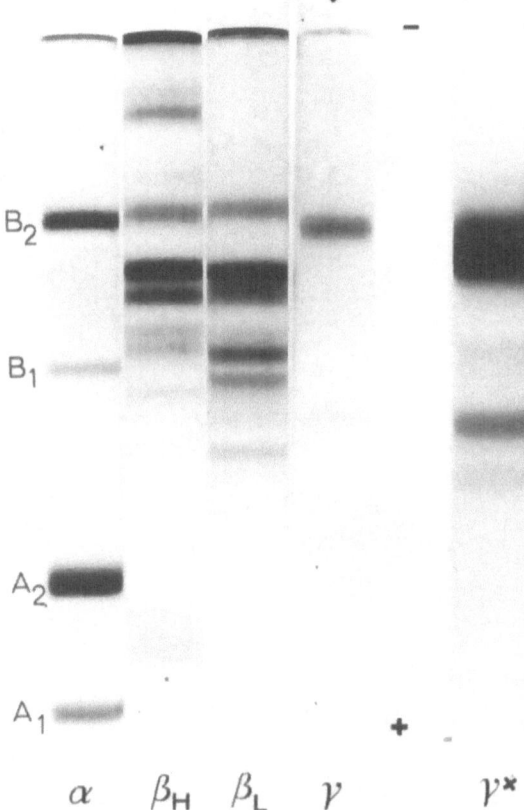

Fig. 5. 6 M urea-polyacrylamide gel electrophoresis at pH 8.9 of the water-soluble crystallins separated on Ultrogel AcA 34. γ^* represents an 'overloaded' gel. In this case additional LM crystallins become visible. – and + indicate the cathode and anode, respectively.

97

gation, whereas for the nucleus 24 h of sedimentation are required to obtain the same ratio. Moreover, a minor β fraction (β_M) becomes separated from β_L after 16 h of centrifugation.

As shown previously by BJÖRK (1964) γ crystallin can be fractionated by SE Sephadex chromatography. Fig. 4 shows the separation by this procedure of the total non-lyophilized γ crystallin fraction obtained after Sephadex G-75 gel filtration. The dashed line indicates the localization of β_s if this component is applied together with the γ crystallin.

The isolated fractions in the experiments described have been identified by 6 M urea-polyacrylamide gel electrophoresis at alkaline pH. Fig. 5 shows the gel pattern of the separated crystallins from the Ultrogel column (compare Fig. 1). In α crystallin only αA_1, αA_2 and αB_2 are quantitatively important. In β_H and β_L at most three polypeptides, in addition to the major

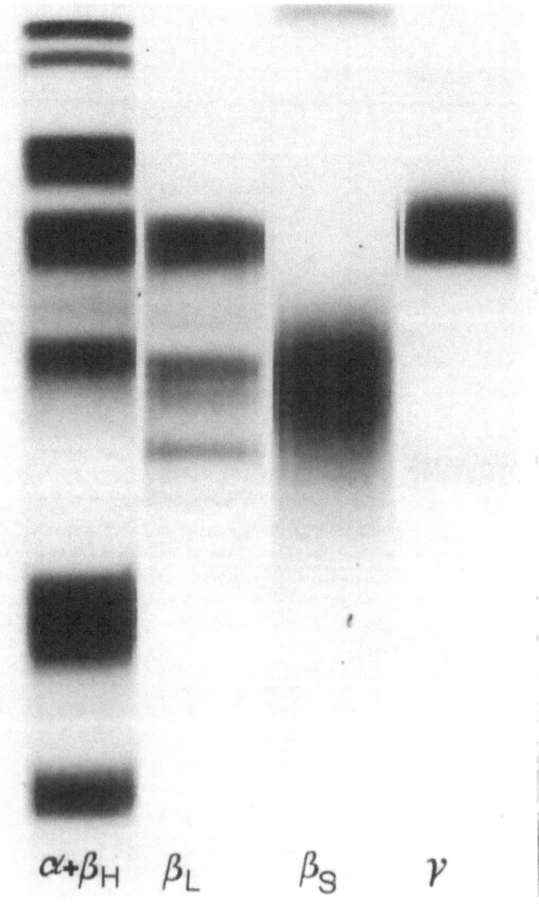

Fig. 6. 6 M urea-polyacrylamide gel electrophoresis at pH 8.9 of the crystallin fraction obtained after gel filtration on Sephadex G-75 (compare Fig. 3).

component βB_p, are quantitatively significant. The gel pattern of the γ crystallin fraction is characterized by one predominant band. In overloaded gels the number of additional faint bands increases (see Fig. 5 γ^*).

We may conclude from the Sephadex G-75 gel filtration experiment (compare Fig. 3) that both β_L and γ actually are not pure fractions. The first one is at least contaminated with β_M, the second one at least with β_s. This is sustained by the gel electrophoretic analysis depicted in Fig. 6. The first gel at the left of this figure is obviously a mixture of α and β_H crystallin (compare Fig. 5). The two highly basic polypeptides are clearly visible, βB_p is situated between αB_2 and αB_1, whereas αA_2 is considerably broadened by the βA component. The β_L appears now somewhat simplified as compared with the corresponding fraction in Fig. 5.

Electrophoretic analysis on polyacrylamide gels without urea gives even

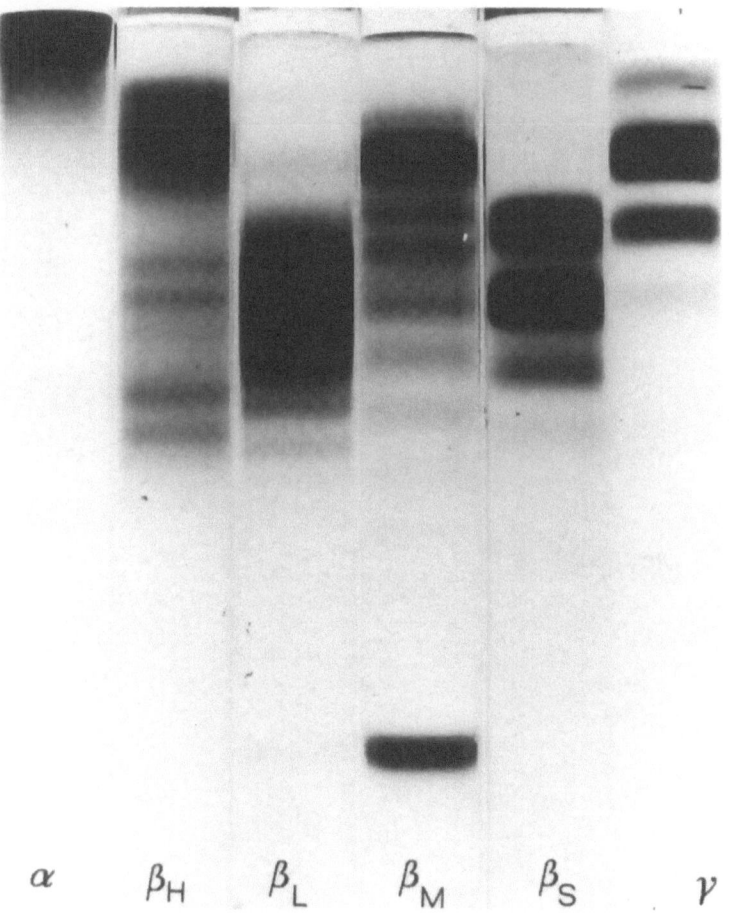

Fig. 7. Polyacrylamide gel electrophoresis (without urea) of various crystallin fractions. α, β_H and β_L were obtained after gel filtration on Ultrogel AcA 34. β_M, β_s and γ were fractionated on Sephadex G-75.

more information about the nature of the fractions from the gel filtration experiments. This is shown in Fig. 7. The first three fractions (at the left side of the figure) are the α, β_H and β_L fractions from the Ultrogel column. The α aggregates do not enter the gel pores: β_H seems to exist as a major aggregate which is, however, apparently contaminated with four discrete proteins whose true nature is as yet unknown. It cannot be excluded that one represents leucine aminopeptidase.

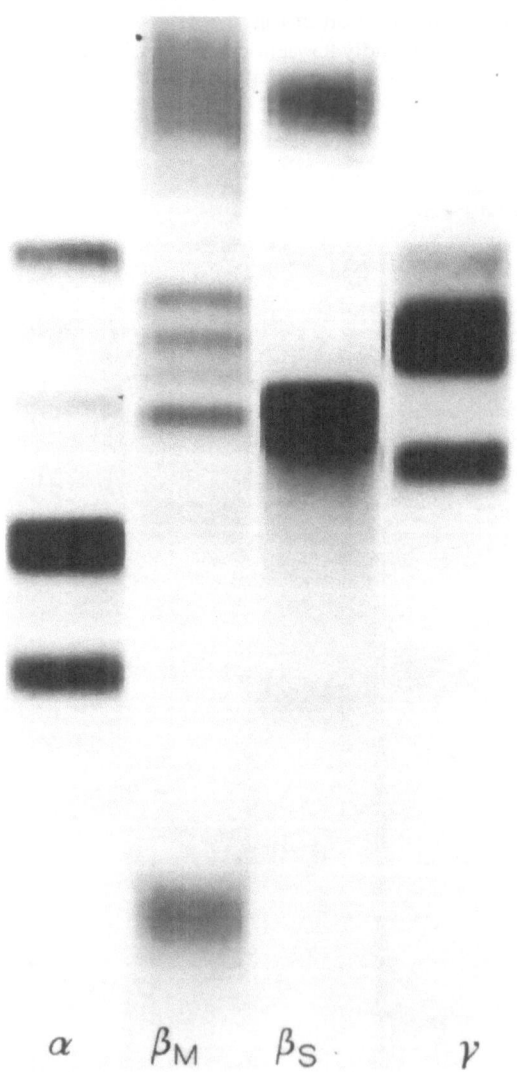

α β_M β_S γ

Fig. 8. 6 M urea-polyacrylamide gel electrophoresis of the separated LM crystallins. For comparison also the pattern of α crystallin is depicted.

This electrophoretic assay is especially useful for the further characterization of LM crystallin. In addition to a slow moving component β_M appears to contain the so-called FM crystallin (VAN DEN BROEK, LEGET & BLOEMENDAL, 1974), whereas also in β_s two major components are detected. The molecular weight of 14,500 estimated earlier after SDS gel electrophoresis of FM crystallin is not in agreement with the position in the β_m fraction upon gel filtration. The discrepancy may be due to changes in conformation.

We have also studied the electrophoretic behavior of fractionated LM crystallins on polyacrylamide gels containing 6 M urea (see Fig. 8). Comparison of Fig. 7 with Fig. 8 shows that there is in principle no difference, This suggests that β_M. β_s and purified γ are no aggregates but mixtures of

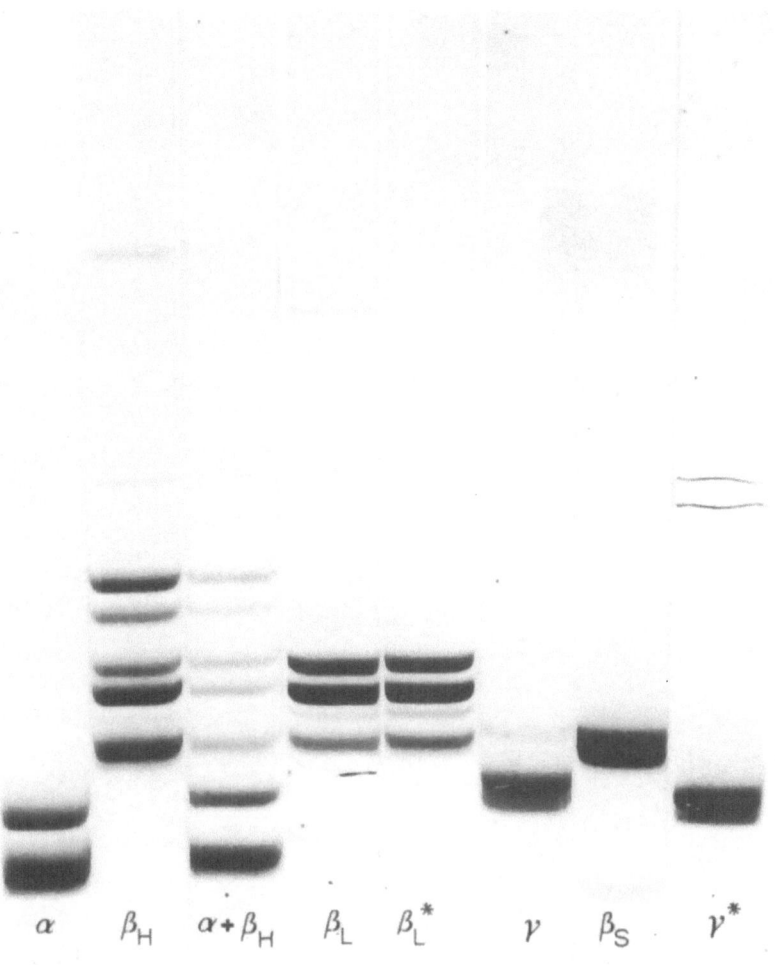

Fig. 9. SDS-polyacrylamide gel electrophoresis of various crystallins. α, β_H, and γ β_L were obtained after gel filtration on Ultrogel AcA 34. $\alpha + \beta_H$, $\beta_L{}^*$, β_s, and γ^* were obtained after gel filtration on a Sephadex G-75 column.

monomeric proteins of different charge. The FM crystallin migrates faster than the fastest α crystallin chain αA_1, reflecting its lower isoelectric point.

Electrophoresis of the separated β_s and γ fraction on 0.1% SDS containing polyacrylamide gels followed by a molecular weight estimation yields an approximate molecular weight of 22,000 for β_s. This value is considerably lower than the 28,000 estimate of VAN DAM (1966) obtained after gel filtration (compare Fig. 9).

Fig. 10 demonstrates that even after SE Sephadex chromatography the separated γ components are not pure single polypeptides.

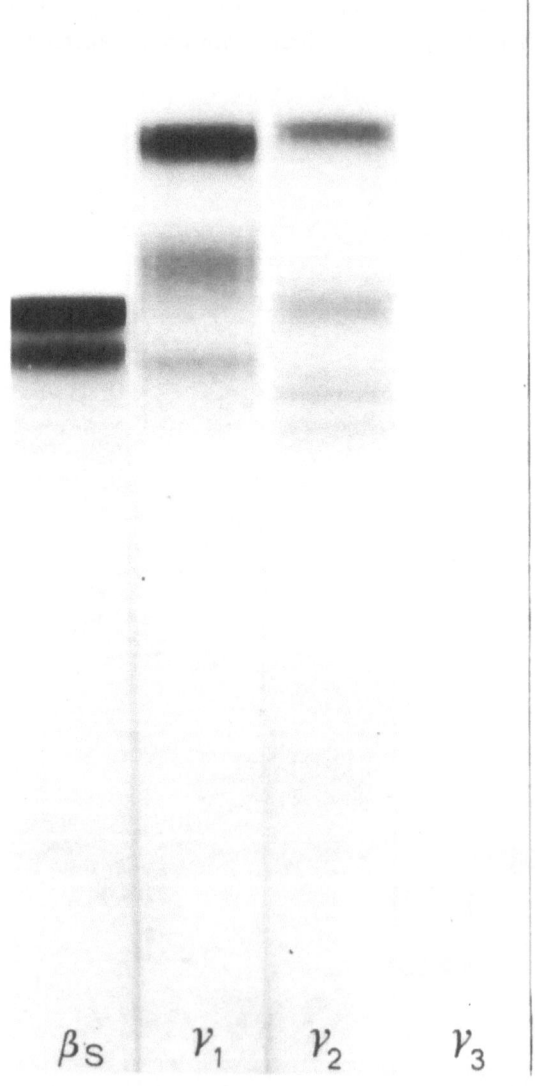

Fig. 10. 6 M urea-polyacrylamide gel electrophoresis of the LM crystallin fractions after SE Sephadex chromatography (compare Fig. 4).

The present communication emphasizes the occurrence of numerous minor components in various 'purified' lens proteins whose meaning and significance remain to be established.

ACKNOWLEDGEMENTS

The authors are grateful to Miss M.C. Potjens for her assistance in preparing the manuscript.

REFERENCES

BJÖRK, I. Studies on γ-crystallin from calf lens. I. Isolation by gel filtration. *Exp. Eye Res.* 1: *145-154* (1961).

BJÖRK, I. Studies on γ-crystallin from calf lens. II. Purification and some properties of the main protein components. *Exp. Eye Res.* 3: *254-261* (1964).

BLOEMENDAL, H. Zone Electrophoresis in Blocks and Columns. Elsevier Publishing Company; Elsevier Monographs: Chemistry Section 28 (1963).

BLOEMENDAL, H. Alpha-crystallin. Structural aspects and biosynthesis. *Acta Morphol. Neerl.-Scand.* 10: *197-213* (1972).

BLOEMENDAL, H., A.J.M. BERNS, F. VAN DER OUDERAA & W.W.W. DE JONG. Evidence for a 'non-genetic' origin of the A_1 chain of α-crystallin. *Exp. Eye Res.* 14: *80-81* (1972a).

BLOEMENDAL, H., T. BERNS, A. ZWEERS, H. HOENDERS & E.L. BENEDETTI. The state of aggregation of α-crystallin detected after large scale preparations by zonal centrifugation. *Eur. J. Biochem.* 24: *401-406* (1972b).

BLOEMENDAL, H. & P. HERBRINK. Growing insight into the structure of β-crystallin. A review. *Ophthal. Res.* 6: *81-92* (1974).

BLOEMENDAL, H., A. ZWEERS, F.L. BENEDETTI & H. WALTERS. Selective reassociation of the crystallins. *Exp. Eye Res.* 20: *463-478* (1975).

BLOEMENDAL, H., A. ZWEERS & H. WALTERS. Self-assembly of lens crystallins *in vitro. Nature* 255: *426-427* (1975).

CROFT, L.R. The amino acid sequence of γ-crystallin (Fraction II) from calf lens. *Biochem. J.* 128: *961-970* (1972).

DE JONG, W.W., F.S.M. VAN KLEEF & H. BLOEMENDAL. Intracellular carboxy-terminal degradation of the αA chains of α-crystallin. *Eur. J. Biochem.* 48: *271-276* (1974).

HARDING, J.J. & K.J. DILLEY. Structural proteins of the mammalian lens: A review with emphasis on changes in development, aging and cataract. *Exp. Eye Res.* 20: *1-73* (1976).

HERBRINK, P. & H. BLOEMENDAL. Studies on β-crystallin. I. Isolation and partial characterization of the principal polypeptide chain. *Biochim. Biophys. Acta* 336: *370-382* (1974).

KABASAWA, I., J.H. KINOSHITA & G.W. BARBER. Aging effects on the bovine lens γ-crystallins. *Exp. Eye Res.* 18: *457-466* (1974).

LAEMMLI, U.K. Cleavage of structural proteins during the assembly of the head of bacteriophage T4. *Nature* (London) 227: *680-685* (1970).

MÖRNER, C.T. Untersuchung der Proteinsubstanzen in den leichtbrechenden Medien des Auges. *Z. Physiol. Chem.* 18: *61-106* (1894).

RABAEY, M., I. RIKKERS & M. DE METS. Low molecular weight protein in the lens of birds. *Exp. Eye Res.* 14: *208-213* (1972).

SPECTOR, A., T. FREUND, L-K. LI & R.C. AUGUSTEYN. Age-dependent changes in the structure of alpha-crystallin. *Invest. Ophthalmol.* 10: *677-686* (1971).

TESTA, M., G. ARMAND & E.A. BALAZS. Separation of the soluble proteins of bovine lenses on polyacrylamide gels. *Exp. Eye Res.* 4: *327-339* (1965).

VAN DAM, A.F. Purification and composition studies of β_S-crystallin. *Exp. Eye Res.* 5: *255-266* (1966).

VAN DEN BROEK, W.G.M., J.N. LEGET & H. BLOEMENDAL. FM-crystallin: a neglected component among lens proteins. *Biochim. Biophys. Acta* 310: *278-282* (1973).

VAN DER OUDERAA, F.J., W.W. DE JONG & H. BLOEMENDAL. The amino-acid sequence of the αA_2 chain of bovine α-crystallin. *Eur. J. Biochem.* 39: *207-222* (1973).

VAN DER OUDERAA, F.J., W.W. DE JONG, A. HILDERINK & H. BLOEMENDAL. The amino acid sequence of the αB_2 chain of bovine α-crystallin. *Eur. J. Biochem.* 49: *157-168* (1974).

VAN KLEEF, F.S.M. & H.J. HOENDERS. Population character and variety in subunit structure of high-molecular-weight proteins from the bovine eye lens. *Eur. J. Biochem.* 40: *549-554* (1973).

VAN KLEEF, F.S.M., W.W. DE JONG & H.J. HOENDERS. Stepwise degradations and deamidation of the eye lens protein α-crystallin in ageing. *Nature* 258: *264-266* (1975).

Authors' address:

Department of Biochemistry
University of Nijmegen
Geert Grooteplein Noord 21
Nijmegen. The Netherlands

CHANGES IN THE SUBUNIT STRUCTURE OF α-CRYSTALLIN FROM BOVINE AND RABBIT EYE LENSES*

H.J. HOENDERS

(Nijmegen, The Netherlands)

ABSTRACT

The subunit structure of α-crystallin varies strongly as a function of its age. Deamidation and specific degradation processes continually alter the structure of the composing polypeptide chains. The composition of bovine α-crystallin in various prenatal stages and in several concentric layers of calf and cow lenses have been studied by gel isoelectric focusing in the presence of 6 M urea. In rabbit lenses the changes in subunit structure of α-crystallin were investigated during development of cataract induced by X-irradiation.

INTRODUCTION

In the past years strong progress has been made with respect to the knowledge of the subunit structure of eye lens proteins. Applying isoelectric focusing in polyacrylamide gels in the presence of 6 M urea it was possible to distinguish between polypeptide chains with small differences in isoelectric point. This is especially advantageous for the investigation of the older, nuclear crystallins which fall apart into many polypeptides in denaturing media. For cataract research at the level of protein structure it is imperative that physiological aging phenomena can be differentiated from possible pathological events. Some findings of our laboratory in the past four years concerning the subunit structure of α-crystallin isolated from clear and cataractous eye lenses are surveyed here.

Bovine lenses

In Fig. 1 the quantitatively important polypeptide bands of α-crystallin, separated by gel isoelectric focusing (IEF) in the presence of 6 M urea and gel electrophoresis in the presence of sodium dodecyl sulphate (SDS), are schematically summarized. The presence or absence as well as the relative proportions of the peptide chains depend on the age of the lenses and on the location of the α-crystallin within the lens.

---

* Dedicated to professor Jean Nordmann at the occasion of his eightieth birthday.

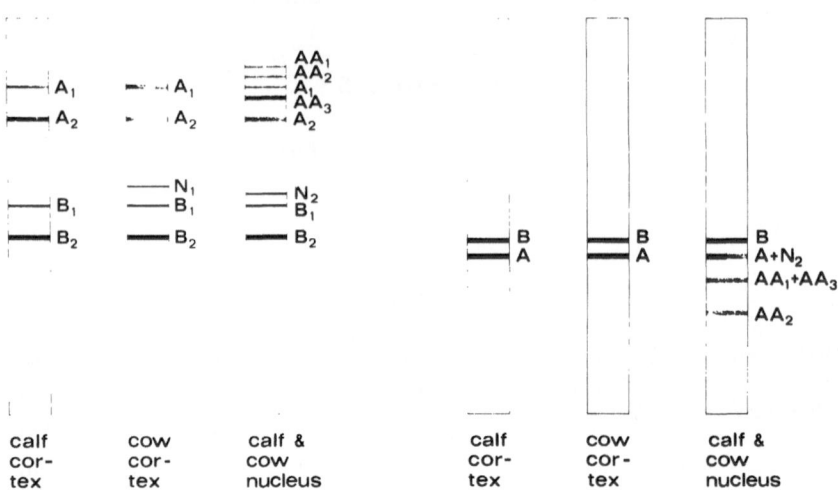

IEF-GELS   SDS-GELS

calf   cow   calf &   calf   cow   calf &
cor-   cor-   cow   cor-   cor-   cow
tex   tex   nucleus   tex   tex   nucleus

Fig. 1. Schematic representation of the subunit analysis of bovine α-crystallin by means of gel isoelectric focusing in the presence of 6 M urea and gel electrophoresis in the presence of 0.1% sodium dodecyl sulphate. Experimental details are given by VAN KLEEF & HOENDERS (1973) and VAN KLEEF (1975). The apparent molecular weights found on SDS gel electrophoresis ranged from 22,000 (B) to 11,000 (AA$_2$).

Prenatal bovine lenses

α-Crystallin from prenatal lenses was investigated by VAN KAMP, STRUY-KER, BOUDIER & HOENDERS (1974) and by VAN KLEEF (1975). Besides the A$_2$ and B$_2$ peptide chains, present in all preparations, the polypeptides A$_1$, AA$_3$, N$_2$ and B$_1$ were found. Their presence or absence with lens age is given in Table I.

Table I. Polypeptide chain composition of α-crystallin at various prenatal stages and from the 3-month-old calf.

Polypeptide chain	Prenatal age (months)						Calf
	1.5	2.5	3.5	4.5	6	8.5	3 months
A$_1$	−	−	−	(+)	+	+	+
AA$_3$, A$_X$	+	+	+	+	+	+	−
A$_2$	+	+	+	+	+	+	+
N$_2$, B$_X$	+	+	+	+	+	−	−
B$_1$	−	(+)	(+)	+	+	+	+
B$_2$	+	+	+	+	+	+	+

Minor proportions are indicated by (+). The designations A$_X$ and B$_X$ were used by VAN KAMP, STRUYKER BOUDIER & HOENDERS (1974).

In order to trace a possible influence of light on the polypeptide chain composition of prenatal α-crystallin, lenses of 6.5- and 8.5-month old fetuses were dissected in the dark. One eye of each animal was then kept dark, whereas the other one was illuminated for 24 hours with a 254 nm ultraviolet lamp. It turned out that only the B_X chain of the 6.5-months prenatal α-crystallin disappeared under the influence of this illumination, whereas no changes could be detected in the α-crystallin of the elder fetus.

Calf lenses

VAN KAMP, SCHATS & HOENDERS (1973) isolated α-crystallin on agarose A-5 m columns from extracts of the epithelium, seven successive concentric layers of the cortex and the nucleus of about 3-month-old calf lenses. Electrophoresis on polyacrylamide gels in 6 M urea at pH 8.9 re-

Table II. Polypeptide chain composition of α-crystallin from concentric calf lens layers.

Polypeptide chain	Outer cortex	Inner cortex	Outer nucleus	Inner nucleus
AA_1	−	−	(+)	+
AA_2	−	−	(+)	+
A_1	+	++	+	+
AA_3	−	(+)	++	++
A_2	++	++	++	+
N_2	+	(+)	+	+
B_1	−	+	+	+
B_2	++	+	+	+

Minor components (relative proportion < 5%) are indicated by (+), major components (relative proportion > 20%) by ++.

Table III. Polypeptide chain composition of cortical α-crystallin from calf lenses after dialysis.
The dialysis buffer, 0.1 M Tris-HCl pH 7.3, containing pentachlorophenol as preservative, was refreshed every 2nd day.

Polypeptide chain	Time span in weeks			
	0	1	3	5
AA_1	−	(+)	(+)	(+)
AA_2	−	−	−	−
A_1	++	++	++	++
AA_3	(+)	+	+	+
A_2	++	++	++	++
N_0	−	−	−	+
N_2	(+)	(+)	+	++
B_1	+	+	+	(+)
B_2	++	++	+	(+)

vealed for the cortical layer four bands, of which it was assumed that they represented the A_1, A_2, B_1 and B_2 polypeptide chains. For the nuclear α-crystallin an additional band, migrating faster than the A_1 chain, was found. This experiment was repeated with 22-week-old calf lenses and some more concentric layers, but now isoelectric focusing in the presence of 6 M urea was applied for the subunit analysis (VAN KLEEF, 1975). The superiority of this method appeared very convincingly from its much better resolution of the peptide chains (Table II).

It was found by chance that considerable changes in subunit structure occurred upon prolonged dialysis of α-crystallin from calf cortex against buffer solution (VAN KLEEF, 1975). The effects could be enhanced by addition of 2% polyethylene glycol 6,000 to the buffer. The results are given in Table III.

Older bovine lenses

Lenses from 6- to 8-year-old cattle were divided into several successive concentric layers. The α-crystallin preparations, obtained by chromatography on agarose A-5 m columns, were submitted to isoelectric focusing in 6 M urea (VAN KLEEF, 1975). The subunit composition of the various lens parts is given in Table IV.

Table IV. Polypeptide chain composition of α-crystallin from concentric cow lens layers.

Polypeptide chain	Outer cortex	Inner cortex	Outer nucleus	Inner nucleus
AA_1	+	+	+	+
AA_2	–	+	+	+
A_1	++	+	+	(+)
AA_3	(+)	+	+	+
A_2	++	++	++	+
N_1	+	(+)	–	–
N_2	–	(+)	+	+
B_1	+	+	+	+
B_2	+	+	+	+

Nature of the polypeptide chains

The structure of the 'new' subunits has recently been elucidated (VAN KLEEF, NIJZINK-MAAS & HOENDERS, 1974; VAN KLEEF, 1975). It could be shown that the *de novo* synthesized A_2 and B_2 chains are not only subject to deamidation, but also to specific and limited C-terminal degradation (VAN KLEEF, DE JONG & HOENDERS, 1975). The various polypeptide chains found in bovine α-crystallin preparations are enumerated in tabel V in the order of increasing isoelectric point. High- and low-molecular-weight α-crystallin fractions, originating from the same lens extract, revealed essentially identical patterns on isoelectric focusing.

Table V. Nature of the polypeptide chains found in bovine α-crystallins.*

Older name(s)	Rationalized name	Number of amino acid residues	Character
AA_1	A_1^{1-151}	151	degraded A_1
AA_2	A^{1-101}	101	degraded A
A_1	A_1	173	deamidated A_2
AA_3, A_X	A_2^{1-151}	151	degraded A_2
A_2	A_2	173	primary gene product
N_0	B_1^{1-170}	170	degraded B_1 (dialysis product)
N_1	B_0	175	deamidated B_1
N_2, B_X	B_2^{1-170}	170	degraded B_2
B_1	B_1	175	deamidated B_2
B_2	B_2	175	primary gene product

* In addition to these polypeptides degraded A chains with 169 and 168 amino acid residues were found by *de Jong, van Kleef, Bloemendal* (1974). These chains do not separate from A_1 and A_2 on isoelectric focusing.

Rabbit lenses

Experimental cataracts were obtained approximately three months after X-irradiation of one eye of 2-month-old rabbits. The irradiated, totally opaque lenses were compared with the completely transparent control lenses (LIEM-THE, STOLS, JAP & HOENDERS, 1975). The polypeptide patterns of low- and high-molecular-weight α-crystallin from the normal and cataractous cortices (outer 40% of the lens) and nuclei (inner 20%) are shown in Fig. 2.

Cortical low-molecular-weight α-crystallin from the normal rabbit lens showed the same, rather simple pattern (comprising the four well-known polypeptide chains A_1, A_2. B_1 and B_2) as cortical α-crystallin from calf lens. The other preparations were much more complex and contained chains with isoelectric points identical to those of A_X and B_X in bovine α-crystallin (cf. Table V) as well as β-crystallin chains (see legend of Fig. 2).

The irradiated lenses and their controls were also studied during the development of the X-ray induced cataracts (LIEM-THE, 1975). A comparison of prenatal α-crystallin (21 days after conception) with α-crystallin from control and irradiated lenses at three stages of development is given in Table VI.

CONCLUDING REMARKS

The polypeptide chain composition of α-crystallin strongly depends upon the age of the molecule and, therefore, upon its location within the eye lens. Moreover, ultraviolet illumination, X-irradiation and prolonged dialysis can alter peptide chains via hitherto unknown mechanisms.

The polypeptides are subject to deamidation and specific C-terminal chain-shortening processes, resulting in more complex subunit compositions.

Table VI. Polypeptide chain composition of α-crystallin from 3-, 4- and 5-month-old rabbit lenses

Polypeptide chain	Prenatal (21 d)	control cortex 3m.	4m.	5m.	control nucleus 3m.	4m.	5m.	irradiated cortex 4m.	5m.	irradiated nucleus 3m.	4m.	5m.
A₁	−	−	+	+	−	+	+	+	+	−	+	+
Ax	−	+	(+)	−	+	(+)	+	+	+	(+)	+	+
A₂	+	+	+	+	+	+	+	+	+	+	+	+
Bx	+	+	+	−	+	+	+	+	+	+	+	+
B₁	−	−	−	+	−	−	(+)	−	−	−	−	−
B₂	−	−	+	+	−	−	+	+	+	−	−	+

110

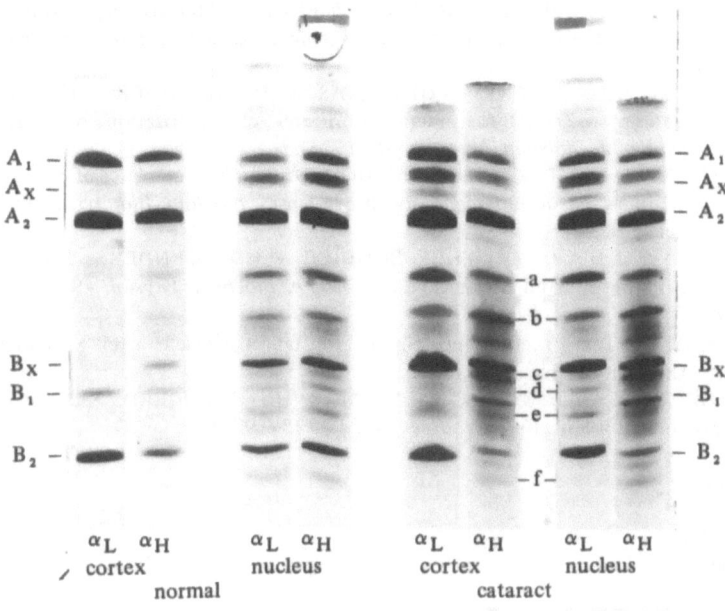

Fig. 2. Isoelectric focusing on polyacrylamide gels in the presence of 6 M urea and 0.04% 1,4-dithioerythritol. From left to right gel patterns of respectively the normal cortical, the normal nuclear, the cataractous cortical and the cataractous nuclear low-(α_L) and high-molecular-weight α-crystallins (α_H). Bands a-f correspond with β-crystallin polypeptides.

These processes coincide with the formation of very high-molecular-weight aggregates and with insolubilization. Whether post-synthetic peptide chain modification and aggregation are interrelated remains as yet obscure.

REFERENCES

JONG, W.W. DE, F.S.M. VAN KLEEF & H. BLOEMENDAL. Intracellular carboxy-terminal degradation of the αA chain of α-crystallin. *Eur. J. Biochem.* 48: *271-276* (1974).

KLEEF, F.S.M. VAN. Post-synthetic modifications of bovine α-crystallin. Thesis, University of Nijmegen (1975).

KLEEF, F.S.M. VAN & H.J. HOENDERS. Population character and variety in sub-unit structure of high-molecular-weight proteins from the bovine eye lens. *Eur. J. Biochem.* 40: *549-554* (1973).

KLEEF, F.S.M. VAN W.W. DE JONG & H.J. HOENDERS. Stepwise degradations and deamidation of the eye lens protein α-crystallin in ageing. *Nature* 258: *264-266* (1975).

KLEEF, F.S.M. VAN, M.J.C.M. NIJZINK-MAAS & H.J. HOENDERS. Intracellular degradation of α-crystallin. Fractionation and characterization of degraded αA-chains. *Eur. J. Biochem.* 48: *563-570* (1974).

KAMP, G.J. VAN, L.H.M. SCHATS & H.J. HOENDERS. Characteristics of α-crystallin related to fiber cell development in calf eye lenses. *Biochim. Biophys. Acta* 295: *166-173* (1973).

KAMP, G.J. VAN, H.A.J. STRUYKER BOUDIER & H.J. HOENDERS. The soluble proteins of the prenatal bovine eye lens. *Comp. Biochem. Physiol.* 49B: *445-456* (1974).

LIEM-THE, K.N. The structural proteins of the rabbit eye lens after X-irradiation. Thesis, University of Nijmegen (1975).

LIEM-THE, K.N., A.L.H. STOLS, P.H.K. JAP & H.J. HOENDERS. X-ray induced cataract in rabbit lens. *Exp. Eye Res.* 20: *317-328* (1975).

Keywords:

Lens protein
α-crystallin
Subunit structure
Polypeptide composition
Aging
Cataract
Isoelectric focusing

Author's address:

Department of Biochemistry
University of Nijmegen
Geert Grooteplein Noord 21
Nijmegen, The Netherlands

Acknowledgment: The author thanks Academic Press for permission to reproduce Fig. 2.

A COMPARATIVE STUDY OF RABBIT LENS PROTEINS

KENSHI SATOH & MASAYASU BANDO

(Chiba/Tokyo, Japan)

ABSTRACT

A comparative study of the water soluble and insoluble proteins isolated from lens of normal rabbit at age of 24 months has been performed by use of animo acid analysis, and of ampholine isoelectric focusing method. Evidence is presented indicating that the urea-soluble fraction of the insoluble protein is formed by a partial combination of beta- and gamma-crystallins. It is also revealed that the sugar moiety seems to be involved in the formation of the insoluble from the soluble proteins in rabbit lens.

INTRODUCTION

By comparing physico-chemical properties, including electrophoretic mobility, immunochemical behavior and amino acid composition, of the water insoluble protein with those of the water soluble proteins, it has been demonstrated that the major component of the insoluble protein is closely similar to, and derived from, alpha crystallin in bovine lens (SIRCHIS et al., 1956; THOMANN, 1962; RAO et al., 1965; RUTTENBERG, 1965), and in human lens (MEHTA & MAISEL, 1967; CLARK et al., 1969). Other lines of evidence, however, has indicated that the water insoluble protein contains small amounts of beta-, and gamma-crystallins in addition to alpha crystallin in bovine lens (MANSKI et al., 1968; MEHTA & MAISEL, 1968). It has also been demonstrated that the water insoluble protein of rat lens is mainly composed of gamma-crystallin (ZIGMAN & LERMAN 1968; LERMAN et al., 1968). A controversial evidence against this finding, however, has been proposed by HARDING (1969) who indicated the insoluble proteins isolated from rat lens be derived from mixture of the soluble proteins rather than from any single crystallin.

The water insoluble proteins isolated from rabbit lens has received less attention, but it has recently been reported that the insoluble protein derived from the central region (lens nucleus) of normal rabbit lens is composed of alpha- and beta-crystallins (LIEM-THE & HOENDERS, 1974). The authors have also indicated that the high molecular weight (HM) crystallin from the rabbit lens is composed of alpha- and beta-crystallins, which led them to the suggestion that the HM crystallin may be an intermediate in the conversion of the water soluble into water insoluble proteins during aging of the lens.

The present paper describes a comparative study of the water soluble and

113

insoluble proteins of normal rabbit lens to delineate the relatedness between the lens proteins. The molecular association that might be involved in the conversion of the soluble to insoluble proteins in the lens will also been discussed.

MATERIALS AND METHODS

Lens proteins

Lenses from albino rabbit (New Zealand white) eyes at age of 24 months were carefully dissected with a posterior approach. Each lens with the capsule intact was weighed and used immediately. The lenses were homogenized individually in ten times their weight of water in a Potter Elvehjem homogenizer in ice. The lens homogenate was then centrifuged for 60 min at 15,000 g, at 4 °C. The precipitate formed was washed twice with 5 ml each of water by 60 min centrifugations at 18,000 g, 4 °C, and the washings were added to the initial supernatant. The pooled supernatant was dialyzed for 48 hr against 200 volumes of 2 mM potassium phosphate buffer, pH 7.2, with three volume changes, and were named as the water soluble protein. While the washed precipitate was named as the water insoluble protein. The insoluble protein fraction derived from each lens was then treated with 8 M urea containing 10 mM Tris-HCl, pH 8.2, in a final volume of 5 ml, and the mixture was left for 60 min at room temperature. The urea-insoluble material was then removed by 60 min centrifugation at 18,000 g, at 10 °C, and was washed twice with 5 ml each of the buffered 8 M urea by 60 min centrifugation, at 10 °C, at 20,000 g. The washings and the initial supernatant were pooled, which was named as the urea soluble (US) fraction. The final precipitate was taken up with 5 ml of 2 mM Tris-HCl, pH 8.2, and was named as the urea insoluble (UI) fraction. Both US- and UI-fractions were dialyzed for 24 hr against 200 volumes of 2 mM Tris-HCl, pH 8.2, with two volume changes.

DEAE-cellulose column chromatography

Alpha-, beta- and gamma-crystallins in rabbit lens soluble protein were fractionated by the method of DEAE-cellulose column chromatography as described previously (SATOH, 1972). Each crystallin fraction thus obtained was dialyzed for 24 hr against 200 volumes of 2 mM Tris-HCl, pH 8.2, with two volume changes.

Ampholine isoelectric focusing

The isoelectric focusing (VESTERBERG & SVENSSON, 1966) of the lens proteins on a pH gradient from 5 to 8 was carried out by use of Ampholine, pH range 5-8, in an isoelectric focusing column having a capacity of 110 ml (LKB-Produkter AB, Stockholm, Sweden). By employing mixing device supplied from LKB, the density gradient was prepared from a 55 ml 50% (W/V) sucrose solution in water containing 0.6 g of the carrier ampholite, and a 60 ml apholite solution containing 0.2 g of the ampholite and protein sample in water. An electric potential applied to the column was 720 volts, and the experiment was run for 24 to 36 hr. The column was kept at 10 °C throughout the experiment by circulating thermostatted water. After completion of each run the column was emptied from bottom at a flow rate of 2 ml/min, and the effluent collected in 2 ml aliquot. pH of each fraction thus collected was measured at 10 °C. 2 ml of water was then added to each tube, absorption of which was measued at 280 nm. The absorption due to ampholine itself was corrected by running the same experiments as the one described above without protein sample.

Amino acid analyses

Amino acid analyses were performed with an amino acid analyzer (JEOL, JLC-5H) by the method of Spackman, et al. (1958). Protein sample (0.3-0.5 mg) was hydrolyzed in constant boiling 6 N HCl (5 ml). Hydrolysis was continued for 24 hr at 110 °C. Tryptophan contents and hydrolysis losses of any amino acid were disregarded in this study.

Sugar assays

The contents of sugar in the lens protein were estimated by the phenol-sulfuric acid method as described by DUBOIS et al. (1956) using D-glucose as standard.

Protein estimations

The content of protein in the lens protein was estimated by biuret method (GORNALL et al., 1949) using bovine serum albumin as standard.

RESULTS AND DISCUSSION

The relative amounts of various protein fractions isolated from lens of rabbit at age of 24 months are given in Table I. The lens protein fractions

Table I. Protein fractions isolated from rabbit lens (643 mg wet wt)

Protein fraction		% of total protein recovered	% of soluble protein*
Water soluble:	alpha		23.6
	beta	78.9	52.7
	gamma		23.7
Water insoluble:	urea soluble	18.4	–
	urea insoluble	2.7	–

* Values presented were estimated by summing up each area corresponding to respective crystallin under the elution profile obtained from the isoelectric focusing as shown in Fig. 1.

115

(305 mg in total) represent 47% of the wet weight of the lens. This value is unusually high in comparison with the ones in rat lens (32% HARDING, 1969), and in human lens (∿32%, SATOH, 1972). The proportion of the water insoluble protein of the rabbit lens is intermediate in value among those found in rat lens (29% of total protein, HARDING, 1969), and in cattle lens (12.5% of total protein, KRAUSE, 1933). The proportion of the US-fraction is higher as compared to that of rat lens (10% of total protein, HARDING, 1969), whereas the proportion of the UI-fraction is lower in rabbit lens than in rat lens (19% of total protein, HARDING, 1969) but is comparable with the value in cattle lens (0-10% of total protein, DISCHE, 1965; MANSKI et al., 1968). The proportion of the water soluble protein in rabbit lens is rather high as compared to the one in rat lens (71% of total protein, HARDING, 1969). It is noteworthy that the proportion of beta-crystallin in the water soluble protein is double that of alpha-, and of gamma-crystallins.

Amino acid compositions of protein fractions of the rabbit lens are given in Table II. The amUS-fraction is the major peak fraction isolated from the US-fraction by the ampholine isoelectric focusing as shown in Fig. 1. Half cystine is found only in the US-fraction and gamma-crystallin. Methionine is found in all the protein fractions except for alpha-crystallin. The result suggest the possibility that the US-fraction may be closely related to beta- and gamma-crystallin but not to alpha-crystallin.

One method by which the relatedness between proteins may be assessed is the use of difference index, which has been proposed by METZGER et al.

Table II. Amino acid compositions of protein fractions of rabbit lens*

| | Residues/1000 residues | | | | | |
	alpha	beta	gamma	US	amUS**	UI
Lysine	66	36	15	41	53	4
Histidine	40	33	37	41	13	23
Arginine	77	84	126	89	47	47
Aspartic acid	89	88	101	93	101	78
Threonine	40	30	20	30	58	43
Serine	106	86	86	86	55	120
Glutamic acid	109	138	117	126	121	120
Proline	71	50	39	57	48	44
Glycine	75	106	89	81	108	191
Alanine	47	62	36	45	113	78
Valine	71	73	60	57	85	94
1/2 cystine	null	null	17	23	null	null
Methinine	null	12	19	18	16	5
Isoleucine	37	43	38	42	42	24
Leucine	81	75	87	84	84	84
Tyrosine	20	33	66	49	24	21
Phenylalanine	72	52	46	39	34	24

* Values presented are average of two determinations.
** Major fraction isolated from the US protein by the isoelectric focusing method as shown in Fig. 1.

116

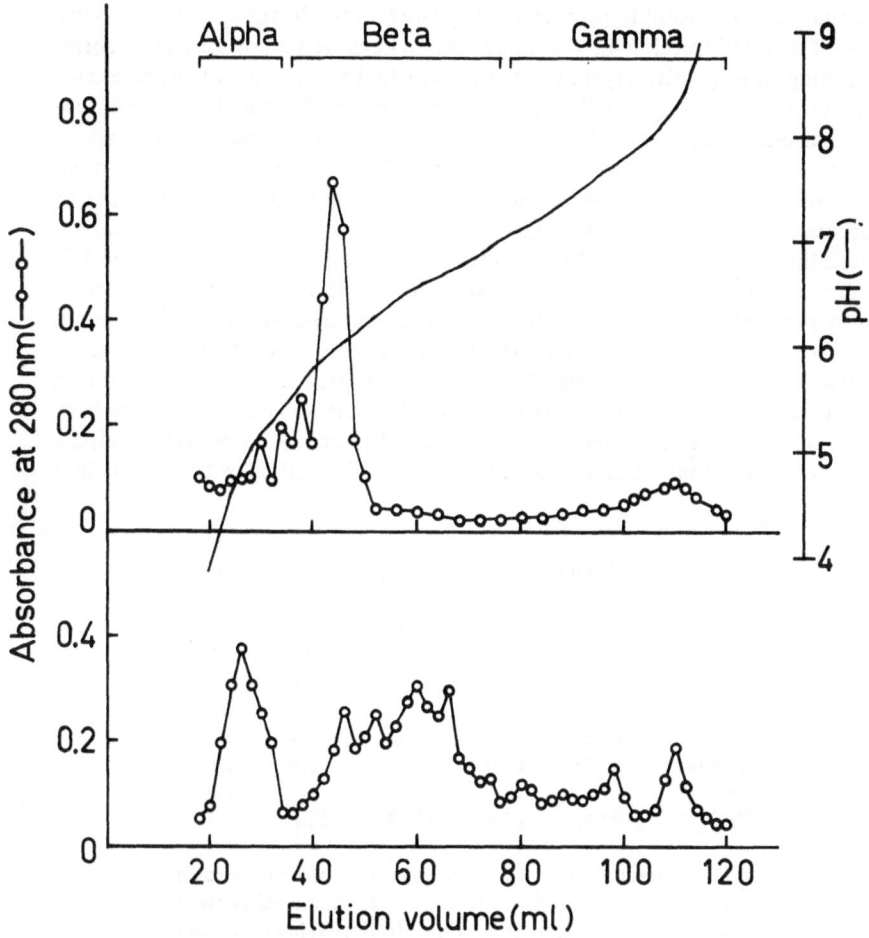

Fig. 1 Isoelectric focusing patterns obtained from the water soluble proteins (lower) and the US-fraction (upper) of the water insoluble protein in rabbit lens. See text for detail.

(1968). The difference indices (DI) were calculated from the amino acid compositions in Table II, and are tabulated in Table III. The DI will be smaller in value (<5) for a pair of proteins that are closely related than for a pair of proteins that are unlike in composition. A distinct relatedness between the protein fractions is hardly assumed because the DI for all combinations listed is too high (~8) to be considered identical. The DI for the combinations of the US-fraction with beta-crystallin, and with gamma-crystallin, however, are lowest in value among other combinations listed, whereas the DI for the UI-fraction are higher in all cases. Nature and origin of the UI-fraction remain to be investigated.

In order to establish the relationship of the US-fraction to the crystallins, the isoelectric focusing patterns of the US-fraction, and of the water soluble protein fraction were compared, and the result is shown in Fig. 1. The profile from the soluble protein is illustrated in the lower part of the figure and of the US-fraction in the upper part. Each group of fractions corresponding to respective crystallins were identified by running the same experiments with each crystallin that is fractionated by the DEAE-cellulose column chromatography. It is seen that bulk of the US-fraction is localized in the region, where one component of beta-crystallin is located. A small portion of the US-fraction is also localized in the region corresponding to gamma-crystallin group. Any group of fractions corresponding to alpha-crystallin, however, is hardly detected but deposits of the beta in the US-fraction. The result seems to indicate that the US-fraction may be derived from particular portions of both beta- and gamma-crystallin, thus relatedness of the US-fraction to two crystallins, assessed by the DI, should be indistinct as noted previously. The results presented also appear to be in a controversy with the observation made by LIEM-THE & HOENDERS (1974) who have indicated the US-fraction be mainly composed of alpha- and beta-crystallins. It is concluded that the US-fraction of the rabbit lens

Table III. Difference indices (D.I.)* for protein fractions of rabbit lens

	alpha	beta	gamma	US	UI
alpha	–	11.5	17.3	11.8	20.8
beta	11.5	–	12.9	8.4	17.9
gamma	17.3	12.9	–	8.5	24.3
US	11.8	8.4	8.5	–	22.8
UI	20.8	17.9	24.3	22.8	–

* The difference index (D.I.) between two proteins is calculated by determining the difference in the fractional contents of each amino acid, the sum of the absolute value of which is multiplied by 50. The calculation is based on the values presented in Table II.

Table IV. The content of sugar in protein fractions of rabbit lens

Protein fraction*	Sugar (μg/mg protein)
whole homogenate	4.4
water soluble	2.3
water insoluble:	
US	4.1
UI	20.5

* The lens protein fractions were extensively dialyzed against 2 mM Tris-HCl, pH 8.2, to remove free sugar present, and the buffer used for the final dialysis was employed as a diluting medium for all the solutions used in the sugar assays.

insoluble protein seems to be formed by a partial combination of beta- and gamma-crystallins, but an exact combination involved is as yet obscure.

Distribution of sugar in protein fractions of rabbit lens has also been investigated. The result is tabulated in Table IV. It appears that most of sugar is concentrated in the UI-fraction, and 1/5 of which is in the US-fraction and 1/10 in the water soluble protein fraction. A portion of sugar found in the UI-fraction may be derived from the lens capsule, which contains a collagen-like protein combined with carbohydrate material (PIRIE, 1951). The increase in the sugar content seems to be in parallel with the decrease in solubility of the lens proteins. This tendency seems to be consistent with the implication as proposed by DISCHE (1965) that the formation of complex between sugar moiety in trace amounts and the soluble proteins might yield material having the gross composition of the crystallins but markedly different solubility characteristics. Nature of the sugar moiety in the lens protein is under an extensive investigation.

ACKNOWLEDGEMENTS

The authors are grateful to Professor Akira Nakajima for suggestions and counsel throughout this work.

REFERENCES

CLARK, R., ZIGMAN, S. & LERMAN, S. Studies on the structural proteins of the human lens. *Exp. Eye Res.* 8: *172-182* (1969).

DISCHE, Z. The glycoproteins and glycolipoproteins of bovine lens and their relation to albuminoid. *Invest. Ophthal.* 4: *759-778* (1965).

DUBOIS, M., GILLES, K.A., HAMILTON, J.K., REBERS, P.A. & SMITH, F. Colorimetric method for determination of sugars and related substances. *Anal. Chem.* 28: *350-356* (1956).

GORNALL, A.G., BARDAWILL, C.J. & DAVID, M.M. Determination of serum proteins by means of biuret reaction. *J. Biol. Chem.* 177: *751-766* (1949).

HARDING, J.J. Nature and origin of the insoluble protein of rat lens. *Exp. Eye Res.* 8: *147-156* (1969).

KRAUSE, A.C. Chemistry of the lens; relation of the anatomic distribution of the lenticular proteins to their chemical compositions. *Arch. Ophthalmol.* (Chicago). 10: *788-792* (1933).

LERMAN, S., ZIGMAN, S, & FORBES, W.F. Insoluble protein fraction of the lens. *Exp. Eye Res.* 7: *444-448* (1968).

LIEM-THE, K.N. & HOENDERS, H.J. HM-crystallin as an intermediate in the conversion of water-soluble into water insoluble rabbit lens proteins. *Exp. Eye Res.* 19: *549-557* (1974).

MANSKI, W., BEHRENS, M. & MARTINEZ, C. Immunochemical studies on albuminoid. *Exp. Eye Res.* 7: *164-171* (1968).

MEHTA, P.D. & MAISEL, H. Albuminoid of human and cynomologus monkey lens. *Am. J. Ophthal.* 63: *967-972* (1967).

MEHTA, P.D. & MAISEL, H. Subunit structure of bovine α-crystallin and albuminoid. *Exp. Eye Res.* 7: *265-268* (1968).

METZGER, H., SHAPIRO, M.B., MOSIMANN, J.E. & VINTON, J.E. Assessment of compositional relatedness between proteins. *Nature* 219: *1166-1168* (1968).

PIRIE, A. Composition of ox lens capsule. *Biochem. J.* 48: *368-371* (1951).

RAO, S., MEHTA, P.D. & COOPER, S. Conversion of α-crystallin of bovine lens into insoluble protein *in vitro. Exp. Eye Res.* 4: *104-107* (1965).

RUTTENBERG, G. The insoluble proteins of bovine crystalline lens. *Exp. Eye Res.* 4: *18-23* (1965).

SATOH, K. Age-related changes in the structural proteins of human lens. *Exp. Eye Res.* 14: *53-57* (1972).

SIRCHIS, J., FROMAGEOT, P. & BERNARD, H. Points communs entre l'α-crystalline et la fraction principale Fl de l'insoluble du crystallin de boeuf. *C. r. Séanc. Acad. Sci. Paris* 243: *2164-2167* (1956).

SPACKMAN, D.H., STEIN, W.H. & MOORE, S. Automatic recording apparatus for use in the chromatography of amino acids. *Anal. Chem.* 30: *1190-1206* (1958).

THEOMANN, H. Struktur chemische Untersuchungen ueber den Aufbau des wasser-unloeslichen Eiweisses klarer Rinderlinsen. *v. Graefes Arch. Ophthal.* 165: *219-226* (1962).

VESTERBERG, O. & SVENSSON, H. Isoelectric fractionation, analysis and characterization of ampholytes in natural gradients. *Acta Chem. Scand.* 20: *820-834* (1966).

ZIGMAN, S. & LERMAN, S. The relationship between soluble and insoluble proteins in the lens. *Biochim. Biophys. Acta* 154: *423-425* (1968).

Keywords:

Water soluble and insoluble proteins
Lens crystallins
Amino acid compositions
Isoelectric focusing
Sugar

Authors' addresses:

Kenshi Satoh*
Department of Applied Biological Science
Science University of Tokyo
Noda, Chiba 278, Japan

Masayasu Bando
Department of Ophthalmology
Jutendo University School of Medicine
Bunkyo-ku, Tokyo 113, Japan

*requests for reprints to be addressed to Dr. Satoh

THE PROTEIN STRUCTURE OF CHICK LENS FIBER CELL MEMBRANES AND INTRACELLULAR MATRIX*

H. MAISEL, J. ALCALÁ & N. LIESKA

(Detroit, Michigan)

SUMMARY

Electrophoretic analysis of the water soluble fraction of chick lens fiber cells, the urea-soluble fraction, and the urea-insoluble plasma membrane fraction was performed in 5.13% polyacrylamide gels containing 1% sodium dodecyl sulfate (SDS). Five polypeptides were identified for the water soluble fraction. One polypeptide of molecular weight 22,500 daltons corresponded to subunits of α-crystallin, three polypeptides of molecular weights 25,000 daltons, 27,500 daltons, and 37,000 daltons corresponded to subunits of β-crystallins, and one polypeptide of 43,000 daltons corresponded to subunits of δ-crystallin. The water insoluble fraction contained twelve additional polypeptides with molecular weights ranging from 41,000 to 200,000 daltons. The 8 M urea soluble fraction (albuminoid) contained the 5 crystallin polypeptides as well as 8 additional bands. The major component of albuminoid consisted of a polypeptide of 41,000 daltons not found in the water soluble fraction of the lens. The urea-insoluble fraction (cell membranes) consisted of only 8 bands, one of which corresponded in molecular size with subunits of δ-crystallin and 2 with subunits of β-crystallin. However, the presence of lipid in the major membrane component (54.0%; with a mobility of a β-crystallin subunit) suggests that this component ist not a β-crystallin polypeptide.

INTRODUCTION

Biochemical studies of the lens have entered a phase of intensive analysis of the water insoluble components of fiber cells with emphasis on the cell membrane (BLOEMENDAL et al., 1972; DUNIA et al., 1974; BROEK-HUYSE & KUHLMAN, 1974; ALCALÁ et al., 1975). BURGER (1974) commented that the surface membrane of a cell is not only involved in the regulation of cell division and development, but that there is also an interrelation between the surface membrane and the interior of the cell. These suggestions are particularly intriguing with respect to the lens since fiber cells do not divide, and rapidly lose their nuclei in the process of differentiation.

The present paper reports the analysis of the water insoluble fractions of the chick lens by sodium dodecyl sulfate (SDS)-polyacrylamide gel electrophoresis.

* This study was supported by Ressearch Grant No. EY-01417 of the National Eye Institute, Bethesda, Maryland.

MATERIALS AND METHODS

Preparation of chick lens fiber cell fractions

Lenses from freshly killed White Leghorn chicks (3 months of post-hatching age) were decapsulated and epithelial and annular pad cells removed from the fiber mass. The lens fiber mass was homogenized in all glass tissue grinders at 4 °C in 9 volumes (w/v) of a standard salt solution containing 0.1 M KCl, 0.005 M $MgCl_2$, 0.006 M sodium phosphate buffer, pH 7.2, to which 0.001 M EDTA and 0.01 M 2-mercaptoethanol were added. The buffer will be referred to as the SEM buffer. The homogenate was centrifuged for 20 minutes at 37,000 g at 4 °C and the supernatant (water-soluble fraction: WSF) and the pellet (P) retained for further studies. The WSF was further centrifuged at 100,000 g for 2 h at 4 °C in an SW 65K rotor in the L3-40 Beckman ultracentrifuge. A pellet (100,000 g pellet) was recovered, washed in SEM and retained.

The pellet (P) was washed repeatedly in SEM buffer with rehomogenization and centrifugation, at 37,000 g for 15 minutes at 4 °C. This washing procedure was repeated until soluble proteins were no longer detected in the washing fluid by immunological and electrophoretic means. For this purpose, the volume of washing fluid was reduced by one-half to maximize the immunologic detection of lens crystallins in the supernatants. The total volume of buffer used in the washing procedure was 350 ml for 2.3 gm of initial pellet material. The thoroughly washed pellet, designated as the water-insoluble fraction (WIF), was retained.

Fractionation of water-insoluble lens fraction (WIF)

The WIF was treated with 8 M urea for the solubilization of albuminoid (RAO et al., 1965). The sample was subjected to repeated treatments by homogenization (50 mg wet weight pellet/ml) in a solution of 8 M urea in SEM buffer at 7 °C with occasional stirring. Following each treatment, the suspension was centrifuged at 77,000 g for 25 minutes at 7 °C. The procedure was repeated until the urea supernatant was immunologically free of crystallins. The supernatant obtained after the first urea treatment was designated as the 8 M urea-soluble fraction (8M-USF). The urea-insoluble pellet (urea-insoluble membrane rich fraction; UIMF) was washed repeatedly with SEM buffer to remove urea. The UIMF, previously shown to be a membrane-rich fraction (MAISEL et al., 1976) and the 8M-USF were retained.

In a separate experiment, the 8M-USF was adjusted to a 4 M concentration of urea with the SEM buffer, allowed to stand for 1 h at 7 °C and then centrifuged at 77,000 g for 30 minutes at 7 °C. A pellet (4 M urea pellet) was recovered and washed with the SEM buffer. A portion of the pellet was fixed for electron microscopy, and the remainder subjected to SDS gel electrophoresis. The supernatant (4M-USF) was retained.

Crystallin fractions were isolated from the WSF by continuous flow electrophoresis (MAISEL & LANGMAN, 1961) and by starch gel electrophoresis (SMITHIES, 1955). Both the two dimensional, combined filter paper-starch gel electrophoresis system (POULIK, 1957) and the one dimensional horizontal starch gel electrophoresis system were used. Protein was eluted from segments of the gel corresponding to specific crystallins (MAISEL et al., 1965).

SDS-polyacrylamide-gel electrophoresis

The sodium dodecyl sulfate-polyacrylamide gel electrophoresis system used was that of HINMAN & PHILIPS (1970), as modified by ALCALÁ et al. (1975) but with the adjustment of the ammonium persulfate: N,N,N′,N′-tetramethylethylenediamine ratio to 6:1 as suggested by FAIRBANKS et al. (1971).

Electrophoresis

Electrophoresis was performed on 9 cm polyacrylamide gel columns (T = 5.13%; C = 2.5%) polymerised by 0.025% N,N,N′,N′-tetramethylethylenediamine and 0.15% ammonium persulfate in a 0.1 M Tris-acetate, 1% sodium dodecyl sulfate, 0.001% EDTA buffer at pH 9.0. The electrophoresis buffer consisted of a 0.1 M Tris-acetate, 1% sodium dodecyl sulfate, 0.01% EDTA, 0.1% 2-mercaptoethanol solution at pH 9.0. Samples were prepared for application by mixing 7 parts of the sample with 2 parts of 30% sucrose and 1 part of 0.05% bromophenol blue. The applications per gel on a dry weight basis consisted of approximately 80 μg WSF, 284 μg WIF, 162 μg UIMF, 36 μg 8M-USF, 80 μg 100,000 g USF, and 4.06 mgs (wet weight) each of the 100,000 g and the 4M-urea pellets. Electrophoresis was at 2 mA/gel column at 25 °C, each gel column being removed when the bromophenol blue front had migrated approximately 80 mm into the gel (approximately 3.5 h).

Protein bands were fixed, in a solution of 7% acetic acid and 40% ethanol, and stained with 1% Amido Black, (in 7% acetic acid, 40% ethanol). Gels were destained in a solution of 75 ml acetic acid, 50 ml ethanol, and 875 ml of water, stored in 7% acetic acid and scanned in a Canalco model G densitometer as previously described (ALCALÁ et al., 1975).

Solubilization of samples

Pellets were homogenized (100 mg wet weight/ml) in a solubilizing solution consisting of 0.01 M Tris-acetate, 1% sodium dodecyl sulfate, 0.001% EDTA, and 0.1% 2-mercaptoethanol (pH 9.0) and incubated with intermittent stirring at 37 °C for 1.5 h. After incubation, the solubilized samples were centrifuged at 6,000 g for 5 minutes at 25 °C to remove any particulate matter; the latter was never more than 2% of the weight of the original pellet. Fluid samples were mixed with the solubilizing solution in the ratio of 1:9.

123

Molecular weight estimations

Molecular weight estimations were carried out according to the method of WEBER & OSBORN (1969) but utilizing the 1% SDS electrophoresis system as described by ALCALÁ et al., 1975. The standard markers consisted of catalase, ovalbumin, pepsin, and myoglobin.

Immunological Methods

The techniques of double diffusion in agar (OUCHTERLONY, 1962) and immunoelectrophoresis (MAISEL et al., 1975) were used. Antisera to total soluble lens proteins and to isolated crystallins were used (MAISEL et al., 1975).

Protein Determinations

Dry weight estimates of various fractions were obtained by direct weighing of their lyophilised products.

Electron Microscopy

All pellets were routinely characterized by electron microscopic analysis according to the method of MAISEL & PERRY, 1972.

RESULTS

Morphological characterization of the lens fractions

It has been shown that the chick lens the WIF consists of the cell membranes and an intracellular matrix (albuminoid) of fibrillar elements (in the form of chains and filaments) and dense granules (MAISEL et al., 1976) After treatment of the WIF with 8 M urea to solubilize the albuminoid, the resultant UIMF was seen to consist only of membranes, because all fibrillar elements and granules had been solubilized by urea as the USF. The 4 M urea pellet also was seen to consist of membranes. The 100,000 g pellet consists primarily of chains and filaments (MAISEL & PERRY, 1972).

Characterization of lens fractions by SDS polyacrylamide-gel electrophoresis

Analysis of the various lens fractions in 5.13% polyacrylamide gels containing 1% SDS yielded a pattern in which at least 16 polypeptide bands, labelled 1-16 were resolved (Fig. 1). The band indicated by the arrow was seen only in the WIF and therefore was not numbered. Components comprising less than 0.3% of the total protein recovered in the fraction were not singled out. Table I summarises the data, including the mobilities (R_F) relative to the bromophenol blue front, estimates of the molecular weights, and relative abundance (as percentage of stain) of the predominant polypeptides of the total protein recovered in the various fractions. No protein bands were found to run ahead of the front when the tracking dye was run only 40 mm into the gel.

124

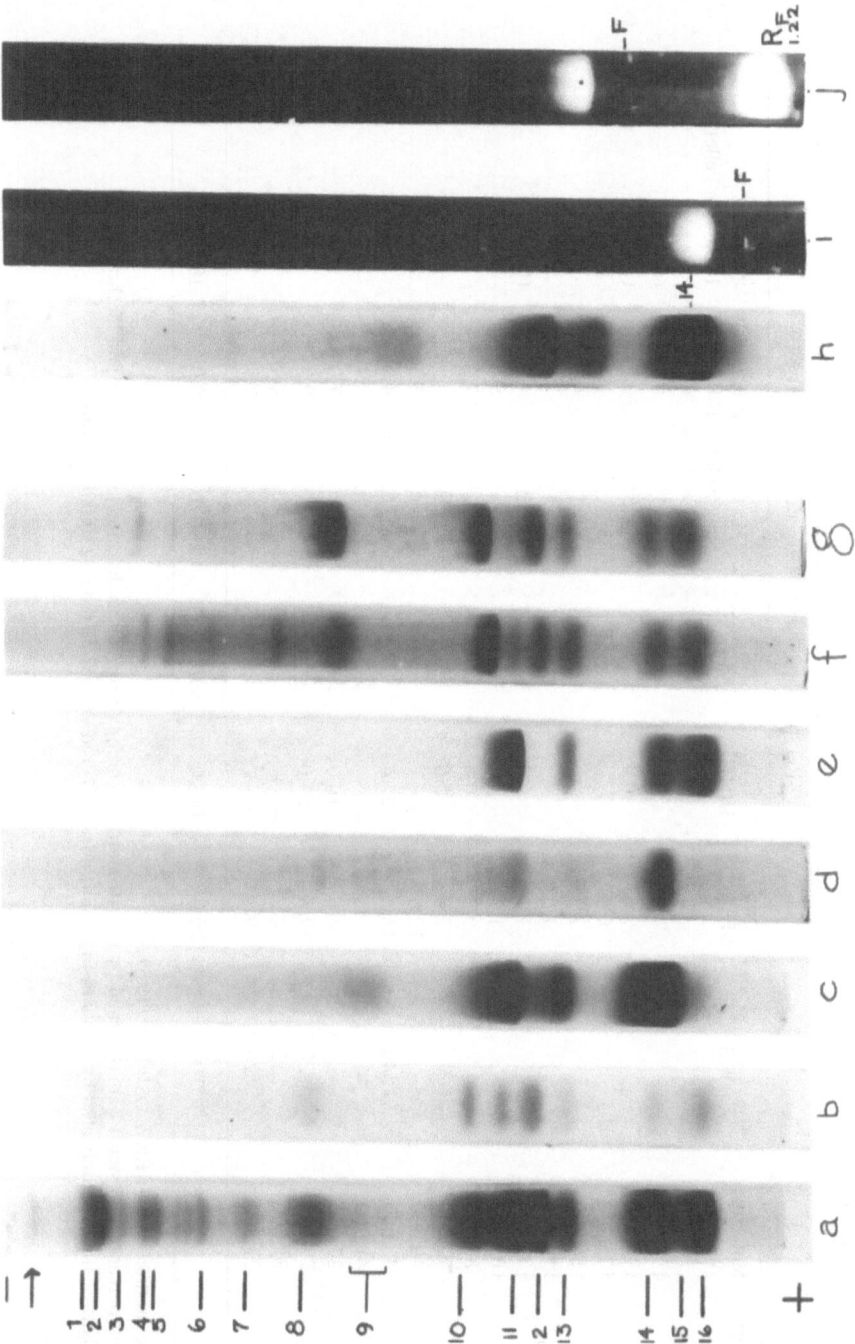

Fig. 1. Electrophoretic patterns of the lens fractions in 5.13% polyacrylamide gels containing 1% sodium dodecyl sulfate (SDS). a – WIF; b – 8M-USF; c – UIMF; d – 4 M-urea pellet; e – WSF; f – 100,000 g pellet; g – 8M-USF of 100,000 g pellet; h – UIMF; i – UIMF, fixed unstained gel to show lipid character of band 14 (F = bromophenol blue front); j – UIMF, unstained gel in which the tracking dye was run only a distance of 70 mm. A second whitish band (R_F 1.22), which did not take up the protein stain, is seen to have run ahead of the front (F).

Table I. Size and abundance of polypeptides of the various lens fractions

Band	Relative Mobility* (R_F)	Estimated* Molecular Weights	Relative Abundance (Percentage of Stain) †						
			WSF	WIF §	UIMF	8M-USF	4M Urea Pellet	Pellet 100,000 g	8M-USF 100,000 g Pellet
1	.169	195,000		4.0	0.6	3.5	1.5	0.5	(trace)
2	.180	190,000		2.6	0.3	1.2	1.5	0.5	(trace)
3	.214	175,000		0.9	---	1.1	---	1.4	1.6
4	.249	160,000		2.2	---	---	---	4.2	---
5	.265	150,000		1.6	---	1.2	---	2.3	0.5
6	.329	130,000		1.1	1.2	1.1	(trace)	4.2	(trace)
7	.400	107,000		1.5	---	---	---	5.6	---
8	.488	85,000		9.3	0.9	14.0	4.5	17.2	27.8
9	.562	72,000		2.8	5.6	---	(trace)	---	---
10	.700	49,000		12.6	---	14.0	---	23.3	23.0
Δ 11	.750	43,000	40	15.8	27.4	11.6	25.8	4.2	2.7
12	.744	41,000	---	9.3	---	24.4	---	8.4	13.9
β 13	.809	37,000	7.3	4.6	10.0	3.5	3.0	7.0	6.4
β 14	.927	27,500	20.0	17.8	54.0	6.9	63.7	9.3	8.6
β 15	.959	25,000	12.7	4.6	---	4.7	---	4.2	4.8
α 16	1.000	22,500	20.0	9.3	---	12.8	---	7.7	10.7
			100.0	100.0	100.0	100.0	100.0	100.0	100.0

* Determined by the method of WEBER & OSBORN (1969).

† Relative peak areas (percentage of stain) were obtained by densitometric scanning of the gels as described in Materials and Methods.

§ The molecular weight of the band indicated by arrow in Fig. 1 but not numbered was estimated at 230,000 daltons.

In order to identify the bands found in the WSF, isolated crystallin fractions were characterized immunologically in agar gel and by electrophoresis in the SDS-gel system (Fig. 2).

Isolated $\propto$ crystallin formed, after dissociation, one band, No. 16, with a molecular weight of 22,500 daltons. Delta crystallin subunits were represented by a single band, No. 11, of molecular weight 43,000 daltons. A mixture of $\propto$ and β crystallins formed, after dissociation, bands 13-16, while a mixture of β and δ crystallins formed bands 11, 13, and 14. Furthermore, an anodal migrating β crystallin formed mainly band 13, while the major cathodal β crystallins formed only bands 14 and 15. It was concluded that bands 13, 14 and 15 represent subunits of β crystallin of molecular weights 37,000, 27,500, and 25,000 daltons respectively. Densitometric scanning of the WSF gel showed that δ crystallin comprised 40%, β crystallin 40%, and $\propto$ crystallin 20% of the total protein recovered in the WSF of the fiber cell mass.

WIF

The washed pellet (WIF), free of soluble crystallins, was resolved into 16 bands (Fig. 1). Bands 11, 13, 14, 15, and 16, corresponding in mobility to crystallin polypeptides, comprised 52.1% of the total WIF protein. Eleven additional bands (1-10 and 12) in the range of 40,000-200,000 daltons accounted for 47.9% of the total protein.

8M-USF and 4M-USF

Immunoelectrophoretic analysis showed that the 8M-USF consisted of $\propto$, β and δ crystallins (Fig. 3). The reason for the retarded mobility of $\propto$ crystallin, and the faint δ crystallin reaction has been noted (MAISEL et al., 1975).

Analysis of the 8M-USF in the SDS-gel system revealed 13 bands (Fig. 1). A comparison with the WIF showed that bands 4, 7 and 9 were absent. All the bands (11, and 13-16) corresponding in molecular weights to crystallin polypeptides were present, comprising 39.5% of the total protein. However, there were quantitative changes in the distribution of the crystallin polypeptides when compared with the WIF pattern. Thus, in the 8M-USF, band 16 ($\propto$ crystallin) comprised 12.8% of the total protein (9.3% in the WIF) while the β crystallin polypeptide band 14 formed only 6.9% of the total protein (17.8% in WIF). The major 8M-USF component (band 12) accounted for 24.4% of the protein, while bands 8 and 10 each accounted for 14% of the 8M-USF protein. The 8M-USF constituted approximately 78% of the dry weight of the WIF.

When the 8M-USF was adjusted to 4 M urea, a pellet (4 M-urea pellet) was obtained after centrifugation. The nature of the pellet is described below. The supernatant was subjected to electrophoresis (not shown) and all bands found in the 8M-USF were present. However, there was a slight decrease in the relative abundance of bands 11 and 14.

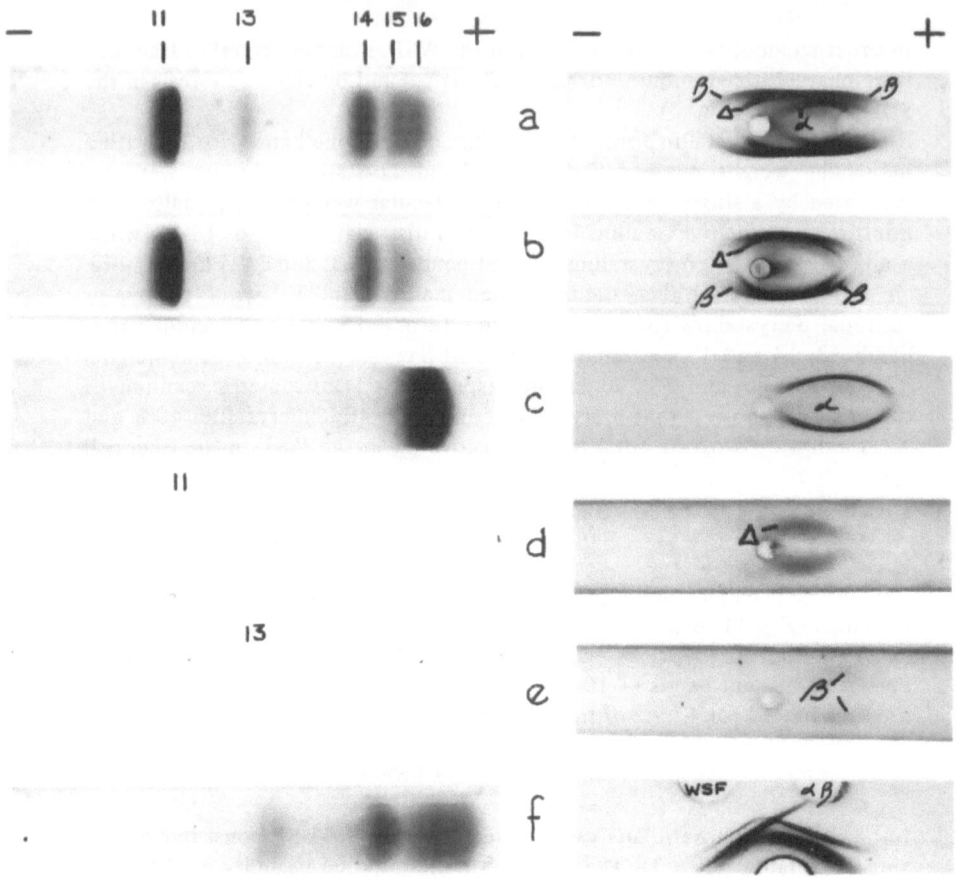

Fig. 2. Electrophoretic analysis of the soluble lens protein fractions in 5.13% poly-acrylamide gels containing 1% SDS (left side) and their corresponding immunoelectro-phoretic patterns utilizing antiserum to total lens crystallins (right side). a = mixture of α, β and δ crystallins; b = β and δ crystallins; c = α crystallin; d = δ crystallin; e = an anodal β crystallin; f = α and β crystallins tested by double immunodiffusion against total crystallins (WSF) with antiserum to total lens crystallins.

100,000 g pellet

The pellet obtained after centrifugation (100,000 g) of the WSF contained all the polypeptides found in the WIF, with the exception of band 9. In contrast to the 8M-USF a higher relative abundance of bands 10 (23.3%) and 8 (17.2%) was noted, while band 11 comprised only 4.2% of the total protein.

The 100,000 g pellet was solubilized by 8 M urea and subjected to elec-trophoresis. The pattern obtained was qualitatively similar to that of the 8M-USF (Fig. 1). Bands 8, 10, 12, and 16 were predominant but there was a considerable reduction in the relative abundance of bands 11 and 12.

128

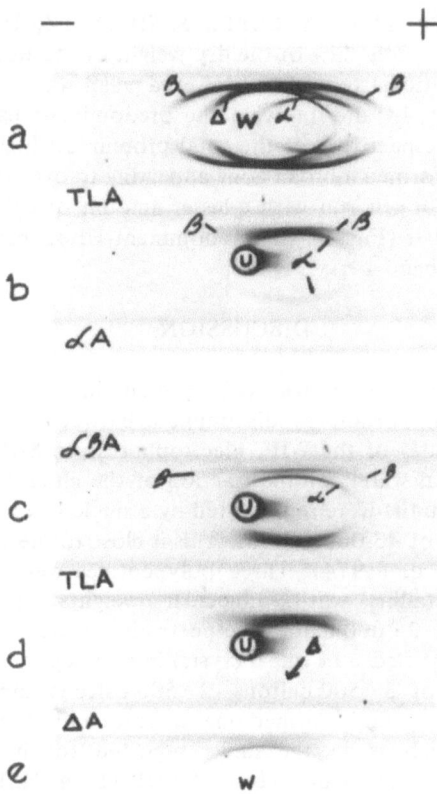

Fig. 3. Immunoelectrophoretic patterns of the 8M-USF. TLA = antiserum to total soluble lens proteins; ∝A = ∝ crystallin antiserum, ∝βA = antiserum to ∝ and β crystallins; δA = δ crystallin antiserum; w = total water soluble proteins; u = 8M-USF.

UIMF and 4 M urea pellet (membrane-rich fractions)

Analysis of the UIMF showed only 8 bands. Bands 14 and 11 were predominant, comprising respectively 54% and 27.4% of the total protein. The molecular weight of polypeptide 14 was estimated at 27,500 daltons and that of polypeptide 11 at 43,000 daltons. A comparison with the 8M-USF showed that band 9 (mol. wt. 72,000) was unique to the UIMF. Bands 15 and 16, corresponding in molecular weight to ∝ and β crystallin polypeptides respectively, were absent. When the gel was viewed against a dark background with indirect light, after fixation but prior to staining, an opaque, whitish band was noted corresponding in position (R_F 0.927) to band 14 (Fig. 1). A second opaque, whitish band formed ahead (R_F 1.22) of the bromophenol blue front when the tracking dye was run only 70 mm into the gel (Fig. 1); this band did not take up the protein stain and migrated in the region corresponding to cell membrane phospholipid (FAIR-

BANKS et al., 1971; MIRA Y LOPEZ & SIEKVITZ, 1973). The UIMF constituted approximately 22% of the dry weight of the WIF.

The electrophoretic pattern of the 4M urea pellet was very similar to that of the UIMF. Bands 14 and 11 were the predominant bands, comprising 63.7% and 25.8% respectively of the total protein. At high concentrations of UIMF, band 14 formed a broad zone appearing to overlap the position of band 15. However, in gels run with a lesser amount of UIMF and in the gel of the 4 M urea pellet (Fig. 1), the predominant UIMF band corresponded in mobility only to band 14.

DISCUSSION

Since lens crystallins are known to be present in the USF (RAO et al., 1965), it became important to discriminate between crystallin and non-crystallin polypeptides of the WIF. Electrophoresis in SDS-polyacrylamide gel resolved the total water soluble fraction of the chick lens into 5 bands. Delta crystallin subunits were represented by a single band corresponding to a molecular weight of 43,000 daltons. This is close to the value reported by PIATIGORSKY et al. (1974). Three polypeptides were identified as belonging to β crystallins with molecular weights of 37,000 daltons, 27,500 daltons and 25,000 daltons respectively. BLOEMENDAL & HERBRINK (1974) identified 6 bovine β crystallin polypeptides, 3 of which had molecular weights of 37,500 daltons, 27,500 daltons and 25,000 daltons respectively. Alpha crystallin formed one subunit band of molecular weigght 22,500 daltons which is in the range reported for bovine and rabbit $\propto$ crystallin polypeptide chains (BLOEMENDAL & HERBRINK, 1974; LIEM-THE & HOENDERS, 1974).

The morphology of the chick lens water-insoluble albuminoid and cell membranes has been described (MAISEL et al., 1976). Albuminoid (intracellular matrix) consists mainly of aggregates of filaments, chains of globular particles, and some dense granules all solubilizable by 8 M urea. The morphology of the urea-insoluble cell membrane fraction appears to be unaltered by the urea treatment. However, BROEKHUYSE & KUHLMAN (1974) speculate that urea probably affects the structure of the isolated membranes to some extent. The structure of the 100,000 g pellet isolated from the lens water-soluble fraction is comparable to that of albuminoid but lacks dense granules (MAISEL et al., 1976).

Analysis of the WIF (cell membranes and albuminoid) resolved 16 bands which were divided into crystallin and non-crystallin components on the basis of mobility in the SDS-gel system. Even after repeated washing crystallin polypeptides still comprised 52.1% of the total WIF protein, while polypeptides 8, 10 and 12 (mol. wts. 85,000, 49,000 and 41,000) comprised 31.2% of the protein.

When the patterns of the 8M-USF and UIMF were compared with that of the WIF, several differences in polypeptide distribution were discerned. Bands 3, 5, 10, 12, 15, and 16 were present in the 8M-USF but absent from the UIMF. The non-crystallin polypeptides 3, 5, 10, and 12 appear to be unique to albuminoid as opposed to the membranes. All polypeptides with molecular weights of crystallin polypeptides were present in the USF.

Bands 14 and 11 (δ and β crystallin subunits) of the 8M-USF were decreased in concentration when compared with the WIF, while the $\propto$ crystallin (band 16) concentration was increased. The polypeptide of band 9, (mol. wt. 72,000), was uniquely associated with the membranes (UIMF).

The 100,000 g pellet, is minimally contaminated with cell membrane (MAISEL & PERRY, 1972), as further substantiated by the absence of band 9 from its gel pattern. Based on its morphology and protein composition, we suggest that this pellet is a more reliable representation of the true nature of lens intracellular matrix, undistorted by the possible effects of the more common albuminoid isolation method (urea extraction). Urea treatment of the 100,000 g pellet results in changes in the gel pattern of a similar order of magnitude to those observed to occur for the urea-extractable material in the WIF (compare the WIF to 8M-USF, and 100,000 g pellet to 100,000 g USF in Table I). The presence of relatively more δ crystallin subuntis (band 11) in the 8M-USF than in the 100,000 g pellet is not readily explicable, especially since the pellet was isolated from a medium (WSF) richer in δ crystallin than the WIF from which the 8M-USF was isolated. It is possible that some δ crystallin subunits are released by urea from the cell membrane in which band 11 is a major component. Both the 8M-USF and the 100,000 g pellet showed a predominance of non-crystallin bands 8, 10 and 12.

The 4 M urea pellet obtained after adjustment of the urea concentration of the 8M-USF to 4 M urea yielded an electrophoretic pattern essentially identical qualitatively to that of the UIMF. Its composition may have been affected by urea as evidenced by only trace amounts of band 9, the polypeptide unique to membrane, and by the decreased concentration of band 11 relative to band 14. The isolation of this fraction results from the lower density of the medium following the adjustment of 4 M urea, and from the specific gravity characteristics of the membranes free of soluble lens proteins (LASSER & BALAZS, 1972).

Analysis of the membrane rich fraction (UIMF) revealed a limited composition (8 bands). The major components, bands 11, 13 and 14 comprised 91.4% of the protein recovered in this fraction and exhibited mobilities identical to those of δ (band 11) and β crystallin polypeptides (bands 13 and 14).

The predominant membrane polypeptide component 14 (mol. wt. 27,500) comprised more than half of the UIMF protein. Its mobility was identical to that of the β crystallin polypeptide. However, when viewed in indirect light prior to staining, this polypeptide band showed evidence of lipid, (MIRA Y LOPEZ & SIEKEVITZ, 1973) suggesting that it is not a soluble β crystallin polypeptide but a different component. The predominant polypeptide in calf lens fiber cell membrane has a molecular weight of 25,500 daltons (BROEKHUYSE & KUHLMAN, 1974), while ALCALÁ et al. (1975) reported a molecular weight of 27,500 daltons for the major polypeptide of the bovine lens fiber cell membrane. However, LIEM-THE & HOENDERS (1974), reported a single band in the 31,000 daltons position for rabbit cortical urea-insoluble material, and 4 additional minor bands ranging from 19,000 to 60,000 daltons in nuclear urea-insoluble material. Other studies of lens cell membranes by SDS-polyacrylamide gel electrophoresis reported a similar single major polypeptide component which migrated in the β crystallin region corresponding to 25,000-37,000 daltons (BLOEMENDAL et al., 1972; DUNIA et al., 1974).

The question remains as to whether UIMF bands 11, 13 and 14 represent crystallin polypeptides intrinsic to the cell membrane, non-crystallin polypeptides with molecular sizes identical to crystallin polypeptides, or a mixture of crystallin and non-crystallin polypeptides. The presence of polypeptides with mobilities identical to crystallin polypeptides even after extensive washing with buffers, treatment with urea, and other agents (BLOEMENDAL et al., 1972; DUNIA et al., 1974; BROEKHUYSE & KUHLMAN, 1974; and ALCALÁ et al., 1975) may indicate that crystallins are intrinsic constituents of the lens plasma membranes. However, similar mobility in gel electrophoresis is not sufficient proof of identity and verification by other methods is needed.

ACKNOWLEDGEMENT

The support of the Capital Poultry Company of Detroit, which provided the chick lenses, is gratefully acknowledged.

REFERENCES

ALCALÁ, J., LIESKA, N. & MAISEL, H. Protein composition of bovine lens cortical fiber cell membranes. *Exp. Eye Res.* 21: *581-595* (1975).

BLOEMENDAL, H. & HERBRINK, P. Growing insight into the structure of β-crystallin. A review. *Opthal. Res.* 6: *81-92* (1974).

BLOEMENDAL, H., ZWEERS, A., VERMORKEN, F., DUNIA, I. & BENEDETTI, E.L. The plasma membranes of eye lens fibers. Biochemical and structural characterization. *Cell. Diff.* 1: *91-106* (1972).

BROEKHUYSE, R.M. & KUHLMAN, E.D. Lens membranes. I. Composition of urea-treated plasma membranes of calf lens. *Exp. Eye Res.* 19: *297-302* (1974).

BURGER, M.M. Role of the cell surface in growth and transformation. In Macromolecules Regulating Growth and Development. Ed. E.D. Hay, T.J. King & J. Papaconstantinou, p. 3-24 (Academic Press, New York 1974).

DUNIA, I., SEN GHOSH, C., BENEDETTI, E., ZWEERS, A. & BLOEMENDAL, H. Isolation and protein patterns of eye lens fiber junctions. *FEBS Letters* 45: *139-144* (1974).

FAIRBANKS, G., STECK, T. & WALLACH, D. Electrophoretic analysis of the major polypeptides of the human erythrocyte membrane. *Biochemistry* 10: *2606-2617* (1971).

HINMAN, N. & PHILLIPS, A. Similarity and limited multiplicity of membrane proteins from rough and smooth endoplasmic reticulum. *Science* 170: *1222-1223* (1970).

LASSER, A. & BALAZS, E. Biochemical and fine structure studies on the water-insoluble components of the calf lens. *Exp. Eye Res.* 13: *292-308* (1972).

LIEM-THE, K.N. & HOENDERS, H.J. HM-crystallin as an intermediate in the conversion of water-soluble into water-insoluble rabbit lens proteins. *Exp. Eye Res.* 19: *549-557* (1974).

MAISEL, H. & LANGMAN, J. An immuno-embryological study on the chick lens. 9: *191-201* (1961).

MAISEL, H., KERRIGAN, M. & SYNER, F. The ontogeny of lactate dehydrogenase in the chick lens. *Invest. Ophthal.* 4: *362-371* (1965).

MAISEL, H., LIESKA, N. & ALCALÁ, J. Effect of urea on chick lens proteins. *Opthal. Res.* 7: *416-419* (1975).

MAISEL, H. & PERRY, M.M. Electron microscopic observations on some structural proteins of the chick lens. *Exp. Eye Res.* 14: *7-12* (1972).

MAISEL, H., PERRY, M.M., ALCALÁ, J. & WAGGONER, P. The structure of chick lens water-insoluble material. *Opthal. Res.* 8: *55-63* (1976).

MIRA Y LOPEZ, R. & SIEKEVITZ, P. SDS-Polyacrylamide gel electrophoresis of membrane proteins: effect of phospholipids. *Anal. Biochem.* 53: *594-602* (1973).

OUCHTERLONY, O. Diffusion-in-gel methods for immunological analysis II. *Prog. in Allergy* 6: *30-154* (1962).

PIATIGORSKY, J., ZELENKA, P. & SIMPSON, R.T. Molecular weight and subunit structure of delta-crystallin from embryonic chick lens fibers. *Exp. Eye Res.* 18: *435-446* (1974).

POULIK, M.D. Starch gel electrophoresis in a discontinuous system of buffers. *Nature* 180: *1477-1479* (1957).

RAO, S., MEHTA, P. & COOPER, S. Antigenic relationship between insoluble and soluble lens proteins. *Exp. Eye Res.* 4: *36-41* (1965).

SMITHIES, O. Zone electrophoresis in starch gels: Group variations in the serum proteins of normal human adults. *Biochem. J.* 61: *629-641* (1955).

WEBER, K. & OSBORN, M. The reliability of molecular weight determinations by dodecyl sulfate polyacrylamide gel electrophoresis. *J. Biol. Chem.* 244: *4406-4412* (1969).

Keywords:

chick lens
cell membrane
sodium dodecyl sulfate
polyacrylamide gel electrophoresis
crystallins
albuminoid
intracellular matrix

Authors' address:

Wayne State University
Department of Anatomy
540 E. Canfield
Detroit, Michigan 48201, USA

133

INVESTIGATION OF PROTEOLYTIC ACTIVITY IN BOVINE LENSES WITH AGE I. THE EXOPEPTIDASES

A.A. SWANSON*, U. HAHN & O. HOCKWIN

(Charleston, S. Car./Bonn, W. Germany)

ABSTRACT

Bovine lens exopeptidases including an esterase, leucine aminopeptidase and a triglycinpeptidase were assayed in lenses ranging in age from a few days old to eighteen years of age. Esterase activity increased in lenses in excess of 15 years. Leucine aminopeptidase showed significant increase during the early postnatal growth phase and again after 15 years of age. Triglycinpeptidase gave similar activities, however, on a much lower level of magnitude.

INTRODUCTION

ABDERHALDEN & HANSON (1938) described a polypeptidase which hydrolyzed the substrate α-leucyl-glycine at pH 8 in bovine lens tissue. This was the first demonstration that leucylaminopeptidase activity was observed in lens tissue. Later other investigators further confirmed the presence of leucylaminopeptidase in mammalian lens tissue (SPACKMAN et al., 1955; HANSON & METHFESSEL, 1958; KLEINE & HANSON, 1962 and GLÄSSER & HANSON, 1962). ZELLER & DEVI (1957) and ZELLER et al. (1960) observed a lens peptidase having chymotrypsin characteristics that Kleine and Hanson described as leucinaminopeptidase. SPECTOR (1961 and 1962) has described peptidase activity in mammalian lenses. SWANSON & TRUESDALE (1974 A&B) have described a human lens esterase I which hydrolyzes α-naphthyl acetate, butyrate, caproate, caprylate, and β-propionate, as well as an arylamidase from human lenses which will hydrolyze leucyl-arginyl and lysyl-β-naphthylamides. Both enzymes were shown to be dependent on metal ions for activity.

The present study reports on mammalian lens exopeptidases which include an esterase, leucine-aminopeptidase and a triglycinpeptidase activity in bovine lenses ranging in age from a few days old to eighteen years of age (mean life expectancy of a cow is about 30 years).

MATERIALS AND METHODS

Fresh bovine eyes were obtained from slaughter houses in Bonn and Köln and the lenses with intact capsule were removed by a posterior approach and used immediately or frozen overnight at −20 °C. Lens age was estimated

---

* Alexander von Humboldt-Stiftung Awardee, 1974-1975.

according to the procedure of SCHMUTTER (1961). Dissection of lenses into equator, anterior and posterior cortex and nucleus was performed as described by HOCKWIN & KLEIFELD (1965). Lenses were homogenized in 15 ml 0.1 M Tris-HCl buffer (pH 7.0 at 4 °C); following centrifugation at 20,000 g for 45 minutes at 0 °C, the supernatant was removed for the enzyme assays.

Esterase activity was determined with the substrate α-naphthyl acetate (Serva 30050, 0.01M in acetone), 0.1M Tris-buffer, pH 7.0, incubated at 37 °C for 60 minutes. The reaction mixture was centrifuged at 20,000 g at

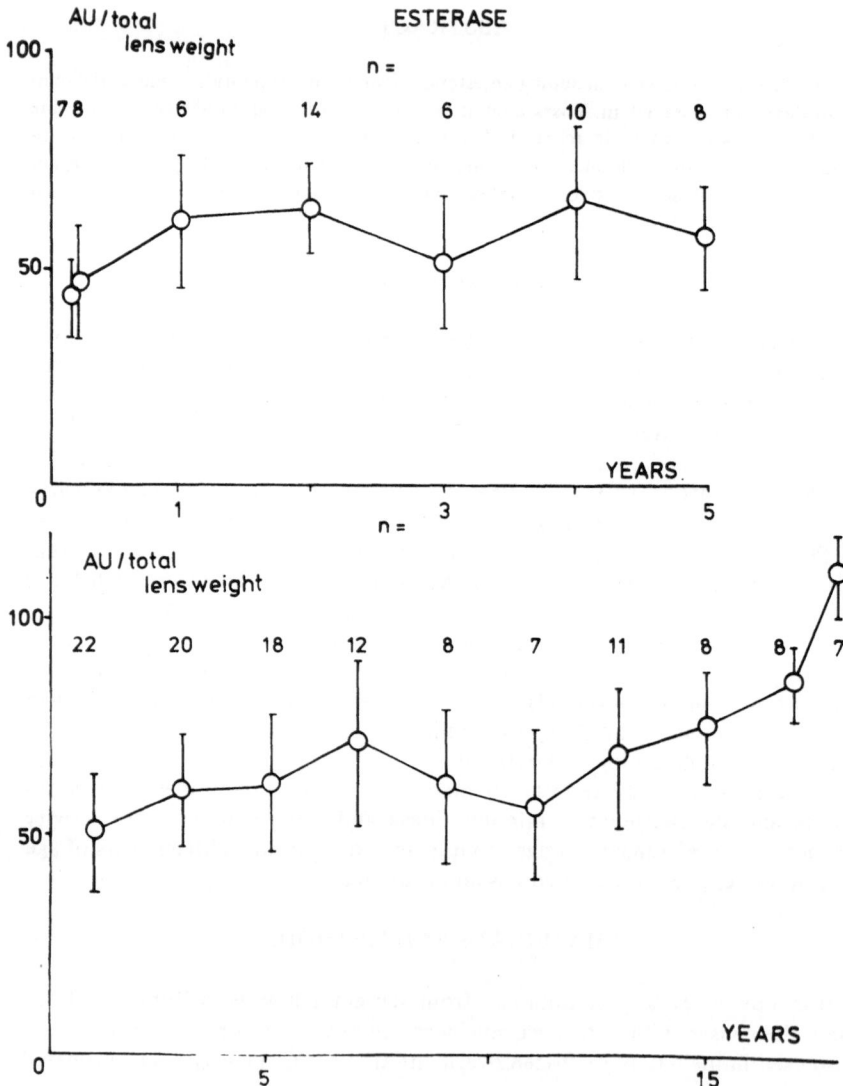

Fig. 1. Esterase activity in units per total lens wet weight in terms of age dependence of the bovine species.

1 °C for 2 minutes and measured spectrophotometrically at 540 nm. Parallel substrate and enzyme blanks were determined with each estimation. Leucine aminopeptide (EC 3.4.1.1) was assayed by its action on L-leucyl-glycine in the presence of ninhydrin according to the principal of MARKS et al. (1968).

Triglycinpeptidase (EC 3.4.1.3) activity was measured by a ninhydrin reaction essentially as described by MATHESON & TATTRIE (1964) using glycyl-glycyl-glycin (Fluka SG 50240) as substrate. The absorbance was measured at 570 nm. The ΔOD is plotted as a function of time. Enzyme concentration as adjusted to give a linear reaction for at least 30 minutes. Activity units of the three exopeptidases are expressed as extinction changes of 0.01 μmol per test assay. Specific activity designates the number of units per milligram of water soluble protein. Protein in the supernatant was determined according to LOWRY et al. (1951). Further experimental details are given by HAHN (in preparation).

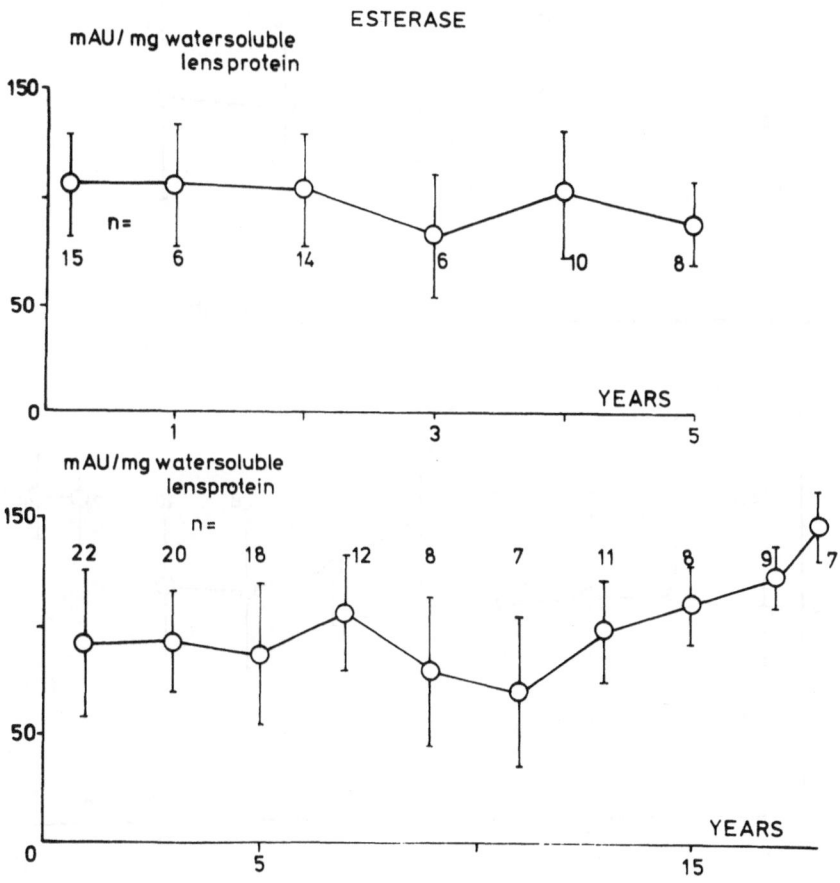

Fig. 2. Specific activities of esterase on age dependence.

RESULTS

The values presented with each figure are based upon means within specific age groups. Standard deviation is given along with the number of lenses belonging to each mean value. The upper region of each figure (Fig. 1-6) presents the data of the early life period in which the growth rate of lens is much higher than in later periods. It should be emphasized that the life expectancy of the bovine species is about 30 years, the time period covered by the present investigations corresponds to about 60% of the life span. The very old age periods (senile phase) are missing for technical reasons. The single curves were based upon the mean values, no additional statistical

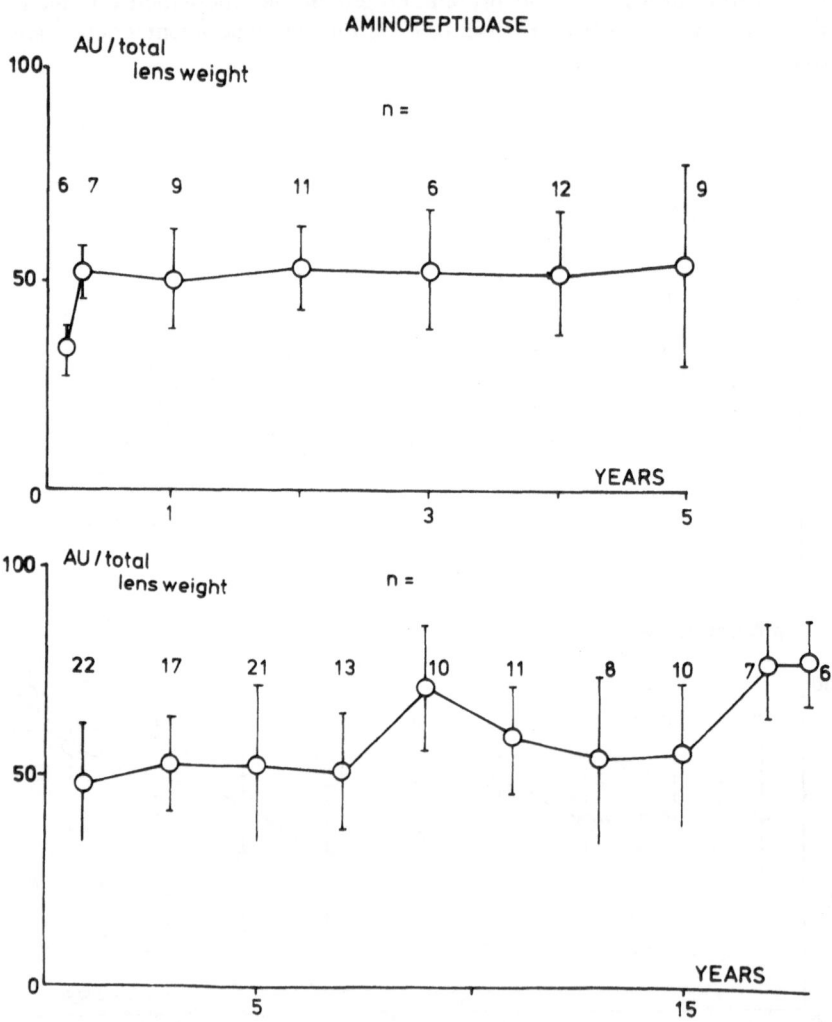

Fig. 3. Aminopeptidase activity in units per total lens wet weight on age dependence of the bovine species.

138

evaluation (regresison coefficient etc.) has been performed. Therefore, the curves may be regarded only as indications for the age trends of the single activities.

Esterase activities shows essentially no great changes in the early life, the values for lenses in excess of 15 years indicate an age related increase (Fig. 1 & 2). With the data including the protein values, one may conclude, that age induced changes on protein composition have little influence on the enzyme over an extended period of the life span. The activity of leucine aminopeptidase shows a significant increase during the early postnatal period, which might correspond to the growth rate (Fig. 3). After reaching a plateau, there is very little change in activity until 15 years of age. From then on the activity shows a dramatic increase, also, this can be shown by plotting the

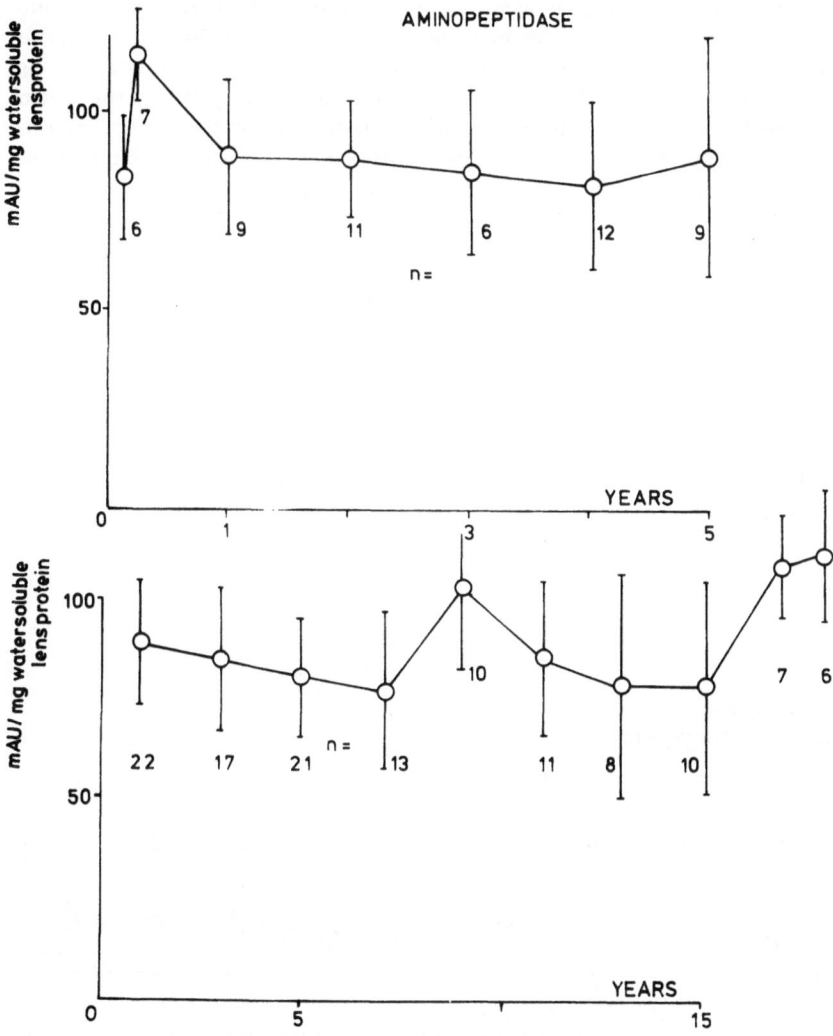

Fig. 4. Specific activities of aminopeptidase on age dependence.

specific activities (Fig. 4). Perhaps the loss of soluble protein does not effect the protein fraction that the leucine aminopeptidase activity belongs to. In contrast to the esterase and aminopeptidase having somewhat comparable activities, the triglycin-peptidase is considerably less active in the bovine lenses of all age groups. There is a slight increase during the growth period, followed by very little enzyme over an extended period of time, then proceeds to increase after 18 years of age (Fig. 5). The specific activities of the triglycin-peptidase, although on a much lower level of magnitude, are somewhat comparable to lens aminopeptidase activities in older age groups, perhaps this may be due to protein changes as the rational for this late increase in activity.

Due to the increase in weight and volume during the course of life, the lens metabolism shows differences dependent on localization. Figure 7 represents each of the enzyme activities in different parts of the lens in 5 and 7 year old bovine lens. The lens sections evaluated include the anterior cortex and epithelium, lens nucleus, posterior cortex and equatorial ring presented in Figure 7. For esterase activity, the equatorial ring for 7 year old bovine lenses contains the highest activity, followed by the anterior cortex and epithelium. The posterior cortex contains appreciable high esterase activity in the 7 year old lens and the lowest activity for esterase was

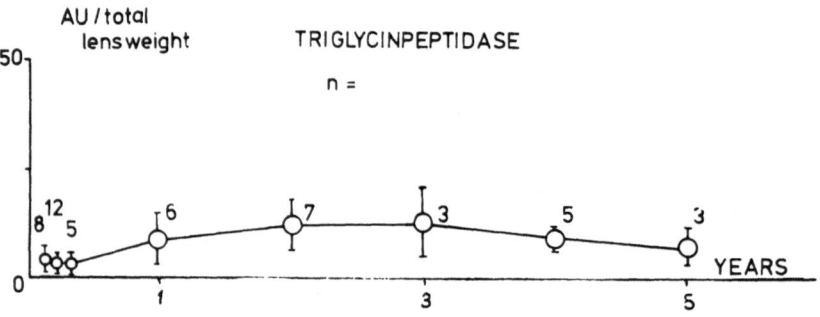

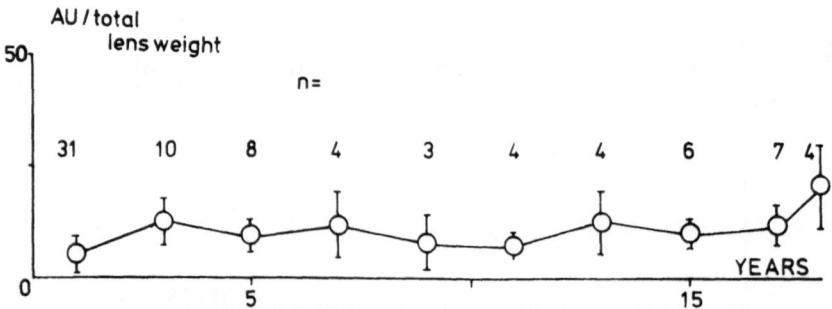

Fig. 5. Triglycinpeptidase activity in units per total lens wet weight on age dependence of the bovine species.

140

observed in the lens nucleus for both age groups. Leucine aminopeptidase activities were lower in all regions of the lens, with the lowest activities noted in the lens nucleus and the highest activity for this enzyme was demonstrated in the equatorial ring area. Hoewver, the lowest order of magnitude was detected with the enzyme triglycin-peptidase in all sections of the lens. This enzyme showed near equal activities in the anterior cortex and epithelium and equatorial ring zones. Likewise, comparable activities were observed in both the lens nucleus and posterior cortex sections in the 5 and 7 year old bovine lenses.

DISCUSSION

The major purpose of this study was to investigate several exopeptidases in a longitudinal study in bovine lenses. The data show a measurable difference between the rate of aging and enzymic activity. The latter generally increasing with age.

The effect of age on lens protein composition in mammalian lens is not only manifested in the accumulation of the insoluble fraction (MEHTA & MAISEL, 1967; MOK & WALEY, 1967; 1968; PIRIE, 1968). Age-related changes in the relative amounts of the crystallins also occur (FRANCOIS & RABAEY, 1957; HOCKWIN et al. 1958; KAMP, 1973). Our results may be

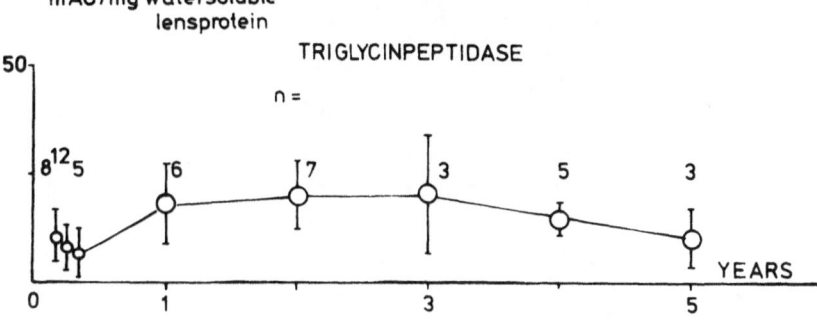

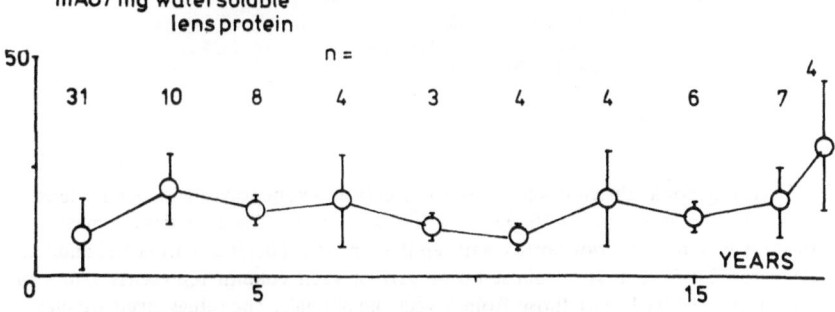

Fig. 6. Specific activities of triglycin-peptidase on age dependence.

of some importance with regards to these lens proteins with aging in terms of proteolysis. However, this study does not describe what proteins may be involved, and the precise state of the protein changes *in situ* is not known. It is tempting to equate exopeptidase activities with structural changes in the lens protein.

One interesting and important conclusion that can be drawn from these studies is that specific enzyme activities can be localized within the various regions in the lens. The highest activities could be demonstrated in the anterior cortex and epithelium and the equatorial regions followed by the posterior cortex. The lowest exopeptidase activities were more pronounced in the lens nucleus. However, because of the magnitude of the observed differences, we may assume that differences in protein content both qualitatively and quantitatively must vary in the different regions of the lens.

Further studies are in progress to determine the specific proteins which may undergo proteolysis or changes involving aggregation with exopeptidases and endopeptidases.

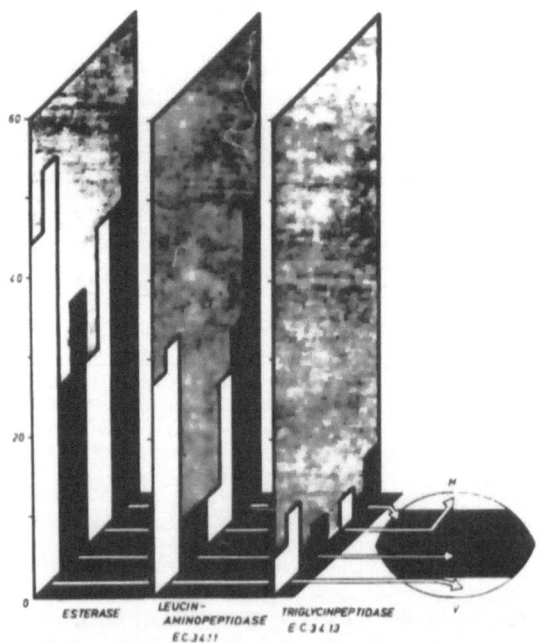

Fig. 7. Topographic distribution of the proteolytic exopeptidases in bovine lenses. Values are given as activity units per 1.4 g lens wet weight. The activities are measured in the lens equator, anterior cortex with epithelium (V), posterior cortex (H) and lens nucleus for 2 different age groups. Front part of each column represents values of 5 year old lenses, back part those from 7 year old animals. The values given are means of 6 single determinations each.

142

REFERENCES

ABDERHALDEN, E. & HANSON, H. Über das Vorkommen von Polypeptidasen in der Linse, in der Hornhaut, im Glaskörper und in Kammerwasser des Auges. *Ferment-forschung* 16: *67-80* (1938).

FRANCOIS, J. & RABAEY, M. On the existance of an embryonic lens protein. Arch. Ophthal. *Chicago 57*: *672-680* (1957).

GLÄSSER, D. & HANSON, H. Einfaches Verfahren zur präparativen Gewinnung hochgereinigter Leucinaminopeptidase aus Rinderaugenlinsen. *Z. Physiol. Chem.* 329: *249-256* (1962).

HAHN, U. Med. Inaug. Diss. Bonn (in preparation).

HANSON, H. & METHFESSEL, J. Zur Spezifität der Peptidaseaktivität der Rinderlinse. *Acta Biol. Med. Germ.* 1: *414-421* (1958).

HOCKWIN, O. & KLEIFELD, O. Das Verhalten von Fermentaktivitäten in einzelnen Linsenteilen unterschiedlich alter Rinder und ihre Beziehung zur Zusammensetzung des wasserlöslichen Eiweisses. In: Die Struktur des Auges. II Symp. Hrsg. J.W. Rohen. S. *395-401* Stuttgart: Schattauer 1965.

KAMP, G.J. VAN. The soluble proteins of the bovine eye lens. Studies on Development and Aging. Proefschrift Universiteit Nijmegen, 1973.

KLEINE, R. & HANSON, H. Untersuchungen zur Frage des Vorkommens von Endopeptidasen in der Rinderaugenlinse. *Acta Biol. Med. Germ.* 9: *606-622* (1962).

LOWRY, O.H., ROSEBROUGH, N., FARR, A.L. & RANDALL, R.J. Protein measurement with Folin-Phenol-reagent. *J. Biol. Chem.* 193: *265-275* (1951).

MARKS, N., LAJATHA, A. & DATTA, R.H. Brain aminopeptidase hydrolyzing leucylglycyl-glycin and similar substrates. *J. Biol. Chem.* 243: *2882-2891* (1968).

METHESON, A.T. & TATTRIE, B.L. A modified ninhydrin reagent for peptidase assay. *Can J. Biochem.* 42: *95-103* (1964).

MEHTA, P.D. & MAISEL, H. Albuminoid of human and cynomolgus monkey lens. *Amer. J. Ophthal.* 63: *967-972* (1967).

MOK, C.C. & WALEY, S.G. Structural Studies on Lens Proteins. *Biochem. J.* 104: *128-134* (1967).

MOK, C.C. & WALEY, S.G. N-Terminal groups of lens proteins. *Exp. Eye Res.* 7: *148-153* (1968).

PIRIE, A. Colour and solubility of the proteins of human cataracts. *Invest. Ophthal.* 7: *634-650* (1968).

SCHMUTTER, J. Untersuchungen über die Altersabhängigkeit des Gewichts und Volumens von Rinderlinsen. Med. Inaug. Diss. Bonn (1961).

SPACKMAN, D.H., SMITH, E.L. & BROWN, D.M. Leucinaminopeptidase IV. Isolation and properties of the enzyme from swine kidney. *J. Biol. Chem.* 212: *255-269* (1955).

SPECTOR, A. Studies on amino acid esterase activity of lens. *Exp. Eye Res.* 1: *60-67* (1961).

SPECTOR, A. A study of peptidase and esterase activity in calf lenses. *Exp. Eye Res.* 1: *330-335* (1962).

SWANSON, A.A. & TRUESDALE, A.W. Some enzymic properties of human lens esterase I. *Invest. Ophthal.* 13: *466-468* (1974)a.

SWANSON, A.A. & TRUESDALE, A.W. Isolation and purification of arylamidase from human lenses. *Ophthal. Res.* 6: *235-244* (1974)b.

ZELLER, E.A. & DEVI, A. On the occurrence of proteolytic enzymes in normal and cataractous lenses. *Am. J. Ophthal.* 44: *281-287* (1957).

ZELLER, E.A., BANERGEE, R. & SCHOCH, D. Enzymology and comparative biochemistry of a new lens peptidase. *Biochem. J.* 76: *49-54* (1960).

143

Keywords:

Age
Bovine lens
Exopeptidases
Esterase
Leucine-aminopeptidase
Triglycin-peptidase

Authors' addresses:

Department of Biochemistry and Ophthalmology
Medical University of South Carolina
80 Barre Street
Charleston, S.C. 29401, USA

Division Biochemistry of the Eye
Klinisches Institut für experimentelle Ophthalmologie
Universität Bonn
Bonn, W. Germany

144

LENS GLUTATHIONE: METABOLISM AND POSSIBLE FUNCTIONS*

WILLIAM B. RATHBUN

(Minneapolis, Minnesota)

Among the exceptional characteristics of the lens is an unusually high GSH content which may exceed 500 mg/100 g of cortex (KUCK, 1970). GSH is especially concentrated in the epithelium (ASGHAR et al., 1975) where, in the rabbit, it may reach 3 g/100 g of epithelium (GIBLIN et al., 1976). This high concentration appears to be a requirement for optical clarity since a low GSH content is not associated with optically clear lenses except in the transition period just prior to opacity formation in certain experimental cataracts. Generally, the GSH concentration decreases dramatically in a variety of experimental and human senile cataracts.

Glutathione is a tripeptide, composed of L-glutamate, L-cysteine and glycine, which contains two important structural components: a sulfhydryl group and a γ-glutamyl peptide bond. The sulfhydryl group is responsible for much of the biological activity of GSH. Lenticular glutathione is largely in the reduced state, the oxidized state comprising only 5-12% of the total (KUCK, 1970). The peptide bond joining glutamate and cysteine utilizes the γ-carboxyl group of glutamate rather than the α-group. This γ-bond is comparatively labile to heat and acidic conditions, but is resistant to hydrolysis by α-peptidases; whereas the second peptide bond formed between cysteine and glycine is the very stable α-peptide linkage. The formation of these two peptide bonds in GSH requires two synthetases, each one utilizing ATP. The cultured rabbit lens incorporated glycine and glutamate into GSH at a rate of 1.8% per hour (REDDY et al, 1966) which was calculated to require approximately 11% of the lens ATP derived from glycolysis (RATHBUN & WICKER, 1973).

BIOSYNTHESIS OF GSH IN THE LENS

Lens GSH is probably entirely synthesized *in situ*, as GSH is undetectable in the aqueous. The glutamate moiety is largely derived from extralenticular glutamine and some glutamate transported into the lens (KERN & HO, 1973), although a small portion may arise from the dismutation of pyruvate (KINOSHITA & MEROLA, 1961; VAN HEYNINGEN, 1965). The source of cysteine is unknown, but it may be derived *in situ* from methionine via

* This work was supported in part by U.S. Public Health Service Grant No. EY-01197.

145

γ-GLUTAMYL CYCLE

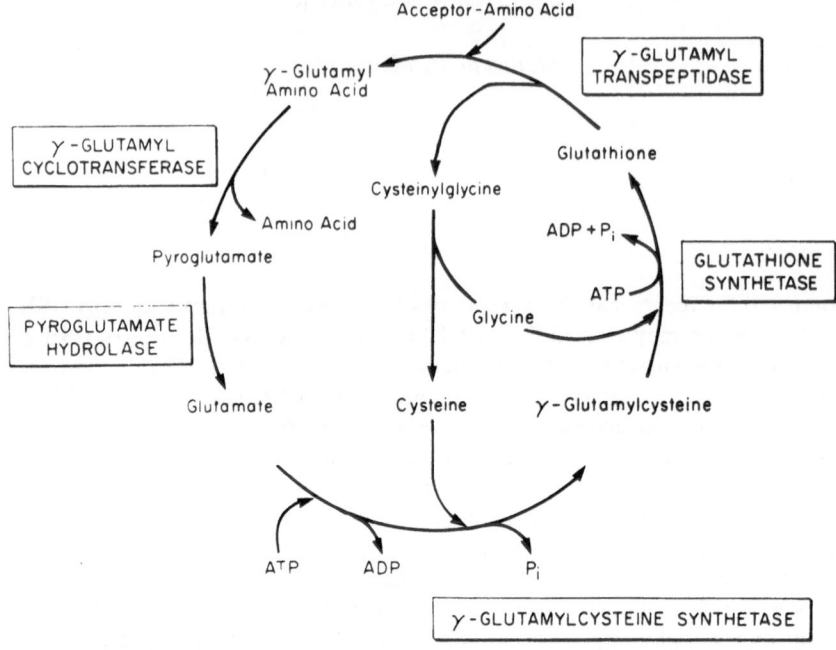

the cystathionase pathway. There is a paucity of free cysteine in the lens (REDDY & KINSEY, 1962). The glycine component is mostly transported from the aqueous although lenticular metabolic pathways may also contribute.

In many mammalian tissues, synthesis and degradation of GSH consists of six discrete steps which form an ordered sequence. When considering only the metabolism of L-glutamate, the scheme may be drawn in the form of a cycle which contains five of the six enzymes (ORLOWSKI & MEISTER, 1970). Of these five steps, four directly involve formation, transfer or hydrolysis of the γ-glutamyl bond, and thus the sequence was termed the *γ-glutamyl cycle* (Fig. 1). All of the component enzymes of the cycle have been demonstrated in the lens, and all but γ-glutamyl cyclotransferase have been purified to some degree.

Formation of the γ-peptide bond is catalyzed by γ-glutamylcysteine synthetase. The bovine lens enzyme, largely confined to the epithelium and cortical regions, has been purified 260-fold. The enzyme is quite specific for L-glutamate and L-isomers of the cysteine moiety (RATHBUN, 1967a), but a variety of L-cysteine derivatives and analogues were found to be reactive with the enzyme (RATHBUN, 1967b), including both optical isomers of β-aminoisobutyrate. This suggests that the enzyme's binding site for the β-substituent of cysteine may be a broad region (RATHBUN & GILBERT, 1973). Specificity for ATP is quite limited, although both ITP and GTP

146

yield low rates of reaction. Manganese is the only divalent metal ion that was found to be an effective substitute for magnesium (RATHBUN et al., 1976). By the use of enzyme kinetics, the reaction mechanism of the lens enzyme was determined to be an ordered bi-uni-uni-bi mechanism in which the enzyme reacts first with L-glutamate, and then ATP (VAN BUSKIRK et al., 1976).

Glutathione synthetase catalyzes the formation of the peptide bond between γ-glutamylcysteine and glycine. The purified lens enzyme exhibits a restricted specificity for its dipeptide and glycine substrates and magnesium, and shows an absolute specificity for ATP. The enzyme activity was increased 10-fold by potassium ion; other alkali metal ions, (lithium, sodium and rubidium) could partially activate the system, but cesium was ineffective. Both GSH synthesis enzymes exhibit isoelectric points of 4.8; thus they are contained in the α-crystallin fraction. The enzymes associated so closely during all stages of the separation procedure that complete separation was not achieved. Such association may reflect physical association within the cell, which would be efficient (RATHBUN et al., 1976).

CATABOLISM OF LENS GSH

Since loss of lenticular GSH and GSSG to the media is minimal, it appears safe to conclude that GSH is entirely degraded within the lens (REDDY et al., 1973). This process requires four enzymes. The only one which reacts effectively with GSH itself is γ-glutamyl transpeptidase. This is a membrane-bound lipoprotein concentrated within the capsule-epithelium (RATHBUN & WICKER, 1973; REDDY & UNAKAR, 1973). The enzyme transfers the γ-glutamyl moiety of GSH and some analogues to a variety of acceptor amino acids, of which L-methionine was the most active with the purified bovine lens enzyme (RATHBUN & WICKER, 1973).

Cysteinylglycinase, an α-peptidase ancillary to the γ-glutamyl cycle, cleaves the α-peptide bond of cysteinylglycine to form the constituent amino acids. The presence of the enzyme in lens can be inferred since in cultured lenses (^{35}S)-GSH gave rise to (^{35}S)-cysteine whose formation requires hydrolysis of the α-peptide bond (REDDY et al., 1973). This peptide bond is not cleaved by lens homogenates prior to removal of the γ-glutamyl moiety (KINOSHITA & MATSURAT, 1957). This suggests that significant GSH disappearance from the lens is initiated only by γ-glutamyl transpeptidase, or by oxidation.

A soluble enzyme, γ-glutamyl cyclotransferase (γ-glutamyl lactamase) cleaves the γ-glutamyl dipeptide products of γ-glutamyl transpeptidase to form pyroglutamate and free amino acid. Many γ-glutamyl dipeptides, including γ-glutamylcysteine, are substrates for the enzyme from brain, but GSH is not reactive (ORLOWSKI et al., 1969). The enzyme was demonstrated in rabbit lens homogenates (CLIFFE & WALEY, 1958, 1961).

Pyroglutamate contains an internal γ-glutamyl peptide bond. This bond is hydrolyzed by pyroglutamate hydrolase (oxoprolinase), a membrane-bound enzyme recently demonstrated in rabbit and bovine lenses by REDDY et al., (1975). The bovine lens enzyme appears to be distinct from that of other sources because it is activated by low concentrations of magnesium ion, does not require ATP for activity, and has a high apparent Michaelis constant ($1 - 2 \times 10^{-2}$) for pyroglutamate. This high value may be responsible for the low reutilization of glutamate in resynthesis of GSH by the lens.

FUNCTIONS OF LENS GSH

GSH acts as a coenzyme in a number of instances. One such system in the lens (VAN HEYNINGEN et al., 1954) is the two enzyme glyoxalase system.

An attractive theory suggesting an amino acid transport function for γ-glutamyl transpeptidase while cleaving GSH was proposed by ORLOWSKI & MEISTER (1970). However, a patient has been recently discovered who has no detectable γ-glutamyl transpeptidase activity in fibroblasts, yet manifests a normal amino acid profile along with glutathionemia and gluta-thionuria (SCHULMAN et al., 1975). Thus far, despite extensive investigation in this laboratory and many others, convincing proof of the transport hypothesis has not been demonstrated.

Reduction of lens protein disulfide links has been suggested to be a possible major function of GSH. AURICCHIO & TESTA (1973) gained supporting evidence, but only by using high oxygen tension and glucose-free media. The lack of glucose has been shown to inactivate hexokinase (CHYLACK, 1973).

It is generally assumed that the vital functions of glutathione in the lens require the reduced form. Several agents have been used to oxidize GSH in cultured lenses. Tyrosine oxidation products formed in the media lowered lenticular GSH content with subsequent loss of GSSG to the media (SRIVASTAVA & BEUTLER, 1968). Intralenticular oxidation of GSH by azoester and diamide was inhibited by glucose. Additionally, diamide caused reduction of ^{86}Rb active transport which was partially reversed by dithio-threitol. Azoester diminished the lenticular ATP concentration (EPSTEIN & KINOSHITA, 1970 a,b). Thus, these authors suggested that GSH might affect the maintenance of membrane integrity via sulfhydryl groups.

Tertiary butylhydroperoxide, a substrate for GSH peroxidase, oxidized GSH in a time-dependent sequence which was initially unaffected by glucose concentration in cultured lenses. Decreases of ^{86}Rb transport, intra-lenticular potassium concentration, Na-K-ATPase activity and lactate production, but increases of intralenticular sodium and water, were observed. The decrease of ATPase activity and transport of ^{86}Rb were not reversible (GIBLIN et al., 1976). Although the authors suggest that this peroxide is a specific oxidant of GSH, the slow nonenzymic oxidation of GSH observed by them, and others, would be nonspecific and might affect sulfhydryl groups in other compounds. Linoleic hydroperoxide inhibits several sulf-hydryl enzymes of intermediary metabolism and other systems (WILLS, 1961; KHANDWALA & GEE, 1973).

The FAD-containing enzyme, GSH reductase, which catalyzes the reduction of GSSG to GSH while using NADPH as a cofactor, has been demonstrated in the lens, and was partially purified (HARDING, 1973). Other disulfides, including mixed disulfides containing GSH and proteins such as lens crystallin, are also substrates (SRIVASTAVA & BEUTLER, 1973).

148

Activity in human cataracts was reported to be inversely related to clarity (KÄRKELÄ & MIETTINEN, 1961), whereas a more recent study indicated enzyme activity was unaffected in any type of senile cataract except the fully mature one (FRIEDBURG & MANTHEY, 1973). Within 18 hours after X-irradiation of rabbit lenses, epithelial cell GSH reductase activity declined dramatically prior to visible clinical manifestations (SWANSON, 1965).

Glutathione peroxidase, which reduces peroxides while oxidizing GSH to GSSG, was first demonstrated in lens by PIRIE (1965a) and is distributed throughout the lens (HOLMBERG, 1968). The purified lens enzyme is quite specific for GSH, but will react with a variety of peroxides, including lipid peroxides (HOLMBERG, 1968). Its occurrence in several rabbit and bovine ocular tissues was reported (REIM et al., 1974). Erythrocyte GSH peroxidase consists of four identical subunits and four atoms of selenium (ROTRUCK et al., 1973; FLOHÉ & GÜNZLER, 1974). The activity of the lens enzyme decreased 85% in a long term deficiency of selenium (LAWRENCE et al., 1974). Long term deficiency of selenium caused cataracts in the third litter of the second generation of rats; selenium deficiency in each successive litter was more severe as the stores of the mother became depleted (SPRINKLER et al., 1971). A decrease of selenium content of human cataracts to approximately 1/6 of controls was reported by SWANSON & TRUESDALE (1971). Glutathione peroxidase, because of its low Michaelis constant as compared to catalase, is widely thought to be the primary agent for removal of low levels of H_2O_2 in cells. Moreover, it is the principal enzyme which acts rapidly on lipid peroxides (O'BRIEN & LITTLE, 1969).

The synergistic interrelationship between α-tocopherol, selenium and the sulfur amino acids in protection against tissue oxidation in deficiency diseases is now better understood. α-Tocopherol probably acts to break free radical chains, preventing peroxide formation, while forms of selenium and the sulfur amino acids combine in the GSH peroxidase reaction to destroy peroxides (CHOW & TAPPEL, 1974). These relationships may be of importance to the lens.

The deleterious effects of radiant energy upon the lens have long been the subject of much speculation and experimentation. A common denominator of peroxide formation appears to exist; this has been well documented for ionizing radiation. It has been suggested that photo-oxidation of organic molecules, especially of certain amino acids and lipids in the presence of oxygen, causes the formation of peroxides (VLADIMIROV et al., 1970; WILLS, 1961). H_2O_2 may be formed nonenzymically in a light-catalyzed oxidation of ascorbate to dehydroascorbate in the aqueous (PIRIE, 1965b). Peroxide increase in the aqueous was also noted in naphthalene and diquat cataracts (PIRIE et al., 1970; VAN HEYNINGEN & PIRIE, 1967). PIRIE (1972) has compared photo-oxidized proteins with those of human cataracts. Ultra-violet light, γ-irradiation, free radicals and H_2O_2 were all shown to cause lysing of isolated lysosome membranes (DESAI et al., 1964). The mechanism of photo-induced lens damage might be related to the production of free radicals; ascorbate, a free radical scavenger, is lost from the lens nucleus during cataract formation (WEITER & FINCH, 1975). It is especially interesting that the actual production of cataracts in mice by use of near ultraviolet light was accomplished by ZIGMAN et al., (1974).

Thus, it appears that the very nature of its primary function, that of light transmission, may subject the lens to the formation of membrane-damaging peroxides. If so, the major function of GSH in the lens may involve the constant destruction of peroxides.

REFERENCES

ASGHAR, K., REDDY, B.G. & KRISHNA, G. Histochemical localization of gluta-thione in tissues. *J. Histochem. Cytochem.* 23: *774-779* (1975).

AURICCHIO, G. & TESTA, M. Factors affecting the sulfhydryl groups of structural proteins of the lens in normal and 'uveitic' eyes. *Ophthal. Res.* 5: *230-235* (1973).

CHOW, C.K. & TAPPEL, A.L. Response of glutathione peroxidase to dietary selenium in rats. *J. Nutr.* 104: *444-451* (1974).

CHYLACK, L.T., Jr. Thermo-instability of rat lens hexokinase. *Expl. Eye Res.* 17: *109-117* (1973).

CLIFFE, E.F. & WALEY, S.G. Acidic peptides of the lens. 4. The biosynthesis of ophthalmic acid. *Biochem. J.* 69: *649-655* (1958).

CLIFFE, E.E. & WALEY, S.G. Acidic peptides of the lens. 6. Metabolism of γ-gluta-myl peptides in subcellular fractions of rabbit liver. *Biochem. J.* 79: *118-128* (1961).

DESAI, I.D., SAWANT, P.L. & TAPPEL, A.L. Peroxidative and radiation damage to isolated lysosomes. *Biochim. biophys. Acta* 86: *277-285* (1964).

EPSTEIN, D.L. & KINOSHITA, J.H. Effect of methylphenyldiazenecarboxylate (azoester) on lens membrane function. *Expl. Eye Res.* 10: *228-236* (1970a).

EPSTEIN, D.L. & KINOSHITA, J.H. The effect of diamide on lens glutathione and lens membrane function. *Invest. Ophthal.* 9: *629-638* (1970b).

FLOHÉ, L. & GÜNZLER, W.A. Glutathione peroxidase, in Glutathione. Proc. of 16th conf. Ger. Soc. Biol. Chem. (ed. Flohé, L., Benöhr, H., Sies, H., Waller, H. & Wendel, A.) Georg Thieme, Stuttgart, 1974, pp 132-145.

FRIEDBURG, D. & MANTHEY, K.F. Glutathione and NADP linked enzymes in human senile cataract. *Expl. Eye Res.* 15: *173-177* (1973).

GIBLIN, F.J., CHAKRAPANI, B. & REDDY, V.N. Glutathione and lens epithelial function. *Invest. Ophthal.* 15: *381-393* (1976).

HARDING, J.J. Affinity chromatography in the purification of glutathione reductase. *J. Chromat.* 77: *191-199* (1973).

HOLMBERG, N.J. Purification and properties of glutathione peroxidase from bovine lens. *Expl. Eye Res.* 7: *570-580* (1968).

KÄRKELÄ, A. & MIETTINEN, P. On the changes in the activity of glutathione reduc-tase on the maturation of senile cataract. *Acta Ophthal.* 39: *411-415* (1961).

KERN, H.L. & HO, C.K. Transport of L-glutamic acid and L-glutamine and their incor-poration into lenticular glutathione. *Expl. Eye Res.* 17: *455-462* (1973).

KHANDWALA, A. & GEE, J.B.L. Linoleic acid hydroperoxide: impaired bacterial up-take by alveolar macrophages, a mechanism of oxidant lung injury. *Science,* N.Y. 182: *1364-1365* (1973).

KINOSHITA, J.H. & MASURAT, T. Studies on the glutathione in bovine lens. *Archs. Ophthal.* 57: *266-274* (1957).

KINOSHITA, J.H. & MEROLA, L.O. The utilization of pyruvate and its conversion to glutamate in calf lens. *Expl. Eye Res.* 1: *53-59* (1961).

KUCK, J.F.R., Jr. in Biochemistry of the eye (ed. Graymore, C.N.) Academic Press, N.Y., 1970. pp 203-206.

LAWRENCE, R.A., SUNDE, R.A., SCHWARTZ, G.L. & HOEKSTRA, W.G. Glutathione peroxidase activity in rat lens and other tissues in relation to dietary selenium intake. *Expl. Eye Res.* 18: *563-569* (1974).

O'BRIEN, P.J. & LITTLE, C. Intracellular mechanisms for the decomposition of a lipid peroxide. II. Decomposition of a lipid peroxide by subcellular fractions. *Can. J. Biochem.* 47: *493-499* (1969).

ORLOWSKI, M., RICHMAN, P.G. & MEISTER, A. Isolation and properties of γ-L-glutamylcyclotransferase from human brain. *Biochemistry.* N.Y. 8: *1048-1055* (1969).

ORLOWSKI, M. & MEISTER, A. The γ-glutamyl cycle: a possible transport system for amino acids. *Proc. natn. Acad. Sci. U.S.A.* 67: *1248-1255* (1970).

PIRIE, A. Glutathione peroxidase in lens and a source of hydrogen peroxide in aqueous humour. *Biochem. J.* 96: *244-253* (1965a).

PIRIE, A. A light-catalyzed reaction in the aqueous humour of the eye. *Nature*, Lond. 205: *500-501* (1965b).

PIRIE, A., REES, J.R. & HOLMBERG, N.J. Diquat cataract: formation of the free radical and its reaction with constituents of the eye. *Expl. Eye Res.* 9: *204-218* (1970).

PIRIE, A. Photo-oxidation of proteins and comparison of photo-oxidized proteins with those of the cataractous human lens. *Israel J. Med. Sci.* 8: *1567-1573* (1972).

RATHBUN, W.B. γ-Glutamyl-cysteine synthetase from bovine lens. I. Purification and properties. *Archs. Biochem. Biophys.* 122: *62-72* (1967a).

RATHBUN, W.B. γ-Glutamyl-cysteine synthetase from bovine lens. II. Cysteine analogue studies. *Archs. Biochem. Biophys.* 122: *73-84* (1967b).

RATHBUN, W.B. & GILBERT, H.D. β-Aminoisobutyrate in the coupled enzymic assay of bovine lens γ-glutamylcysteine synthetase. *Analyt. Biochem.* 54: *153-160* (1973).

RATHBUN, W.B. & WICKER, K. Bovine lens γ-glutamyl transpeptidase. *Expl. Eye. Res.* 15: *161-171* (1973).

RATHBUN, W.B., SETHNA, S.S. & VAN BUSKIRK, G.E. Purification and properties of glutathione synthetase from bovine lens. *Expl. Eye Res.* In Press (1976).

REDDY, D.V.N. & KINSEY, V.E. Studies on the crystalline lens. IX. Quantitative analysis of free amino acids and related compounds. *Invest. Ophthal.* 1: *635-641* (1962).

REDDY, D.V.N., KLETHI, J. & KINSEY, V.E. Studies on the crystalline lens. XII. Turnover of glycine and glutamic acid in glutathione and ophthalmic acid in the rabbit. *Invest. Ophthal.* 5: *594-600* (1966).

REDDY, D.V.N., VARMA, S.D. & CHAKRAPANI, B. Transport and metabolism of glutathione in the lens. *Expl. Eye Res.* 16: *105-114* (1973).

REDDY, D.V.N. & UNAKAR, N.J. Localization of gamma-glutamyl transpeptidase in rabbit lens, ciliary process and cornea. *Expl. Eye Res.* 17: *405-408* (1973).

REDDY, D.V.N., CHAKRAPANI, B., RATHBUN, W.B. & HOUGH, M.M. Evidence for lens oxoprolinase, an enzyme of the gamma-glutamyl cycle. *Invest Ophthal.* 14: *228-232* (1975).

REIM, M., HEUVELS, B. & CATTEPOEL, H. Glutathione peroxidase in some ocular tissues. *Ophthal. Res.* 6: *228-234* (1974).

ROTRUCK, J.T., POPE, A.L., GANTHER, H.E., SWANSON, A.B., HAFEMAN, D.G. & HOEKSTRA, W.G. Selenium: biochemical role as a component of glutathione peroxidase. *Science,* N.Y. 179: *588-590* (1973).

SCHULMAN, J.D., GOODMAN, S.I., MACE, J.W., PATRICK, A.D., TIETZE, F. & BUTLER, E.J. Glutathionuria: inborn error of metabolism due to tissue deficiency of gamma-glutamyl transpeptidase. *Biochem. biophys. Res. Commun.* 65: *68-74* (1975).

SPRINKLER, L.H., HARR, J.R., NEWBERNE, P.M., WHANGER, P.D. & WES-

151

WIG, P.H. Selenium deficiency lesions in rats fed vitamin E supplemented rations. *Nutr. Rep. Int.* 4: *335-340* (1971).

SRIVASTAVA, S.K. & BEUTLER, E. Permeability of normal and cataractous rabbit lenses to glutathione. *Proc. Soc. exp. Biol. Med.* 127: *512-514* (1968).

SRIVASTAVA, S.K. & BEUTLER, E. Cleavage of lens protein – GSH mixed disulfide by glutathione reductase. *Expl. Eye Res.* 17: *33-42* (1973).

SWANSON, A.A. The effect of radiation on lenticular epithelial enzymes in young rabbits. *Expl. Eye Res.* 4: *231-236* (1965).

SWANSON, A.A. & TRUESDALE, A.W. Elemental analysis in normal and cataractous human lens tissue. *Biochem. biophys. Res. Commun.* 45: *1488-1496* (1971).

VAN BUSKIRK, G.E., GANDER, J.E. & RATHBUN, W.B. Bovine lens γ-glutamyl-cysteine synthetase: reaction mechanism. To be published elsewhere (1976).

VAN HEYNINGEN, R., PIRIE, A. & BOAG, J.W. Changes in lens during the formation of X-ray cataract in rabbits. 2. *Biochem. J.* 56: *372-379* (1954).

VAN HEYNINGEN, R. The metabolism of glucose by the rabbit lens in the presence and absence of oxygen. *Biochem. J.* 96: *419-431* (1965).

VAN HEYNINGEN, R. & PIRIE, A. Metabolism of naphthalene and its toxic effect on the eye. *Biochem. J.* 102: *842-52* (1967).

VLADIMIROV, Y.A., ROSHCHUPKIN, D.I. & FESENKO, E.E. Photochemical reactions in amino acid residues and inactivation of enzymes during u.v.-irradiation. A review. *Photochem. Photobiol.* 11: *227-246* (1970).

WILLS, E.D. Effect of unsaturated fatty acids and their peroxides on enzymes. *Biochem. Pharmac.* 7: *7-16* (1961).

WEITER, J.J. & FINCH, E.D. Paramagnetic species in cataractous human lenses. *Nature*, Lond. 254: *536-537* (1975).

ZIGMAN, S., YULO, T. & SCHULTZ, J. Cataract induction in mice exposed to near UV light. *Ophthal. Res.* 6: *259-270* (1974).

Keywords:

glutathione
lens
γ-glutamyl cycle

Author's address:

Department of Ophthalmology
Box 376 Mayo Building
University of Minnesota
Minneapolis, Minnesota 55455, USA

PROTEIN-BOUND GLUTATHIONE IN MAMMALIAN LENSES AND IN GALACTOSE CATARACT

V.N. REDDY & R.F. HAN*

(Rochester, Mich., U.S.A.)

ABSTRACT

Protein-bound glutathione in various mammalian lenses and in galactose cataracts in the rat has been determined using a specific method for the assay of reduced form of glutathione (GSH). In bovine lens the concentration of protein-bound GSH accounts for only 1-2% of total GSH in the lens. In rabbit and rat lenses the concentration of bound GSH is nearly 10% of the total tripeptide while in the human lens it is as high as one third of the total GSH. Bovine lens nucleus was found to contain a slightly higher concentration of protein-bound GSH than the cortex. In contrast to human cataractous lenses, which have been reported to show an increase in the concentration of protein-bound GSH, the concentration of bound tripeptide in galactose cataractous lenses was found to be actually lower than that in normal rat lenses.

INTRODUCTION

Lens contains an unusually large concentration of glutathione (GSH), the bulk of which is in the reduced form although a small but significant amount of oxidized glutathione (GSSG) is also present. The reason for the high concentration of GSH in the lens is not understood at the present time. It has been suggested that the tripeptide may serve to protect protein sulfhydryl groups (PSH) in the lens from undergoing oxidation (KINOSHITA, 1964). Assuming that thiol groups of proteins are involved in the interaction with GSH, the following reactions could lead to the formation of protein-bound GSH.

$$PSSP + GSH \rightleftharpoons PSH + PSSG$$
$$PSH + GSSG \rightleftharpoons GSH + PSSG$$

Evidence for the presence of protein-bound GSH in the lens has been provided previously (HARDING, 1970). This evidence is based on the observation that when disulfide bonds of lens proteins are reduced, there is an increase in non-protein thiol groups, presumably due to the splitting of mixed disulfide of protein and GSH. The methods employed, however, do not distinguish whether the liberated thiols are GSH, cysteine and/or other sulfhydryl compounds that may also be bound to the proteins by disulfide linkages. As part of a broader study of the role of GSH in the lens, we have determined the concentration of protein-bound GSH in several mammalian lenses by a more direct method involving ion exchange chromatography.

* Recipient of NSF Undergraduate Fellowship from a grant awarded to the Department of Biological Sciences

153

The possibility that the decrease in GSH in galactose cataract may in part be due to the formation of mixed disulfides has also been examined.

METHODS

Bovine lenses were obtained from a local abattoir an hour after the animals were killed while rabbit (2 kg) and rat (50-60 g) lenses were removed immediately after sacrifice. Human lenses were obtained from a local eye bank (Kresge Eye Institute, Detroit, Michigan). Galactose cataracts were induced by feeding a 50% galactose diet to Sprague-Dawley rats weighing 50-60 g as described earlier (REDDY, SCHWASS, CHAKRAPANI & LIM, 1976). All animal lenses were removed by posterior approach, rolled on absorbent tissue and weighed prior to homogenization. In some instances bovine lenses were separated into nuclear and cortical fractions. For this purpose the lenses were frozen in dry ice and separated into the peripheral portion and central core with a cork borer. The nuclear fraction, amounting to 25% of the total weight of the lens, was removed from the central core by dissecting off the anterior and posterior sections (REDDY, KLETHI & KINSEY, 1966). The procedure followed for the reduction of disulfide bonds was similar to that of HARDING (1970) with minor modifications. Tissues were homogenized in distilled water (6 ml/g wet weight) and placed in Thunberg tubes*, evacuated and treated with iodoacetic acid, sodium bicarbonate and a sufficient amount of urea to make the homogenate 7 M with respect to this compound. The reaction was allowed to proceed for 24 hours in the dark and the contents of the tube were dialyzed against 4 l of 7 M urea adjusted to pH of 4.0 for 36 hours at 4 °C with one change of urea solution.

The contents of the dialysis bag were removed and the pH adjusted to 8.8 with sodium hydroxide and treated with sodium borohydride (40 mg/g wet tissue) for 2 hours at room temperature to cleave the disulfide bonds. Trichloracetic acid (TCA) was then added to precipitate the proteins and destroy excess borohydride and centrifuged at 12,000 g for 40 minutes. The supernatants were collected and the precipitates washed 3 times with small amounts of TCA and recentrifuged. The supernatants and the washings were combined and extracted 4 times with 3 volumes of ice-cold ether to remove TCA. Traces of ether in the aqueous phase were removed by bubbling nitrogen gas through the solution. The resultant extracts were concentrated *in vacuo* to a small volume and chromatographed on a Sephadex Column (G-10) to separate urea and GSH. The effluents containing GSH and GSSG were collected, concentrated to a small volume and made up to 2 ml with .01 N HCl. Experiments to test the adequacy of the procedure indicated complete separation of urea and GSH and that more than 95% of added GSH could be recovered.

---

* Dr. Frank Giblin in our laboratory has shown that a better procedure is to dissolve the lens in a nitrogenated solution of 6 M guanidine hydrochloride containing 0.2 M Tris and 0.025 M EDTA directly in the Thunberg tube. The lens extract after treatment with iodoacetic acid is then dialyzed against 7 M urea. This method has the advantage of preventing any oxidation of thiol groups during the initial homogenization of lens.

154

RESULTS AND DISCUSSION

Lens extracts prepared in the manner described above and chromatographed using an automatic amino acid analyzer showed only traces of GSSG but no GSH (Fig. 1a). The possibility existed that there was no significant amount of bound GSH or that GSH cleaved from proteins was being oxidized to GSSG or recombining with protein -SH groups or with other unknown sulfhydryl compounds to form mixed disulfides. Earlier studies of MOORE, COLE, GUNLACH & STEIN (1958) have shown that removal of excess of sodium borohydride by acidification can lead to reoxidation of -SH groups which are initially cleaved by this reducing agent. Also, formation of mixed disulfides which are either retained on the Dowex column or whose position on the chromatogram is unknown could explain the absence of GSH. If

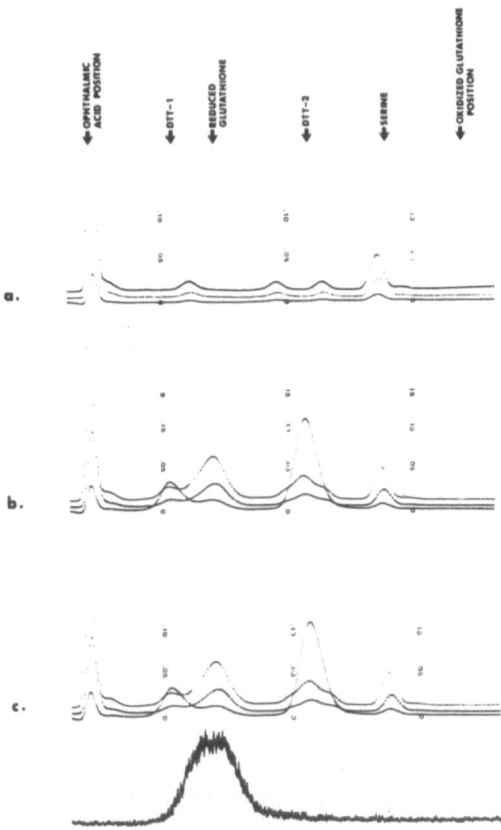

Fig. 1. Chromatographic separation of protein-bound glutathione (GSH) from lens extracts prepared as in Scheme 1. (a) lens extracts without dithiothreitol (DTT) treatment, (b) lens extracts treated with excess of DTT, (c) lens extracts treated with DTT but a trace amount of ^{35}S-labeled GSH was added to extracts after borohydride reduction. Lower tracing was obtained by simultaneous monitoring of the effluent from the amino acid analyzer by a flow detector; the radioactive peak corresponds to the position of GSH on the chromatogram. See text for additional details.

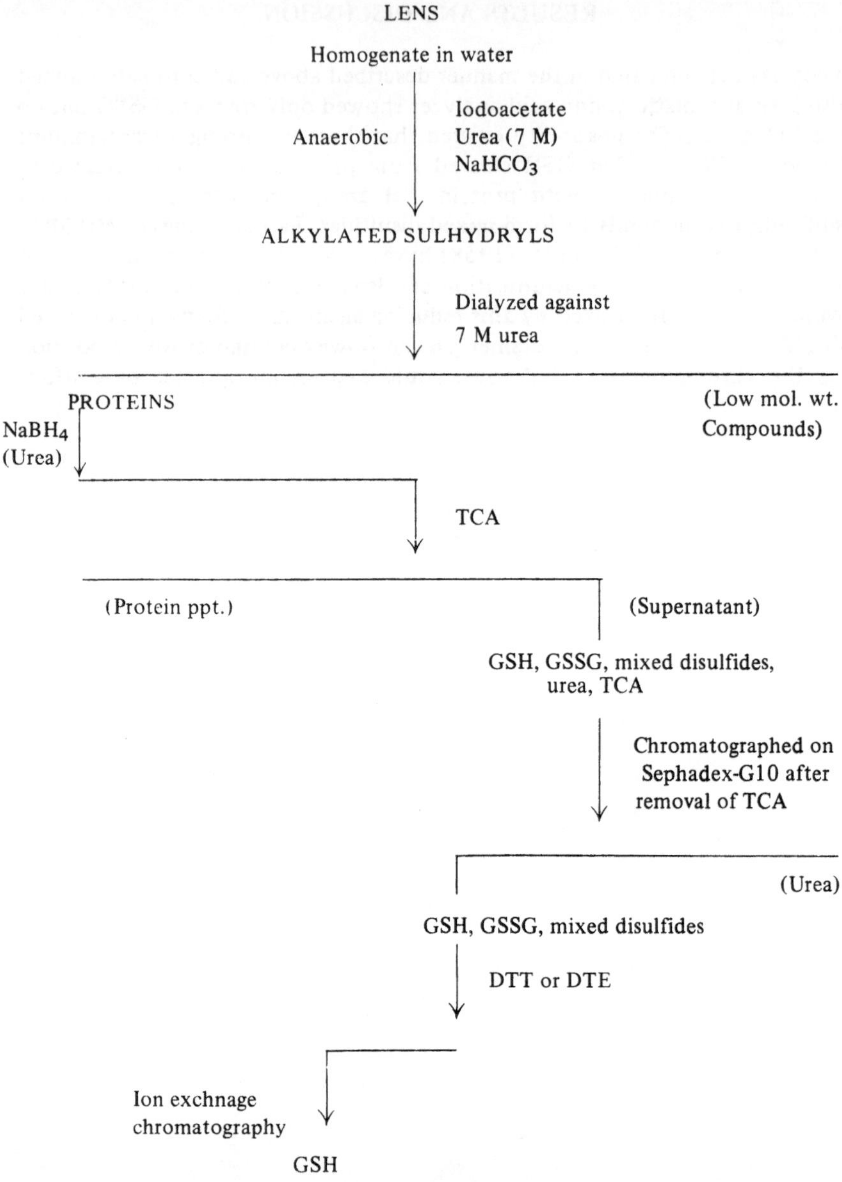

LENS

Homogenate in water

	Iodoacetate
Anaerobic	Urea (7 M)
	NaHCO$_3$

↓

ALKYLATED SULHYDRYLS

| Dialyzed against |
| 7 M urea |

↓

PROTEINS   (Low mol. wt.

NaBH$_4$ Compounds)

(Urea) ↓

TCA

↓

(Protein ppt.)   (Supernatant)

GSH, GSSG, mixed disulfides,
urea, TCA

| Chromatographed on |
| Sephadex-G10 after |
| removal of TCA |

↓

(Urea)

GSH, GSSG, mixed disulfides

| DTT or DTE |

↓

Ion exchnage
chromatography

↓

GSH

Scheme 1. Scheme for isolation of protein-bound glutathione. Experimental details given in text.

mixed disulfides are in fact formed, it should be possible to bring about their reduction by further treatment with dithiothreitol (DTT). Accordingly, the lens extracts were treated with DTT at a pH of 8.5 for one hour and then analyzed by column chromatography following the adjustment of pH to 2.2. The resulting analyses showed that the addition of DTT to lens extracts results in the appearance of a peak in the same position as that of

156

GSH (Fig. 1b). The addition of increasing amounts of DTT resulted in a further increase in the height of GSH peak until a maximum value was reached. Under these conditions two additional peaks absorbing maximally at 440 millimicrons also appeared on the chromatogram. To rule out the possibility that one or both of these peaks may have been due to mixed disulfides of GSH and DTT, a trace amount of ^{35}S-labeled GSH was added to the lens extract after borohydride reduction and treated in the usual manner and subsequently chromatographed. Radioactivity was monitored simultaneously with a flow detector unit attached to the amino acid analyzer. The chromatogram (Fig. 1c) illustrating the presence of a single peak of radioactivity corresponding to the position of reduced GSH suggests that the '440 mμ peaks' do not contain any GSH. These peaks apparently are due to DTT and its derivatives since they appear even when a solution of DTT alone is chromatographed. Additional studies showed that dithioerythritol (DTE) is a reagent of choice since its peak is farther removed from that of GSH on the chromatogram. In all experiments in which protein-bound GSH was determined, lens extracts were treated with excess of DTE prior to chromatographic determination of GSH (Scheme 1).

Table I shows the concentration of protein-bound GSH in various mammalian lenses. For comparison, the values of free GSH in these lenses determined in another series of experiments is also included. It is evident that a small but significant amount of GSH is present in the bound form in all of the mammalian lenses studied. In bovine lens, protein-bound GSH represents the smallest fraction of total lens GSH (1-1.5%), while in the rabbit and rat lenses the concentration of bound GSH is nearly 10% of total GSH. The values now found for normal human lenses appear to be slightly higher than those of HARDING (1970) but within range of those reported by SRIVASTAVA & BEUTLER (1973). Although free GSH was not determined in the same human lenses, its concentration in 2 other lenses of approximately the same age was found to be 2 and 2.34 μmoles/g lens. HARDING (1970) has observed that the concentration of GSH in human

Table I. Concentration of free and protein-bound GSH in some mammalian lenses

		μmoles/g wet weight	
		Free GSH	Protein-bound GSH
Bovine		14.0	0.20* (0.14 – 0.28)
Rabbit		12.0	1.30* (0.80 – 1.50)
Rat		7.9	0.96* (0.90 – 1.04)
Human**	1		0.89
	2		1.52
	3	2.3	–
	4	2.0	–

*   Average of 3 experiments.
**   Normal lenses from the eye bank: (1) 41 year-old, (2) 44 year-old, (3) 40 year-old. (4) 41 year-old.

Table II. Distribution of free and protein-bound GSH in bovine lens

Lens fraction	% of lens weight	μmoles/g wet weight	
		Free GSH	Protein-bound GSH
Anterior cortex	9.8	13.1	Not determined
Posterior cortex	8.4	13.1	Not determined
Equatorial cortex	56.3	17.4	0.20
Nucleus	25.4	2.4	0.53

Values are averages of 2 experiments.

Table III. Concentration of free and protein-bound GSH in the lenses of normal and galactose-fed rats (μmoles/g wet weight)

Number of days on diet	Free GSH		Protein-bound GSH	
	Control	Galactose-fed	Control	Galactose-fed
4	7.6	0.39	1.4	0.40
11	8.2	0.22	1.0	0.26
21	Not Determined	Trace	1.0	Trace

Values are averages of 3 experiments consisting of 6 pooled lenses each.

lenses is age-dependent and that it is approximately 2.5 μmoles/g lens for the age group between 40 and 45 years. Thus, it appears that the concentration of protein-bound GSH in the human lens represents nearly a third of total GSH and is a much higher fraction than that found in lenses of other species.

The concentration of protein-bound GSH in the nucleus of bovine lens appears to be slightly higher than in the cortex (Table II) and confirms our earlier observations (REDDY & HAN, 1972). Its concentration in the nucleus, however, does not account for the low concentration of free GSH found in this portion of the lens. While it is not clear at the present time which of the cyrstallins of the lens participate in mixed disulfide formation, it is possible that the higher concentration of protein-bound GSH in the nucleus may be related to the higher level of protein thiols present in the nucleus compared to that in the cortex (KINOSHITA & MEROLA, 1958).

In accordance with the previous observations, free GSH decreases very rapidly in lenses of galactose-fed rats (Table III). There is also a decrease in protein-bound GSH but to a lesser extent than that of the free tripeptide. There appears to be a lag period between the loss of free GSH and protein-bound GSH but at the end of 21 days following galactose feeding little GSH, either free or protein-bound, is found in the lens. It is clear that the loss of free GSH in galactose cataract cannot be accounted for on the basis of mixed disulfide formation. In fact, protein-bound GSH actually decreases in these lenses. It is interesting to note that in contrast to galactose cataracts, human senile cataracts have been reported to have increased protein-bound GSH (HARDING, 1970).

The mechanism by which GSH becomes bound to proteins in the lens is unknown although it is conceivable that if GSSG increases at the expense of GSH, glutathione may become bound to protein in a manner analogous to the binding of GSH to hemoglobin in the red blood cell (HUISMAN & DOZY, 1962; SRIVASTAVA & BEUTLER, 1970). This hypothesis, however, remains to be tested. Recent studies in this laboratory have failed to demonstrate any increase of GSSG in galactose cataractous lens. Whether there is an increased formation of oxidized tripeptide in human cataractous lens remains to be established.

ACKNOWLEDGMENT

The expert technical assistance of Mr. B. Chakrapani and Miss Ching Peng Lim is gratefully acknowledged. We thank Dr. John Cowden of Kresge Eye Institute for providing the human lenses and Dr. Frank J. Giblin for confirming the results of protein-bound glutathione in rat lens using the procedure of dissolving the lenses directly in guanidine hydrochloride.

This work was supported in part by research grant EY-00484 from the National Eye Institute, U.S. Public Health Service and the U.S. Atomic Energy Commission Contract AT (11-1)-2012-30.

REFERENCES

HARDING, J.J. Free and protein-bound glutathione in normal and cataractous human lenses. *Biochem. J.* 117: *957-960* (1970).

HUISMAN, T.H.J. & DOZY, A.M. Studies on the heterogeneity of hemoglobin. V. Binding of hemoglobin with oxidized glutathione. *J. Lab. & Clin. Med.* 60: *302-319* (1962).

KINOSHITA, J.H. Annual review. Selected topics in ophthalmic biochemistry. *Arch. Ophthal.* 72: *554-572* (1964).

KINOSHITA, J.H. & MEROLA, L.O. The distribution of glutathione and protein sulf-hydryl groups in calf and cattle lenses. *Amer. J. Ophthal.* 46: *36-41* (1958).

MOORE, S., COLE, R.D., GUNLACH, H.G. & STEIN, W.H. On the cleavage of disulfide bonds in proteins by reduction. *Proc. Fourth Intern. Congr. Biochem.* 8: *52-62* (1958).

REDDY, V.N. & HAN, R.F. Studies on protein-bound glutathione in normal and cataractous lens. Abstracts of the Proc. of Symp. on Lens and Development, Utrecht, 1971. *Ophthalmic Res.* 3: *13,* 1972.

REDDY, D.V.N. & KINSEY. V.E. Studies on the crystalline lens. IX. Quantitative analysis of free amino acids and related compounds. *Invest. Ophthal.* 1: *635-641* (1962).

REDDY, D.V.N., KLETHI, J. & KINSEY, V.E. Studies on the crystalline lens. XII. Turnover of glycine and glutamic acid in glutathione and ophthalmic acid in the rabbit. *Invest. Ophthal.* 5: *594-600* (1966).

REDDY, V.N., SCHWASS, D., CHAKRAPANI, B. & LIM, C.P. Biochemical changes associated with the development and reversal of galactose cataracts. *Exp. Eye Res.* (in press).

SRIVASTAVA, S.K. & BEUTLER, E. Glutathione metabolism of the erythrocyte. The enzymic cleavage of glutathione-haemoglobin preparations by glutathione reductase. *Biochem. J.* 119: *353-357* (1970).

SRIVASTAVA, S.K. & BEUTLER, E. Cleavage of lens protein-GSH mixed disulfide by glutathione reductase. *Exp. Eye Res.* 17: *33-42* (1973).

Keywords:

Glutathione
Protein-bound glutathione
Lens
Bovine
Rabbit
Rat
Human
Galactose cataract

Authors' address:

Institute of Biological Sciences
Oakland University
Rochester, Michigan 48063, USA

160

THE EFFECT OF OXIDANTS ON THE MEMBRANE
SULFHYDRYL GROUPS OF THE LENS

H.N. FUKUI, L.O. MEROLA & J.H. KINOSHITA

(Bethesda, Maryland)

ABSTRACT

The effects of -SH oxidants, iodosobenzoate and diamide, on lens membrane function were studied. Both oxidants decrease the ability of the rabbit lens to concentrate rubidium (Rb) ions. Diamide is more effective than iodosobenzoate. Under the conditions used, diamide affects both the uptake and the leak out processes. While iodosobenzoate affects Rb uptake but does not affect the leak out process to a significant extent. These effects are observed in the absence of glucose. The presence of glucose in the medium abolishes the effects of the -SH oxidants. A marked increase in the oxidation of carbon one atom of glucose is observed in the lens incubated with diamide suggesting the stimulation of the pentose shunt mechanism to provide TPNH necessary to maintain the sulfhydryl groups in the reduced form.

INTRODUCTION

We have been concerned in learning more about the requirements of sulfhydryl (-SH) groups of the lens membrane involved in electrolyte balance and the cation transport mechanism in the lens. For this reason we have been studying the effects of different sulfhydryl oxidants on the membrane function of the rat lens. Diamide and azoester were -SH reagents previously studied (EPSTEIN & & KINOSHITA, 1970a, EPSTEIN & KINOSHITA, 1970b). These studies revealed that -SH groups may influence the uptake process presumably those associated with Na-K ATPase, and -SH groups on the surface membranes that regulate permeability to cations. A similar situation also exists in red cells as ROTHSTEIN, 1970, has demonstrated that membrane -SH groups are involved in cation pumping and in determining the degree of permeability.

Since -SH oxidants usually affect both the uptake and leak out processes in the lens the question arises as to whether there is any difference in the susceptibility of the two different types of -SH groups to oxidation. In the course of this study we found that iodosobenzoate is an oxidant that is useful in shedding light on this question. This report deals with a comparison of the action of diamide and iodosobenzoate (IBA) on the membrane function of the rabbit lens.

METHODS

The incubation procedures for rabbit lenses weighing 175 mg and chemical and isotopic methods used have been previously described (KINOSHITA,

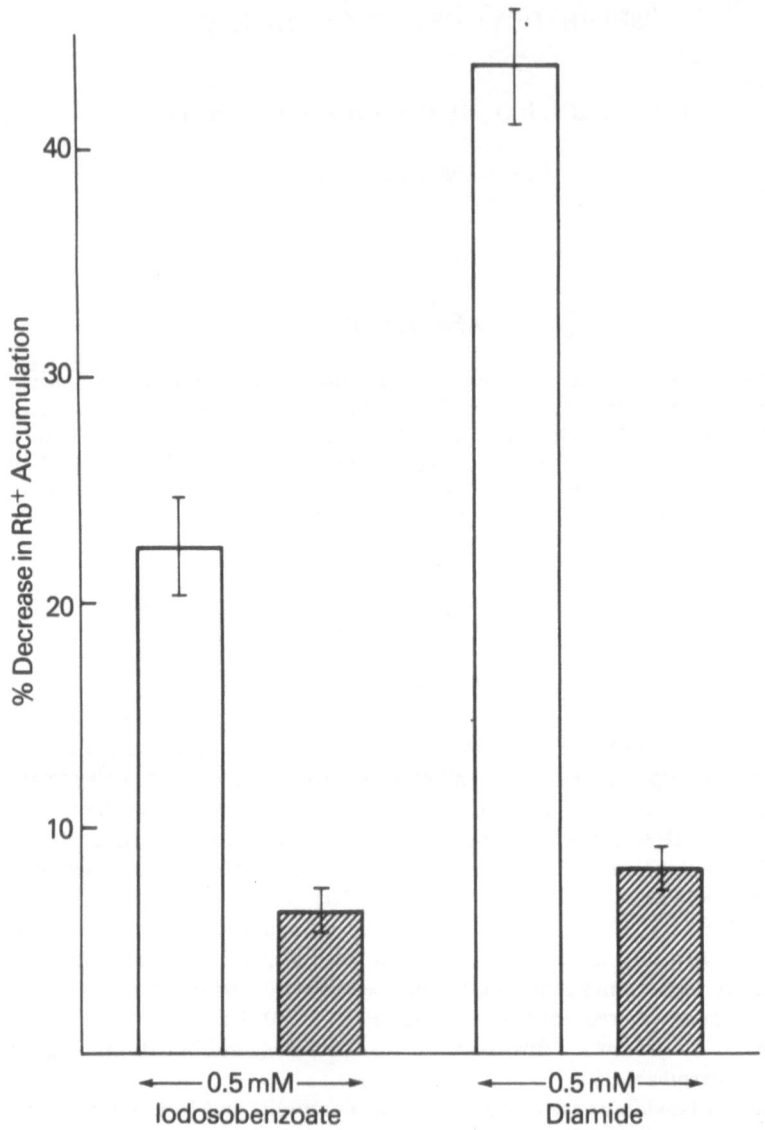

Fig. 1. Effects -SH oxidants on Rb accumulation
open bar – in medium without glucose
hatched bar – in medium with 5.5 mM glucose
Lenses were exposed to oxidants for a 3 hour period and Rb[86] uptake followed for
2 hour period. Results are given as mean ± S.D.

MEROLA & TUNG, 1968, KINOSHITA, FUTTERMAN, SATOH & MERO-LA, 1963 and IWATA & KINOSHITA, 1971). The medium used was a balanced salt mixture containing 135 mM Na^+, 5.5 mM K^+, 0.6 mM Mg^{++} 1.0 mM Ca^{++} with the principal anion Cl^- and 29 mM HCO_3^-. The incubating medium was equilibrated with 5% CO_2 and 95% Air to give a pH between 7.5-7.6 and a tonicity of 295-300 milliosmolal.

The rubidium (Rb) uptake and runout studies were patterned after the experiments described by KINOSHITA, MEROLA & TUNG, 1968. After the lenses were exposed to -SH oxidants for a period varying from 3 to 20 hours, ^{86}Rb was added and the incubation was carried out for an additional 2 to 4 hours. In the Rb runout studies the rabbit lenses were first preloaded with ^{86}Rb for an overnight period after which the medium was replaced by a medium free of ^{86}Rb containing the oxidant and $10^{-4}M$ ouabain. The runout was followed for a period up to 6 hours.

RESULTS

In these studies a medium deficient in glucose was required to produce the desired effects on the -SH groups. The lens, obviously, cannot maintain normal parameters if the incubation is carried on for any protracted period without glucose. We found that 30 mM fructose in the absence of glucose is capable of maintaining transparency, glutathione level and normal electro-

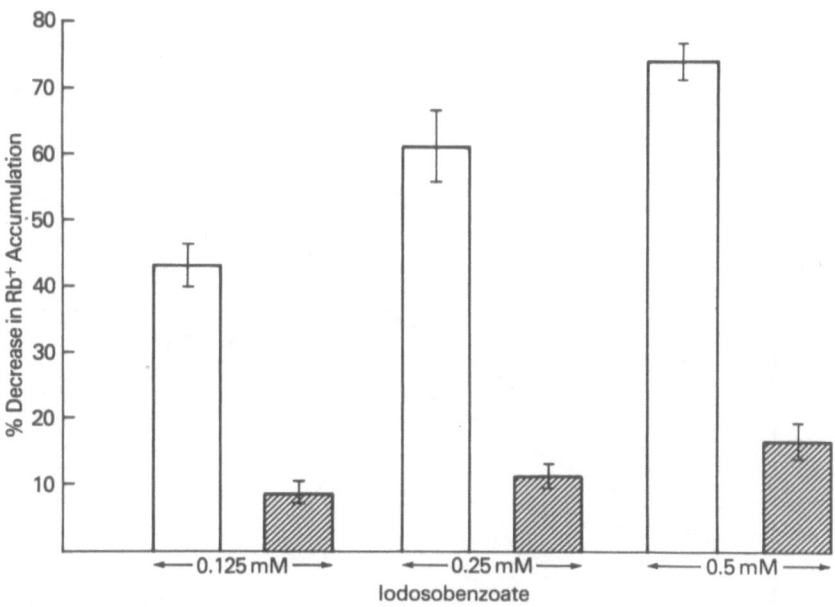

Fig. 2. Effects of Iodosobenzoate on Rb Accumulation. Lenses were exposed to IBA for an overnight period and Rb uptake followed for 2 hour period.
hatched bar indicates lens in medium with 5.5 mM glucose;
open bar without glucose

lyte content for an overnight period. Apparently, the low rate of metabolism through the glycolytic pathway of fructose is sufficient to marginally sustain the lens.

Iodosobenzoate (IBA) appeared to be a mild -SH oxidizing agent as compared to diamide. For example, as shown in Fig. 1, when rabbit lenses were incubated for 3 hours in the presence of 0.5 mM diamide there was a 45% decrease in the accumulation of rubidium ions (Rb+), while in 0.5 mM IBA for the same period there was only a 22% decrease in Rb accumulation. The decrease in the ability of the lens to accumulate Rb was observed in the absence of glucose. When glucose was included in the incubation medium the effects of diamide and iodosobenzoate were minimal. The incubation of the lenses under these conditions also brought about a 20% loss in glutathione (GSH) with diamide but only a slight loss with IBA.

To study further the effects of IBA, longer exposure periods were instituted. As shown in Fig. 2 an overnight exposure of the lens to IBA brought about a more pronounced effect. At 0.125 mM IBA a substantial decrease in Rb accumulation was observed. At higher concentrations the decrease in Rb accumulation became even more striking. The protective action of glucose was again demonstrated. In those lenses incubated in IBA

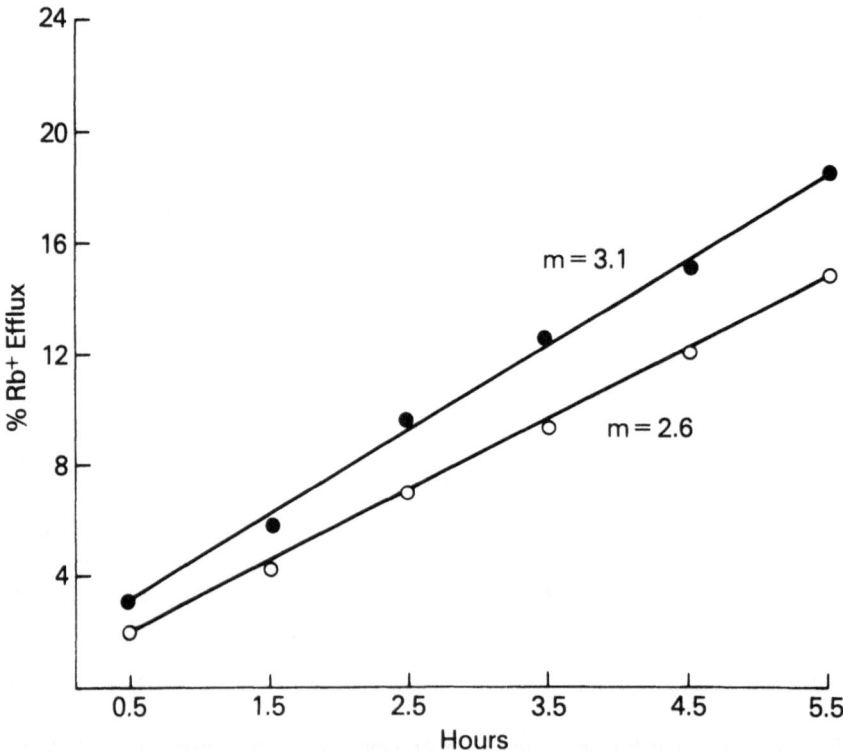

Fig. 3. Effects of Iodosobenzoate on Rb run-out
See Methods for details.

at 0.125 and 0.25 mM for an overnight period no gain in water, some loss in potassium and gain in sodium was observed. At the lower concentration no loss in GSH was observed while at the higher concentration a 15-20% loss in GSH was observed. At 0.5 mM IBA there were marked gains in water and Na, loss in K and about a 70% loss in GSH. Obviously when the lens is exposed for an overnight period in 0.5 mM IBA the damage to the lens membranes appeared severe as the lens was cloudy. At the lower two concentrations, however, the lenses did not gain much water and appeared only slightly hazy.

To determine whether the loss in the ability of the lens to concentrate Rb was due to a defect in the uptake or to an increase in cation permeability, the Rb efflux properties of the IBA exposed lenses were studied. At 0.125 mM and 0.25 mM IBA the rate of Rb runout was no different in the IBA exposed lens as compared to the control lens. At 0.5 mM IBA the Rb efflux was only slightly elevated as shown in Fig. 3. In contrast the rabbit lens exposed to 0.5 mM diamide showed a marked increase in Rb efflux (Fig. 4). The slope of the curve which is a measure of the rate of Rb runout was almost doubled in the diamide treated lens as compared to the control lens.

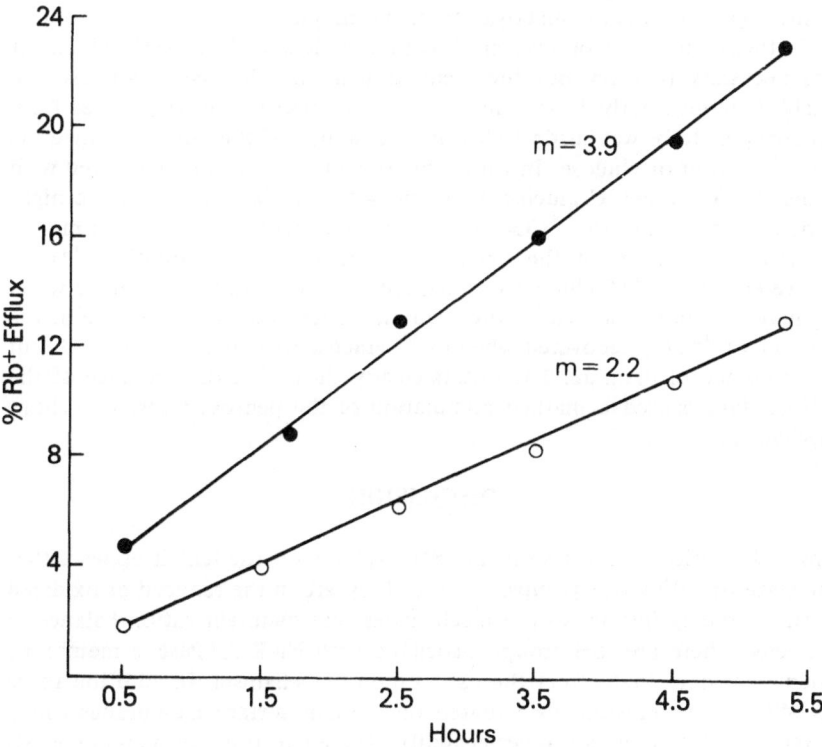

Fig. 4. Diamide on Rb run-out
See Methods for details.

Table I.   Lens Na-K ATPase Inactivation by Iodosobenzoate

IBA (mM)	Incubation Period (hrs)	Glucose 5mM	% Decrease in Enzyme Activity
0.125	20	(−)	22
0.25	6	(−)	44
	20	(−)	85
0.25	20	(+)	0

These results suggest that the effects of IBA are considerably different from that of diamide. In the rat lens it has already been shown that although both the uptake and the leak-out processes were affected, the effects on the leak-out process appeared to occur earlier (EPSTEIN & KINOSHITA, 1970a).

In the case of IBA it appears the effect is not on the run-out process but rather on the uptake mechanism. Further supporting this interpretation are the effects of IBA on the Na-K ATPase of the rabbit lens. As shown in Table 1 the lens incubated in 0.125 mM IBA for an overnight period showed a loss of 22% in its Na-K ATPase activity. At 0.25 mM IBA the loss in Na-K ATPase was 44% after 6 hours of incubation and 85% at 20 hours. The protective action of glucose is shown in that at 0.25 mM IBA the presence of the sugar prevents the inactivation of the enzyme.

In these studies to observe an effect on the lens with the -SH oxidants it was necessary to carry out the incubation in the absence of glucose. To establish more clearly how glucose is able to prevent these changes from occurring a study was made following the ability of the lens to oxidize the carbon 1 atom of glucose. In these experiments lenses were incubated with either $1\text{-}^{14}C$ or $6\text{-}^{14}C$ glucose with and without diamide for an overnight period. The amount of $^{14}CO_2$ recovered after incubation was determined. As shown in Fig. 5, in the presence of diamide the amount of $^{14}CO_2$ recovered from $1\text{-}^{14}C$ glucose was markedly higher than that observed when diamide was not included in the medium. There was no difference in the amount of $^{14}CO_2$ recovered when $6C^{14}$ glucose was used with and without the presence of diamide. The results clearly show that the presence of the -SH oxidant caused a marked stimulation of the pentose phosphate shunt mechanism.

DISCUSSION

From the series of studies on the -SH oxidants on the lens it appears that the state of sulfhydryl groups, whether they are in the reduced or oxidized form, markedly influences the mechanisms that maintain cation balance in the lens. There are -SH groups associated with Na-K ATPase, a membrane bound enzyme, that affect the cation pump mechanism. In addition there are -SH groups presumably situated on the lens surface membranes which govern the degree of cation permeability. These two types of membrane -SH groups are susceptible to oxidation but can be reversibly reduced through the interaction with glutathione. The experiments dealing with the oxidation of 1-^{14}C glucose clearly demonstrates that in the presence of diamide the oxidation carbon 1 of glucose is markedly increased.

The most likely explanation of this phenomena is described in Fig. 6. The -SH oxidant, such as diamide, oxidizes the membrane -SH to disulfide bonds. Glutathione is also oxidized either directly by the oxidant or by interaction with the -S-S- groups as shown in Fig. 6. There is an increased

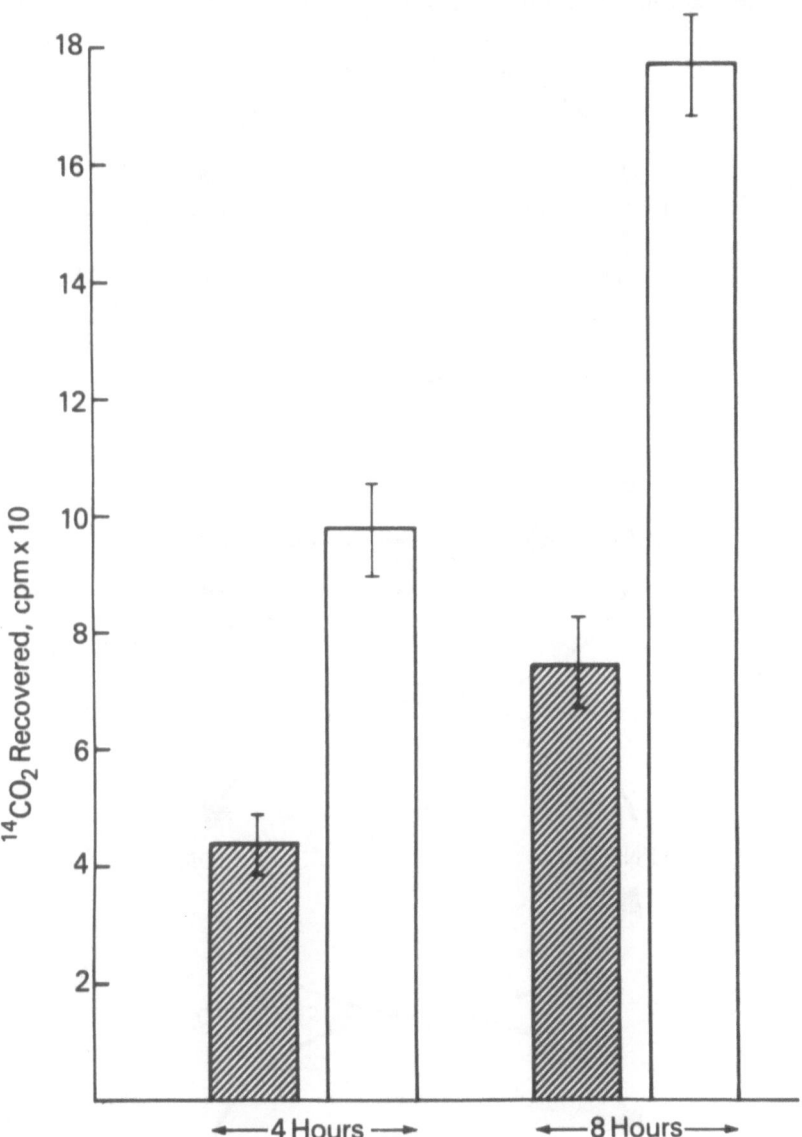

Fig. 5. Glucose Oxidation via shunt pathway.
(1-^{14}C glucose) oxidation in rabbit lens with (open bar) and without (hatched bar) diamide.

167

demand for TPNH since this nucleotide is necessary for the conversion of oxidized glutathione to GSH through the glutathione reductase reaction. The need for an increase rate in the regeneration of TPNH is fulfilled by accelerating the pentose phosphate shunt mechanism. One alternative possibility is the direct interaction of TPNH with the membrane -S-S- group, bypassing the glutathione stage. This alternate route may be catalyzed by glutathione reductase. The main source of TPNH is the pentose phosphate shunt mechanism. Thus the increased demand for TPNH accelerates the

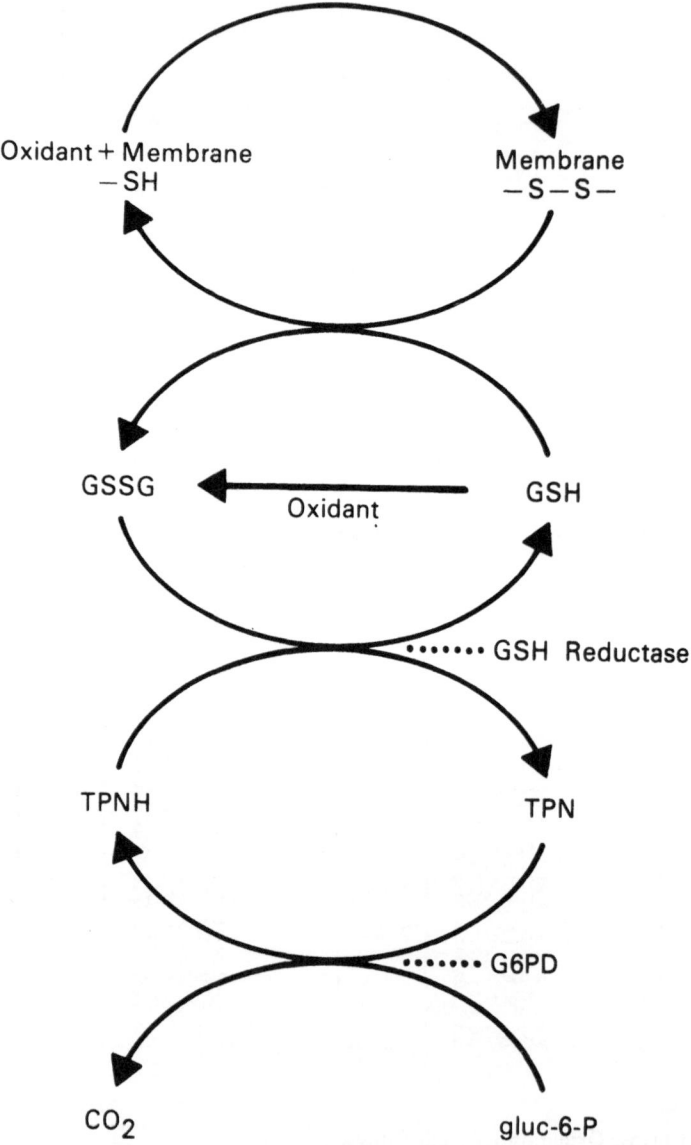

Fig. 6. Coupled oxidation and reduction reactions.

oxidation of glucose-6-phosphate involving glucose-6-phosphate dehydrogenase and 6-phosphogluconate dehydrogenase. The oxidation through these 2 enzymes results in the cleavage of the carbon one atom of glucose leading to CO_2 production.

The study with iodosobenzoate indicates that it is a milder -SH oxidizing agent than diamide. From the results obtained in the IBA experiments, it appears that the -SH groups associated with Na-K ATPase is much more susceptible than the -SH groups involved with governing the degree of cation permeability. However it would be erroneous to conclude that IBA only oxidizes the -SH groups of the ATPase. If the incubation is carried out for longer periods or at higher concentrations of IBA the permeability also becomes affected. This change was quite apparent when the lens was incubated for an overnight period in 0.5 mM IBA. Thus the selectivity of IBA can be demonstrated under certain conditions.

In the rat lens experiments with diamide (EPSTEIN & KINOSHITA, 1970a). There is the suggestion that under certain conditions it can be shown that diamide oxidizes the -SH groups governing the runout process before the -SH groups of the uptake mechanism. The evidence for the existence of these 2 different types of membrane -SH groups is further supported in this study. More data are needed to conclusively establish this point in the lens as it has been in the red cells (ROTHSTEIN, 1970).

The studies with the -SH oxidants suggest the possibility that the cation transport mechanism and permeability of the lens can be regulated by the state of oxidation or reduction of the -SH groups. The fact that the -SH groups of the uptake mechanism appear more susceptible to oxidation with IBA suggests further discrimination of the balance between the leakout process and the transport of cations. These -SH groups, furthermore, appear to interact with the GSH-GSSG system and are intimately linked to glucose metabolism.

REFERENCES

EPSTEIN, D.L. & J.H. KINOSHITA. The effect of diamide on lens glutathione and lens membrane function. *Invest. Ophthalmol.* 9: *629-638* (1970a).

EPSTEIN, D.L. & J.H. KINOSHITA. Effect of methyl phenyldiazene carboxylate (azoester) on lens membrane function. *Exp. Eye Res.* 10: *228-236* (1970b).

IWATA, S. & J.H. KINOSHITA. Mechanisms of development of hereditary cataract in mice. *Invest. Ophthalmol.* 10: *504-512* (1971).

KINOSHITA, J.H., S. FUTTERMAN, K. SATOH & L.O. MEROLA. Factors affecting the formation of sugar alcohol in ocular lens. *Biochim. Biophys. Acta* 74: *340-350* (1963).

KINOSHITA, J.H., L.O. MEROLA & B. TUNG. Changes in cation permeability in the galactose-exposed rabbit lens. *Exp. Eye Res.* 7: *80-90* (1968).

ROTHSTEIN, A. In: Current topics in membrane transport (Eds. F. Bonner & A. Kleinzeller). Academic Press, New York (1970).

Authors' address:

Laboratory of Vision Research   Department of Health, Education and Welfare
National Eye Institute   Bethesda, Maryland 20014, USA
National Institutes of Health

SOME ASPECTS OF HUMAN LENS METABOLISM: GLYCOLYSIS AND PROTEIN SYNTHESIS

KEITH J. DILLEY & RUTH VAN HEYNINGEN

(Oxford, England)

ABSTRACT

Glycolysis by the adult human lens was at the rate of about 2.0 μmoles lactic acid formed /g. wet weight/hour. This rate is of the same order as that of the adult cow, rabbit and rat lens. The average rate of glycolysis by foetal human lenses was 4.1 μ-moles /g lens/hour.

There was negligible incorporation of radioactivity into the proteins of the nucleus of adult human lenses, incubated in a medium containing ^{14}C amino-acids.

INTRODUCTION

Information about metabolism by the human lens is scarce. In this study two separate aspects of lens metabolism were investigated — glycolysis and protein synthesis.

MATERIALS

Foetal eyes (12-20 weeks) were obtained not more than six hours, and the infant and adult lenses between 4 and 22 hours, after death.

[U-^{14}C] tyrosine (> 405 mCi/m-mol) and [U-^{14}C] mixed amino acids (protein hydrolysate; > 45 mCi/milliatom of carbon) were from Radiochemicals, Amersham, Bucks., U.K., HEPES (N-2-hydroxyethyl-piperazine-N'-2-ethanesulphonic acid) was bought from Stuart, Kinney & Co. Ltd., 11 Argyle St., London W1A 4ES.

METHODS

Lenses were incubated at 37°, usually for 22 hours, in tissue culture medium TC199, buffered with HEPES, and with the concentration of glucose and calcium brought to 10 mM and 1.6 mM respectively (VAN HEYNINGEN & LINKLATER, 1975). One ml medium was used for two foetal lenses and 5 ml for each young or adult lens. [U-^{14}C] amino acids were added to the medium at concentrations from 1.5 to 4 μCi/ml.

After incubation the medium was stored frozen until required for enzymic assay of lactic acid (HOHORST, 1963) and the lenses were rinsed and divided into three weighed portions by the method of WANNEMACHER & SPECTOR (1968). Each portion was treated with trichloroacetic acid (10% w/v) and the precipitated protein was dissolved in NaOH to remove acyl

Table I. Glycolysis in the human lens. Production of lactic acid

Type of lens	No. of incubations	μ moles lactic acid per lens per 22h	μ moles lactic acid per g. wet weight/hr*
Foetal	4	1.8 ± 0.2 (1.6 to 2.0)	4.1
Adult	6	8.6 ± 2.5 (5.9 to 11.8)	2.0

The values are expressed as average ± standard deviation (range)

* taking the average wet weight of the foetal lens as 20 mg and of the adult lens as 200 mg.

amino acids (WALEY, 1964; VAN HEYNINGEN, 1965). The protein was reprecipitated with trichloroacetic acid and (30% w/v) and washed on the centrifuge with trichloroacetic acid (10%) at least five times, followed by acetone and ether and then dried. The radioactivity of the resulting preparations of protein was determined using a Beckman scintillation counter.

RESULTS AND DISCUSSION

Glycolysis

The amount of lactic acid formed from glucose by the lens, and diffusing into the medium, is a measurement of the extent of glycolysis during the period of incubation (Table I). As the lenses were not weighed before incubation, the weight of a single foetal lens was taken as 20 mg. and that of an adult lens 200 mg., in order to calculate the approximate amount of lactic acid formed, per g. wet weight per hour.

The six adult lenses (Table I) were 65 years old or more. The approximate value of 2 μmoles lactic acid/g. wet weight/hour formed by these lenses is similar to the values in the literature of 1.3, 2.5, and 6.7 μmoles/g/hour formed by the adult cow, rabbit and rat lens (see VAN HEYNINGEN, 1969).

We can find no values for glycolysis by foetal animal lenses to compare with the value of about 4.1 μmoles lactic acid formed /g wet weight/hour by the foetal human lens. The *young* cow, rabbit and rat lens glycolyse at the rate of 5.5, 9.6 and 20.0 μmoles lactic acid formed /g lens/hour (see VAN HEYNINGEN, 1969).

Although glycolysis by the intact rabbit lens was measured nearly fifty years ago (KRONFELD & BOTTMAN, 1928) these are apparently the first measurements of glycolysis by the human lens (see NORDMANN, 1954, 1962; HOCKWIN 1971).

Protein synthesis

Incorporation of ^{14}C into the proteins of the excised lens, incubated in a medium containing [U-^{14}C] amino acids, gives an indication of their rate of synthesis. After incubation, we divided the lens into three layers, the periphery consisting of the epithelial cells and some adhering fibres, the cortex and

172

the nucleus. Table II gives the results of five experiments in which the radioactivity in the protein in the three layers of lens, and in the cell water was measured. It shows that the labelling of protein decreased very sharply from epithelium to cortex, and that there was probably no protein synthesis in the lens nucleus. We used ^{14}C tyrosine in four of the five experiments because it is not metabolised by the human lens, apart from its incorporation into protein (VAN HEYNINGEN, unpublished). In the fifth experiment, where we used a ^{14}C amino-acid mixture, there was a risk that the glutathione co-valently bound to lens proteins (HARDING, 1970) might become labelled to give a misleading result. However, the radioactivity in the lens nucleus in this experiment was also negligible (Table II).

It has often been postulated that the proteins in the nucleus of the human lens are synthesised in embryonic life or childhood and have remained there without turnover for the following half century or more (see HARDING & DILLEY, 1976). WANNEMACHER & SPECTOR (1968) found no evidence of significant protein synthesis in the nucleus of the *calf* lens, incubated with [^{14}C]-leucine in experiments similar to those of Table II. YOUNG & FULHURST (1966) injected ^{35}S methionine into young *rats* and studied the incorporation of radioactivity into lens proteins *in vivo* for the following four weeks. They concluded from their findings that protein synthesis in the rat lens is largely due to the growth of new

Table II. Incorporation of ^{14}C-amino acids into proteins of the human lens in vitro

Expt. No.	Age (yrs)	uCi/ml of incubation medium	Part of lens	Counts/min non-protein per μl cell water	protein per mg.
1	86	4	Epithelium	8600	lost
			Cortex	1300	1143
			Nucleus	1100	7
2	38	2	Epithelium	3000	150x10^4
			Cortex	4800	661
			Nucleus	3100	31
3	38	2	Epithelium	6200	390x10^4
			Cortex	9000	630
			Nucleus	3200	26
4	5	1.5	Epithelium	3100	9x10^4
			Cortex	4800	4427
			Nucleus	1400	11
5	5	2	Epithelium	4200	15x10^4
			Cortex	11000	2085
			Nucleus	4700	9

Lenses were incubated for 22hr (expt. 1, 2 & 3) or 14hrs (expts. 4 & 5) with [U-^{14}C] tyrosine (expts. 1.2, 3, & 4) or [U-^{14}C] amino acid mixture (expt. 5). The epithelium preparation was 8-10% of the wet weight of the lens after incubation, the cortex 39-48% and the nucleus 42-52% (except for expt. 4 where the values were 5, 30 & 65 respectively).

fibres, though they could not exclude the possibility of a low level of protein turnover.

The nucleus of the bovine and rat lens becomes increasingly dehydrated with age, as new fibres grow at the periphery, whereas that of the adult human lens retains an unaltered degree of hydration (NORDMANN, 1973; VAN HEYNINGEN, 1972). Since the human lens increases in weight and protein content throughout life we thought that a mechanism involving protein turnover, with an excess of breakdown over synthesis, might exist to limit protein concentration in the nucleus. However, although it is not possible to rule out the existence of a slow turnover of protein in the lens nucleus, over a period of decades rather than hours, the present experiments give no indication of protein synthesis.

ACKNOWLEDGEMENTS

We thank Jane Linklater and Joy Rosser for excellent technical assistance; and the Medical Research Council for financial support (K.J.D.), and for the scintillation counter.

Le Professeur Jean Nordmann m'a encouragé et soutenu moralement (R. van H.) dans mon travail de recherche pendant de nombreuses années. Je tiens à lui exprimer ma gratitude et mon affection.

REFERENCES

HARDING, J.J. Free and Protein-Bound Glutathione in Normal & Cataracts Human Lenses. *Biochem. J.* 117: *957-960* (1970).

HARDING, J.J. & DILLEY, K.J. Structural Proteins of the Mammalian Lens: A Review with Emphasis on Changes in Development, Aging and Cataract. *Exp. Eye Res.* 22: *1-73* (1976).

HOCKWIN, O. Age Changes of Lens Metabolism. In: Age Changes in the Eye. F.K. Schattauer Verlag, Stuttgart, New York. *95-129* (1971).

HOHORST, H.J. In: Methods of Enzymatic Analysis. (ed. Bergmeyher, H.V.) Verlag Chemie Weinheim. Academic Press, New York. pp. *266-70* (1963).

KRONFELD, P. & BOTTMAN, L. Zur Frage den Linzenatmung. *Zeits für Augenheilk.* 65: *41-62* (1928).

NORDMANN, J. Biologie du Cristallin. Masson et Cie, Paris (1954).

NORDMANN, J. Acquisitions Recentes dans le Domaine de la Biologie du Cristallin. *Progr. Ophtal.* 12: *1-264* (1962).

NORDMANN, J. Le Noyan du Cristallin. I. La teneur en eau. *Arch. d'Ophthalmol.* 33: *81-86* (1973).

VAN HEYNINGEN, R. The Lens, in The Eye, Vol. 1, 2nd Ed. Ed. H. Davson, Academic Press. P. *387* (1969).

VAN HEYNINGEN, R. & LINKLATER, J. The Metabolism of the Bovine Lens in Air and Nitrogen. *Exp. Eye Res.* 20: *393-396* (1975).

WALEY, S.G. Metabolism of Amino Acids in the Lens. *Biochem. J.* 91: *576-583* (1964).

WANNEMACHER, C.F. & SPECTOR, A. Protein Synthesis Within the Lens of the Rat. *Exp. Eye Res.* 7: *623-625* (1968).

YOUNG, R.W. & FULHURST, H.W. Regional Differences in Protein Synthesis Within the Lens of the Rat. *Invest. Ophthalmol.* 5: *288-297* (1966).

Keywords:

Lens
Human lens
Metabolism
Glycolysis
Protein synthesis

Authors' address:

Oxford University
Nuffield Laboratory of Ophthalmology
Walton Street
Oxford OX2 6AW, England

COMPETITION FOR GLUCOSE-6-PHOSPHATE BY ENZYMES OF BOVINE LENSES

CHRISTIAN OHRLOFF, FRIEDHELM BOUS & OTTO HOCKWIN

(Bonn, W. Germany)

ABSTRACT

Phosphoglucoisomerase (EC 5.3.1.9. PGI), phosphoglucomutase (EC 2.7.5.1. PGM) and glucose-6-phosphate-dehydrogenase (EC 1.1.1.49. G6PDH) compete for the substrate G6P. Besides others it depends on these enzymes in which direction G6P is metabolized (glycolysis, glycogen-cycle, pentose-pathway). G6P concentration was measured in intact bovine lenses as well as in single lens parts in dependence on age. Moreover, the specific activities of the 3 enzymes and their K_m-values were determined. PGM and G6PDH show almost identical K_m-values (1.5 to 3.5 x 10^{-5}M) in intact lenses as well as in all parts investigated, with the exception that G6PDH is not present in the lens nucleus. The special activity with 1 to 3 mU per total lens is also similar in both enzymes. PGI shows a K_m of 1.5 x 10^{-4}M with a specific activity of 300 mU per total lens. Neither PGI nor PGM seems to be rate-limiting even in the aging lens, whereas the decreasing G6PDH activity effects the pentose pathway and thus the NADP/NADPH ratio mainly in the lens nucleus.

INTRODUCTION

Phosphoglucoisomerase, phosphoglucomutase and glucose-6-phosphate-dehydrogenase compete for the substrate glucose-6-phosphate. The preferred metabolic pathway depends, besides regulating factors, largely on these enzymes (Fig. 1). While phosphoglucoisomerase catalyses the first step in glycolysis, glucose-6-phosphatedehydrogenase is the initial enzyme of the pentosephosphate-shunt, and phosphoglucomutase plays an important role in glycogen synthesis and breakdown. While glycolysis is requisite for the energy metabolism, the importance of the pentosephosphate-pathway lies in providing the pentoses necessary for the synthesis of DNA and RNA, i.e. the pentose-phosphate pathway is essential for growth processes, especially of the young lens. Moreover, the pentose-phosphate-pathway also reduces NADP to $NADPH_2$. The glycogen metabolism, on the other hand, is responsible for storing and supplying glucose respectively.

Investigations were performed to elucidate the behaviour of the 3 enzymes in the course of aging, and to compare their capacities in view to the 3 metabolic pathways mentioned.

For this purpose the special activities in whole lenses as well as in certain lens parts of different age groups were determined, and so was the concentration of glucose-6-phosphate. In addition, the activity of the enzymes in dependence on substrate concentration (G6P) and the Michaelis-Menten constant were determined.

177

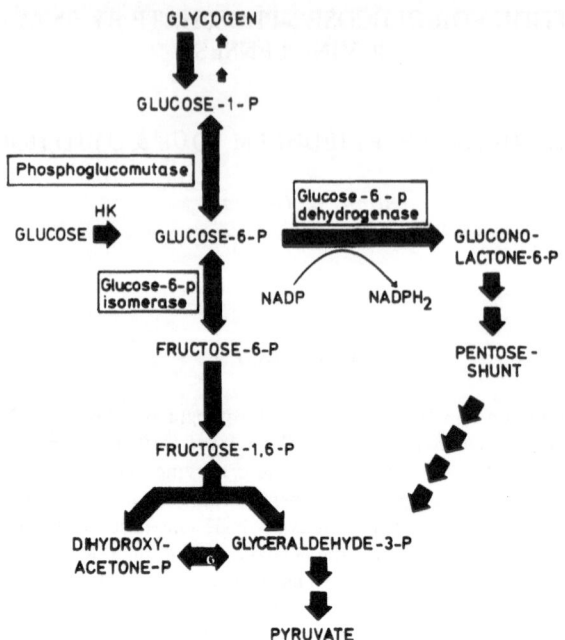

Fig. 1. Scheme of carbohydrate metabolism.

MATERIAL AND METHODS

Material

Chemicals: Merck Chemicals, high purity grade
Biochemicals: Substrates, enzymes and coenzymes purchased from Boehringer, Mannheim (Biochemicals Boehringer)

Methods

All investigations were performed with fresh lenses. For the determination of enzymes 1 g lens was homogenized in 5 ml aqua bidest (Ultra Turrax Jahnke + Kunkel, Freiburg) and zentrifuged for 60 min. at 20.000 x g in an ultrazentrifuge (Spinco L 80, Fa. Beckmann).

Measurements of enzyme activities were performed by subjecting 0.2 ml of the supernatant to enzyme optical test.

For the determination of phosphoglucoisomerase the supernatant was deluted 40 fold with H_2O, and 0.2 ml were subjected to enzyme optical test.

Determination of phosphoglucomutase was performed according to OHRLOFF (1973). Determinations of substrate dependence were performed with glucose-6-phosphate concentrations of $5 \times 10^{-5}M$ to $5 \times 10^{-3}M$. Glucose-6-phosphate-dehydrogenase determination was performed after BERGMEYER (1974).

The substrate glucose-6-phosphate was used in concentrations between 9×10^{-6} M and 9×10^{-4} M. The following test solution was employed for the determination of phosphoglucoisomerase (concentrations used in test): tris-buffer pH 8.80 mM, NADP o.4 mM and glucose-6-phosphate-dehydrogenase 3.5 U. The substrate fructose-6-phosphate was used in concentrations of 1×10^{-5} M to 3×10^{-3} M. Measurements of the single lens parts were performed after separation of the lenses into the respective regions (HOCKWIN & KLEIFELD, 1965).

Glucose-6-phosphate determinations: 1 g lens was homogenized in 3 ml of a 6% perchloric acid, the precipitated protein was separated by 30 min. zentrifugation at 12 000xg, and measurements were made after the supernatant was brought to pH 7 with 1 N KOH (BERGMEYER, 1974).

RESULTS

The specific activity of glucose-6-phosphate-isomerase in whole bovine lenses is considerably high (300 mU) compared with other enzymes of lens metabolism. The distribution of the above enzyme in the individual lens parts is rather uniform, with the exception of the nucleus of older lenses which shows a slight decrease in activity (Fig. 2, I). On the whole, there is only a slight decrease in activity in the course of aging.

In contrast to the values found for glucose-6-phosphate-isomerase, the specific activity of phosphoglucomutase in whole bovine lenses amounts to

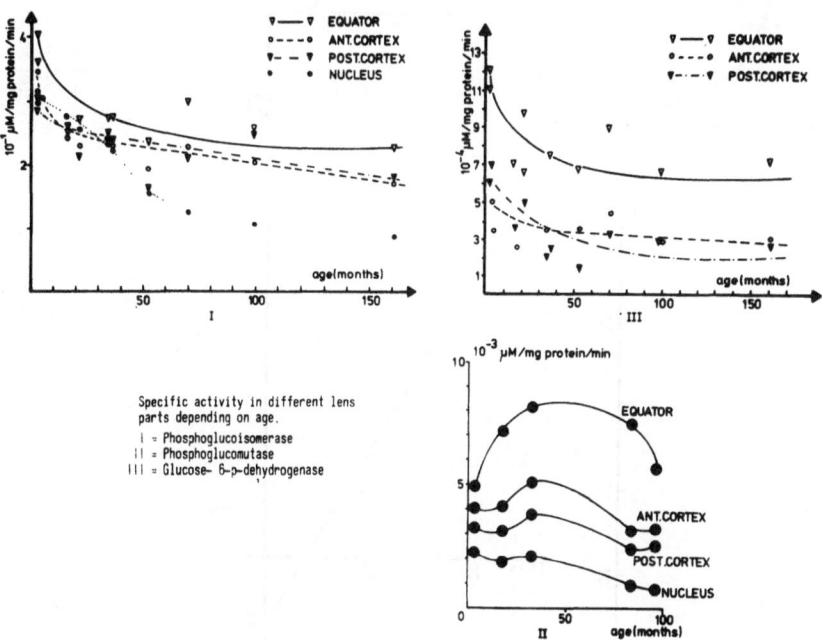

Fig. 2. Specific activity in different lens parts depending on age.
I = Phosphoglucoisomerase; II = Phosphoglucomutase; III = Glucose-6-phosphate-dehydrogenase

179

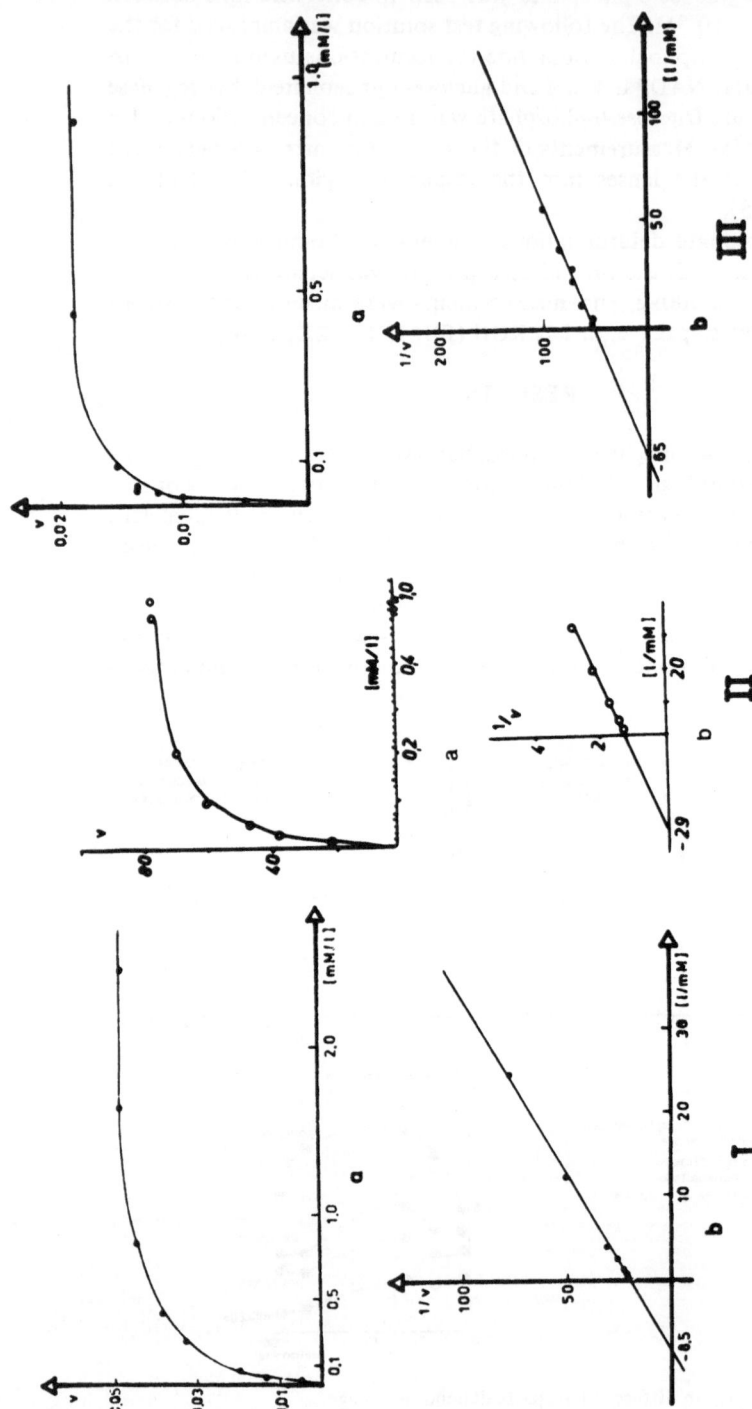

Fig. 3. Enzyme activity in bovine lenses depending on substrate concentration.
a = Michaelis Menten; b = Lineweaver Burk
I = Phosphoglucoisomerase, $K_m = 1.5 \times 10^{-4}$ M
II = Phosphoglucomutase, $K_m = 3.5 \times 10^{-5}$ M
III = Glucose-6-phosphate-dehydrogenase, $K_m = 1.5 \times 10^{-5}$ M

about 3 mU. Highest activity is found in the equator; anterior and posterior region as well as the nucleus show less activity, although even in the nucleus the activity is still measurable in old age (Fig. 2, II.). Phosphoglucomutase activity, too, is only slightly affected by aging processes.

As concerns the glucose-6-phosphate-dehydrogenase activity, it is, compared with other enzymes, remarkably low with 1 mU. Distribution in the individual lens parts is not uniform (Fig. 2, III), for instance, activity found in the equator is twice as high as in the anterior and posterior cortical region. In the nucleus of young lenses measurable activity was only found occasionally, while the nuclei of older lenses showed a total lack in activity. In all investigated lens parts a distinct dependence on age can be observed, the high activity of the first months leveling to uniform values at about the 2nd year.

Fig. 3, I shows the values of glucose-6-phosphate-isomerase in dependence on substrate concentration. The Michaelis — Menten diagram shows a slow initial velocity and the Lineweaver-Burk-plot gives the corresponding K_m-value of $1.5 \times 10^{-4}M$. This value is found for all lens parts in all periods of aging. Although this value has been determined using fructose-6-phosphate as substrate, the results of NOLTMANN (1954) confirm its validity also for glucose-6-phosphate.

Measurements of phosphoglucomutase in dependence of substrate concentration showed higher initial velocity with a K_m-value of $3.5 \times 10^{-5}M$ according to the Lineweaver-Burk diagram, (Fig. 3, II). This value, too, is uniform for all age periods and all lens parts investigated. This holds also true for the K_m-value of glucose-6-phosphate-dehydrogenase. Here, too, the Michaelis-Menten diagram shows a high initial velocity and an early maximal rate. K_m-value is $1.5 \times 10^{-5}M$ (Fig. 3, III).

Concentrations of glucose-6-phosphate ranged from 4.5 to $9.0 \times 10^{-5}M$ in the single lens parts of lenses of different age (Fig. 4).

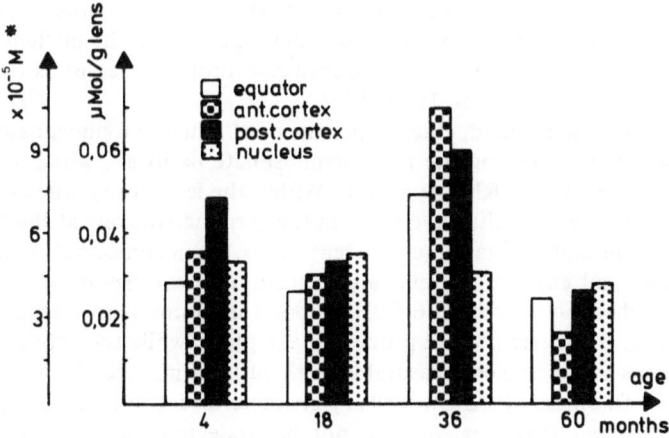

Fig. 4. Glucose-6-phosphate concentration in different lens parts dependent on age. *Molar concentration related to the water content of the lens.

Table 1. Specific activity and K_m-values of the measured enzymes. Comparing the proportion of specific activity and of K_m-values allows an estimation of the proportion with respect to the overall capacity.

| | spec.act. (mU) | K_M – value | proportion of | | resulting capacity |
			spec.act.	K_M – values	
Phosphoglucoisomerase	300	1.5×10^{-4}	100	1	100
Phosphoglucomutase	3	3.5×10^{-5}	1	4	4
Glucose–6–p–dehydrogenase	1	1.5×10^{-5}	0.3	10	3

DISCUSSION

Comparing the K_m-values found for phosphoglucoisomerase and glucose-6-phosphate-dehydrogenase, it is evident that the latter shows a 10 times higher substrate affinity, reaching maximal turnover already at the rather low G6P concentrations present in the lens. The lower substrate affinity of glucose-6-phosphateisomerase is, however, compensated by the high specific activity of the enzyme, which is, in the whole lens, about 100 to 300 times as high as that of G6PDH. The activity of phosphoglucomutase and glucose-6-phosphate-dehydrogenase are rather in the same order of magnitude, the affinity to glucose-6-phosphate is for PGM, however, only half that of G6PDH.

Considering specific activity and K_m-value, the proportion of capacities is 100:4:3 (PGI:PGM:G6PDH) (Table 1), i.e. the greater amount of glucose-6-phosphate joins glycolysis by way of glucose-6-phosphate-isomerase. An age-dependent bottleneck at this part of the glucose breakdown may certainly be excluded. This holds true also for the enzyme phosphoglucomutase and the glycogen metabolism. Although its part in glucose-6-phosphate consumption is considerably lower, the activity of the enzyme is present in all areas, and it is well known that especially in the nucleus of the older bovine lens glycogen is synthesized and probably serves as carbohydrate pool (OHRLOFF et al. 1973, 1976).

As already mentioned, the importance of glucose-6-phosphate-dehydrogenase lies in initiating the pentose-phosphate pathway, which provides pentoses for DNA and RNA synthesis. Within the lens this synthesis mainly takes place in the epithelial layers and in the germinative zone at the time of differentiation and elongation of the lens fibers, when considerable amounts of structure and enzyme proteins are formed. This corresponds to the fact that the highest activity of G-6-PDH is found in young lenses, especially in the outer layers, where growth processes take place, while the activity in the lens nucleus is no longer measurable with progressing age. In accordance with these findings, GLÄßER (1971) characterized G-6-PDH as a growth specific enzyme. However, it must not be neglected that glucose-6-phosphate dehydrogenase plays an important role in supplying $NADPH_2$.

PIRIE's investigations (1965) ascertained that $NADPH_2$ and glutathion form a redox system. One of the possible functions of this system may be the protection of the SH-groups of the proteins and to intercept toxic amounts of H_2O_2, since there is practically no catalase in the lens (ZELTER, 1953, BHUYAN et al., 1973). For the lens with its large amount of protein, this protecting mechanism could be of special importance. If, due to lack of $NADPH_2$, this redox system fails, it is to be expected that especially in the lens nucleus the protection of the SH-groups is no longer guaranteed and that the proteins are likely to lose their initial configuration. Posttranslational changes in the lens nucleus, which might finally lead to opacities, may thus be due to lack of $NADPH_2$, as was confirmed by investigations of ZINKHAM (1961) and WESTRING (1966). They examined patients suffering from congenital haemolytic anaemia due to primaquine-sensitive erythrocytes. A typical criterium with these patients is the decrease in GSH, caused by glucose-6-phosphate-dehydrogenase deficiency, which is also found in patients with the same disease combined with a premature onset of cataracta senilis. KINOSHITA (1964) also pointed out the similarity of the erythrocyte and of the lens fiber metabolism found with this disease. There is every indication that G-6-PDH is not only to be considered as a growth-specific enzyme, but is also requisite to guarantee well-balanced metabolic processes in the aging lens.

REFERENCES

BERGMEYER, H.U. Methoden der enzymatischen Analyse, 3. Auflg. Bd. I u. II, Verlag Chemie, Weinheim 1974.

BHUYAN, K.C., BHUYAN, D.K. & KATZIN, H.M. Amizol-induced cataract and inhibition of lens catalase in rabbit. *Ophthal. Res.* 5: *236-247* (1973).

GLÄßER, D. Enzymologische und enzymimmulogische Untersuchungen zur Zelldifferenzierung von Augenlinsen. Nova acta Leopoldina, Nr. 197, Bd. 36 (1971).

HEYNINGEN, R. VAN Some glycolytic enzymes and intermediates in the rabbit lens. *Exp. Eye Res.* 4: *298-301* (1965).

HOCKWIN, O. & KLEIFELD, O. Das Verhalten von Fermentaktivitäten in einzelnen Linsenteilen und ihre Beziehung zur Zusammensetzung des wasserlöslichen Eiweißes. In Struktur des Auges, II. Symp. Hrg. J.W. ROHEN, F.K. SCHATTAUER Verlag, Stuttgart 1965, S. *395-401.*

KINOSHITA, J.H. Selected topics in ophthalmic biochemistry A.M.A. *Arch. Ophthal.* 72: *554-572* (1964).

NOLTMANN, E. BRUNS, F.H. Reindarstellung und Eigenschaften von Phosphoglucoisomerase aus Hefe. *Biochem. Z.* 331: *436-445* (1959).

OHRLOFF, C., HOCKWIN, O. & KASKEL, D. Glycogen metabolism in bovine lenses. *Ophthal. Res.* 5: *222-229* (1973).

OHRLOFF, C., HOLSTEGE, A., & HOCKWIN, O. Studies on enzymes involved in the glycogen metabolism of the lens in relation of age, topographic distribution and affiliation to water soluble proteins. Ophthal. Res. 8: *227-232* (1976).

PIRIE, A. Glutathione peroxidase in lens and a source of hydrogen peroxidase in aqueous humour. *Biochem. J.* 96: *244-253* (1965).

PIRIE, A. A light-catalysed reaction in the aqueous humour of the eye. *Nature* (Lond.) 205: *500-511* (1965).

WESTRING, D.W. & PISCIOTTA, A.V. Anaemia, cataracts and seizures in patients with glucose-6-phosphate dehydrogenase deficiency. *Arch. Int. Med.* 118: *385-490* (1966).

ZELLER, E.A. Contributions to the enzymology of the normal and cataractous lens. III. On the catalase of the crystalline lens. *Amer. J. Ophthal.* 36, part II: *51-53* (1953).

ZINKHAM, W.H. A deficiency of glucose-6-phosphate dehydrogenase activity in lens from individuals with primaquine-sensitive erythrocytes. *Bull. John Hopkins Hosp.* 109: *206-216* (1961).

Keywords:

Aging
Bovine lens
Glucose-6-phosphate
Phosphoglucoisomerase
Glucose-6-phosphatedehydrogenase
Phosphoglucomutase
K_m-value

Authors' address:

Institute of Experimental Ophthalmology
University of Bonn
Division of Biochemistry of the Eye
Abbestrasse 2
D-5300 Bonn-Venusberg, W. Germany

Acknowledgement: This work was supported in part by Deutsche Forschungsgemeinschaft (Ho 249/8).

EFFECT OF AGING ON TRANSPORT OF AMINO ACIDS BY BOVINE LENS*

H.L. KERN, S.A. OSTROVE & C.-K. HO

(Bronx, New York)

ABSTRACT

The effects of aging of the bovine lens have been evaluated on transport *in vitro* of five neutral amino acids and the dibasic amino acid, arginine. Data were obtained for five systems of transport. A significant decrease in the uptake of all the amino acids was observed with increasing age. Transport was studied at both the anterior and posterior faces of the lens in order to determine the effects of aging on physiological function of both the anterior epithelium and the posterior fiber cells which are formed on differentiation from the epithelium. Transport activity was always greater in the epithelium, but approximately proportionate decreases with age were observed at both surfaces. The A-component of sarcosine appeared to be exceptional in that it was not detected at the posterior surface of the bovine lens. The Non-saturable component of uptake was found to increase at both faces of the lens with age.

INTRODUCTION

SIPPEL, 1968, examined the uptake of α-aminoisobutyric acid (AIB) by the rat lens, and reported that the influx of this amino acid decreased with increasing age both on the basis of unit weight and of unit surface, though there was a plateau in the curve depicting the latter relation from 2 days to about 30 days of age. A remarkable decline in activity of transport was found by SIPPEL, amounting to 80-90% over the age span of 2 days to 1 year. Since the transporting systems in plasma membranes are proteins (PENROSE et al., 1968) and since a number of provocative theories of aging of animal cells are concerned with transcriptional and translational activities of the genetic material (HAYFLICK 1975), it is reasonable to seek alteration in transport with aging.

This laboratory has presented evidence for the existence of four systems of transport for amino acids in the bovine lens-A, L, Ly^+, and Gly (BRASSIL & KERN, 1968), and has since verified the presence of two more-ASC and *Beta* (KERN, unpublished observations). It is possible experimentally to determine the proportion of the total uptake of a given amino acid at each of these systems provided a suitable substrate is chosen for evaluation. It was also of interest to compare the effects of aging at the anterior, epithelial surface, AS, with those at the posterior, fiber cell surface, PS, since pronounced changes in transport of animo acids have been noted on

* This work was supported by Grant No. EY 00268 from the National Institutes of Health.

Table I. Uptake in 1 hr of 0.15 mM Sarcosine by Bovine Lens*

| Animal | Average Wt., mg | Total Uptake | | | A-Component[+] |
		nMoles/Gm	nMoles/Lens	nMoles/Cm²	nMoles/Cm²
Calf	1504	37.5 ± 2.9	56.0 ± 0.7	8.97 ± 0.69	2.53 ± 0.24
Steer	2010	26.9 ± 0.8	54.3 ± 1.7	7.31 ± 0.23	1.27 ± 0.17
Cow	2486	25.2 ± 0.5	62.6 ± 1.2	7.30 ± 0.14	1.33 ± 0.40

* In these double label experiments, the extracellular space determined with D-mannitol-1-H³ (1 mM) was 3.25%, 3.83% and 6.65% for the calf, steer and cow respectively.
[+] The A-component was determined as the uptake inhibitable by 10 mM N-methyl-α-aminoisobutyric acid.

differentiation (KERN, in preparation). An analysis of transport of several amino acids in the bovine lens with increasing age is presented.

MATERIALS AND METHODS

Eyes were obtained from the abattoir within two hours of death, and stored in ice during transport to the laboratory. Calf lenses were from animals 3-6 months of age, steer lenses, 1-2½ years, bull or cow lenses, 4-8 years. Paired lenses were incubated for 1 hr at 37° in modified Ringer-bicarbonate containing 5 mM D-glucose (KERN, 1970). To measure uptake of amino acids by the entire lens, incubation was done in 10-15 ml of medium in wide mouth stoppered 25 ml Erlenmeyer flasks in a shaker operating at 40 RPM. Tetraethylammonium chloride (TEAC) replaced an equivalent amount of NaCl when a sodium-free medium was required; $KHCO_3$ replaced $NaHCO_3$, and the lenses were preincubated for ½ hour in TEAC to remove Na^+ from the outer cortical region. To evaluate transport at the anterior surface (AS) or posterior surface (PS), the lenses were incubated in 85-95% relative humidity on 13 mm I.D. glass vials containing radioactive amino acid in contact with about 6 ml stirred medium (KERN & HO, 1973). Aliquots of the medium and the protein-free filtrate from the lens, prepared from dispersions in 7.5% sulfosalicylic acid, were counted, and the data expressed as nanomoles of amino acid taken up per hour ± S.E.M. of three to six lenses. The surface of the lens was estimated by a photographic method to convert the data to a basis of unit area after determining the curvature at the two surfaces (KERN & HO, 1973). All the data were corrected for extracellular space in double label experiments with 1 mM D-mannitol-1-H³ as extracellular indicator.

Sarcosine-1-C¹⁴ and L-serine-U-C¹⁴ were obtained from California Bionuclear Corp., 7654 San Fernando Road, Sun Valley, Calif. 91352; L-arginine.HCl (guanido-C¹⁴) and L-arginine-U-C¹⁴, from Schwarz/Mann; l-aminocyclopentane-1-C¹⁴-carboxylate (ACPC) and glycine-1-C¹⁴, from Amersham/Searle Corp.; D-mannitol-1-H³, from New England Nuclear. The C¹⁴-compounds were used at a level of 0.04 to 0.28 μCi/ml in the medium

186

and the mannitol-H^3 at a level of 0.4 to 2 μCi/ml. Alcohol present in the tracers was removed by evaporation *in vacuo* at 5° prior to use.

ACPC was purchased from the California Corp. for Biochemical Research. N-Methyl-α-aminoisobutyric acid was synthesized by a modification of the method of GREENSTEIN & WINITZ, 1961, employing methylamine in place of ammonia. The product was recrystallized from ethanol.

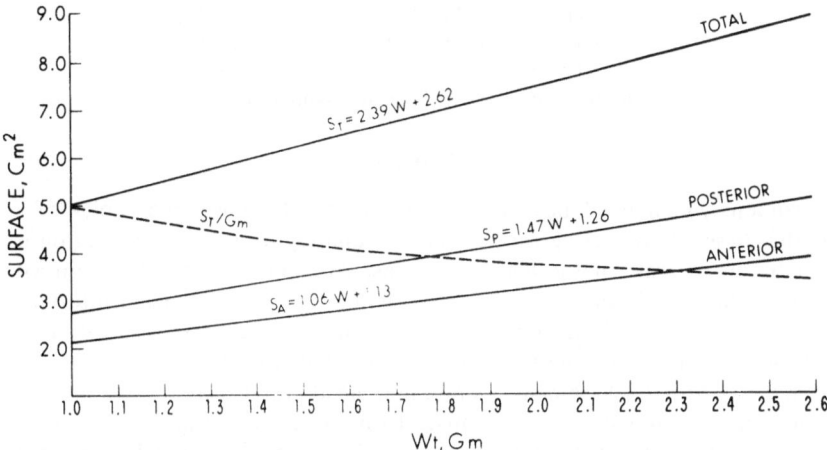

Fig. 1. Dependence of surface of bovine lens on fresh weight. The linear relations represent the area of the anterior surface, the posterior surface and the total surface. The dashed line is the ratio of total surface to weight.

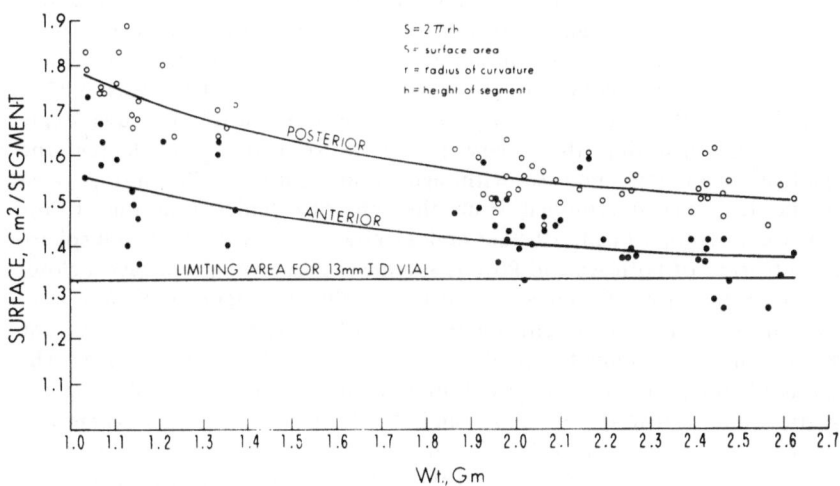

Fig. 2. Dependence of area of central 13 mm diameter segments of anterior and posterior faces of bovine lens on fresh weight.

187

Table II. Uptake of 0.1 mM Sarcosine at Anterior and Posterior Surfaces of Bovine Lens

Surface	Animal	Total $nMoles/Cm^2 \cdot Hr$	A-Component* $nMoles/Cm^2 \cdot Hr$
Anterior	Calf	7.17 ± 0.52	2.77 ± 0.50
	Steer	2.55 ± 0.22	0.39 ± 0.23
	Bull	1.78 ± 0.20	−0.38 ± 0.12
Posterior	Calf	1.61 ± 0.11	−0.01 ± 0.09
	Steer	1.11 ± 0.06	−0.27 ± 0.06
	Bull	0.91 ± 0.09	−0.31 ± 0.12

* Uptake inhibitable by 10 mM N-Methyl-α-aminoisobutyric acid.

RESULTS

A problem which must be addressed in studies of aging is the choice of a suitable basis for reporting the results. Fortunately, a convenient solution is available in the case of the lens since transport can be expressed per unit or surface-area. This is appropriate as it is the biologically significant interface between the lens and its environment, the most superficial layer of cells, with which we are primarily concerned in evaluating transport. The lens capsule, a form of basement membrane, need not be considered in this connection because it does not appear to interfere with transport of small solutes (KERN, 1970). A comparison of various ways of expressing the data for uptake of sarcosine in the aging bovine lens is given in Tabel I. Uptake per lens was little altered by aging, whereas uptake per gram and uptake per square centimeter decreased significantly. Since it is change at the surface (plasma membrane) with which we are concerned, results will be presented on the basis of unit area. The A-component of uptake (17-28% of the total) was more sensitive to aging than the total uptake, and decreased by about 50% as shown in the last column of Table II. The extracellular space, expressed as a percentage of the total water in the lens, was 3.25%, calf, 3.83%, steer, and 6.65%, cow. Since more difficulty was experienced in separating the ciliary processes from the older lenses, the significance of this increase with age is not known. The surface area of the lens was determined from the relations depicted in Fig. 1, for which data from 19 calf, 19 steer and 18 cow lenses were used, and spherical curvature of both AS and PS was assumed. This assumption gave a closer fit for PS than for AS, but appeared to be valid. The figure also shows that the surface per unit weight decreased with increasing weight, and the findings are in agreement with those of SIPPEL, 1965, for the rat lens. The radius of curvature, R, was also found to increase with age, obeying the relation, R = 1.76W + 7.97, at AS and R = 1.56W + 5.99, at PS, where R is expressed in mm and the weight in gm. These results are in contrast to those of BROWN, 1974, who found that the radius of curvature at both surfaces of the human lens decreased with age. The uptake of sarcosine was also determined at the anterior and posterior faces of the lens and the results are summarized in Tabel II. It is apparent that total uptake declined with age in the central segments of either AS or PS, falling more rapidly at AS than at PS. The A-component of uptake at AS was markedly decreased in the steer's lens and disappeared in the bull's lens. No A-component was detected at PS. Differences in the data in Tabels I and II may be attributed in part to transport activity of the peripheral epithelial and fiber cells. Data describing uptake of L-serine, L-arginine, glycine and ACPC are presented in Tables III-VI. In general, it can be stated that uptake declined with increasing age though, in a few instances, it appeared to level off in the steer as compared with the cow (ASC-component of L-serine, L-component of ACPC at PS). On the other hand, the Non-saturable component, NS, at PS (CHRISTENSEN & LIANG, 1966) was consistently observed to increase with age, whereas it remained relatively constant at AS. The non-saturable component is defined as the uptake remaining when all saturable uptake is blocked by appropriate competitors. It increases linearly with concentration of amino acid. It may also be noted that transport activity is greater at AS than at PS as indicated by the ratio, AS/PS, and that this applies to both saturable and Non-saturable components with the possible exception of NS for L-arginine in the cow.

Table III. Uptake of 0.1 mM Glycine by Bovine Lens

Surface	Animal	Total nMoles/Cm^2.Hr	Gly-Component* nMoles/Cm^2.Hr	AS/PS	NS-Component nMoles/Cm^2.Hr	AS/PS
Anterior	Calf	4.80 ± 0.35	1.76 ± 0.23	1.03	0.84 ± 0.07	2.5
	Steer	3.61 ± 0.19	1.69 ± 0.15	1.41	1.20 ± 0.04	2.7
	Cow	2.27 ± 0.28	0.71 ± 0.03	1.16	0.97 ± 0.14	1.3
Posterior	Calf	2.18 ± 0.29	1.71 ± 0.20		0.34 ± 0.06	
	Steer	1.57 ± 0.18	1.20 ± 0.20		0.44 ± 0.10	
	Cow	0.98 ± 0.02	0.61 ± 0.06		0.75 ± 0.16	

* Uptake inhibitable by 10 mM sarcosine in presence of 10 mM L-methionine.

Table IV. Uptake of 0.1 mM L-Arginine by Bovine Lens

Surface	Animal	Total nMoles/Cm^2.Hr	Ly$^+$-Component* nMoles/Cm^2.Hr	AS/PS	NS-Component nMoles/Cm^2.Hr	AS/PS
Anterior	Calf	8.00 ± 0.40	7.57 ± 0.40	4.04	0.40 ± 0.05	1.3
	Steer	5.08 + 0.18	4.41 ± 0.18	4.01	0.63 ± 0.03	2.3
	Cow	2.36 ÷ 0.15	1.62 ± 0.17	3.00	0.74 ± 0.07	0.7
Posterior	Calf	2.18 ± 0.11	1.87 ± 0.12		0.31 ± 0.04	
	Steer	1.37 ± 0.22	1.10 ± 0.22		0.27 ± 0.03	
	Cow	1.51 · 0.11	0.54 ± 0.19		1.05 ± 0.21	

* Uptake inhibitable by 10 mM L-lysine or 10 mM L-homoarginine.

Table V. Uptake of 0.1 mM 1-Aminocyclopentane-1-carboxylate by Bovine Lens

Surface	Animal	Total nMoles/Cm².Hr	L-Component* nMoles/Cm².Hr	AS/PS	NS-Component nMoles/Cm².Hr	AS/PS
	Calf	22.60 ± 0.93	20.70 ± 0.95	16.1	1.89 ± 0.21	9.5
Anterior	Steer	12.70 ± 0.50	10.80 ± 0.53	21.6	1.88 ± 0.17	5.7
	Cow	8.88 ± 0.83	7.57 ± 0.81	13.8	1.32 ± 0.04	2.6
	Calf	1.49 ± 0.27	1.29 ± 0.28		0.20 ± 0.02	
Posterior	Steer	0.83 ± 0.16	0.50 ± 0.17		0.33 ± 0.05	
	Cow	1.05 ± 0.09	0.55 ± 0.06		0.51 ± 0.10	

* Uptake inhibitable by 20 mM L-methionine.

A summary of some of the data in Tables II-VI is given in Table VII, in which transport of the amino acids by various systems is compared in the steer and cow versus the calf. The data illustrate that, aside from the rapid disappearance of the A-component of sarcosine from the central polar regions of the lens on aging, there is a rather uniform decline of transport activity with aging of the Ly^+-, Gly-, ASC- and L-systems, with uptake falling to 40-80% in the steer, and 20-40% in the cow as compared with the calf. The NS-component appears to increase with age, especially at the posterior surface.

DISCUSSION

Data presented for five amino acids show that there is a significant loss in transport activity per unit of surface on aging of the bovine lens. Both total uptake and the component of uptake at various systems of transport declined with increasing age. It was also noted that transport activity was greater at the epithelial surface than at the fiber cell surface as indicated by the values, AS/PS, in Tables III-VI. These ratios, furthermore, did not change appreciably with age, since transport activity generally decreased proportionately at the two faces of the lens. The A-component of sarcosine was exceptional in that it apparently disappeared more rapidly with age from the anterior and posterior poles than did the other systems of transport. Reports on the effects of aging on transport of amino acids by various cells and tissues either indicate no change in liver (YATVIN et al., 1974), intestine (PÉNZES, 1974; PÉNZES & BOROSS, 1974), fibroblasts in culture (HAY & STREHLER, 1967), brain (FINCH et al, 1975) and young vs. adult kidney (SEGAL et al, 1971), or a modest decrease in senescent kidney (BEAUCHENE et al, 1965) and in skeletal muscle and heart (YATVIN et al, 1974). On the other hand, our findings are in agreement with those of SIPPEL, 1968, who noted a pronounced fall in the uptake of AIB by the rat lens over the age range 2 days to 1 year. The range of ages we have examined is probably comparable to SIPPEL's since cows are reported to live to 30 years and it is doubtful that we have investigated any lenses older than

10 years (HOCKWIN et al, 1975). Therefore, this work does not include a study of the sennescent lens.

Determination of transport at AS and PS of the lens has the advantage that two populations can be compared in the same tissue — the anterior epithelial cells and the tips of the posterior fiber cells, which are the products of differentiation of the epithelium. The data in Table VII indicate that the decrement in transport activity which occurs with aging at four of the five systems (Ly^+, Gly, ASC, L) is approximately equivalent in the two populations. This may signify that a similar age-dependent controlling event(s) is operating at AS and at PS, though it is not possible to state whether this involves the genetic material (i.e., synthesis of membrane proteins), the presence of membrane-bound inhibitors, altered lipid composition of the plasma membrane, or structural alteration of the transporting molecules.

REFERENCES

BEAUCHENE, R.E., D.D. FANESTIL & C.H. BARROWS. The effect of age on active transport and sodium-potassium-activated ATPase activity in renal slices of rats. *J. Geront.* 20: *306-310* (1965).

BRASSIL, D. & H.L. KERN. Characterization of the transport of neutral amino acids by the calf lens. *Invest. Ophth.* 7: *441-451* (1968).

Table VI. Uptake of 0.1 mM L-Serine by Bovine Lens

Surface	Animal	Total nMoles/Cm².Hr	ASC-Component* nMoles/Cm².Hr	AS/PS
Anterior	Calf	33.10 ± 2.50	13.20 ± 2.40	1.76
	Steer	18.10 ± 0.92	10.80 ± 1.50	2.80
	Cow	13.70 ± 2.20	10.30 ± 1.70	2.30
Posterior	Calf	9.75 ± 0.66	7.50 ± 0.59	
	Steer	5.36 ± 0.82	3.86 ± 0.57	
	Cow	4.26 ± 1.06	4.40 ± 1.00	

* Na^+-dependent uptake in presence of 10 mM sarcosine.

Table VII. Effect of Aging on the Component of Uptake of Amino Acids at Various Transport Systems in the Bovine Lens

Amino Acid (0.1mM)	Transport System	Steer/Calf (×100) Anterior	Posterior	Cow/Calf (×100) Anterior	Posterior
Arginine	Ly^+	58	59	21	29
Glycine	Gly	96	70	40	36
Serine	ASC	82	51	31	43
ACPC	L	52	39	37	43
Sarcosine	A	14	–	–	–
*	NS	133	127	124	271

* Average for arginine, glycine and ACPC.

BROWN, N. The change in lens curvature with age. *Exp. Eye Res.* 19: *175-183* (1974).

CHRISTENSEN, H.N. & M. LIANG. On the nature of the 'non-saturable' migration of amino acids into Ehrlich cells and into rat jejunum. *Biochim. Biophys. Acta* 112: *524-531* (1966).

FINCH, C.A., V. JONEC, G. HODY, J.P. WALKER, W. MORTON-SMITH, A. ALPER & G.J. DOUGHER, JR. Aging and the passage of L-tyrosine, L-DOPA, and inulin into mouse brain slices *in vitro. J. Geront.* 30: *33-40* (1975).

GREENSTEIN, J.P. & M. WINITZ. In: Chemistry of the Amino Acids; vol. 3. John Wiley & Sons, Inc., New York. pp. *2559-2561* (1961).

HAY, R.J. & B.L. STREHLER. The limited growth span of cell strains isolated from the chick embryo. *Exper. Geront.* 2: *123-135* (1967).

HAYFLICK, L. Current theories of biological aging. *Fed. Proc.* 34: *9-13* (1975).

HOCKWIN, O., H. FINK, H. SCHALLENBERG & F. RAST. Carbohydrate metabolism of the lens depending on age. V. Problems of mathematical approach and graphical presentation. *V. Graefes Arch. Klin. Exper. Ophth.* 195: *17-26* (1975).

KERN, H.L. Efflux of amino acids from the lens. *Invest. Ophth.* 9: *692-702* (1970).

KERN, H.L. & C.-K. HO. Localization and specificity of the transport system for sugars in the calf lens. *Exp. Eye Res.* 15: *751-765* (1973).

PENROSE, W.R., G.E. NICHOALDS, J.R. PIPERNO & D.L. OXENDER. Purification and properties of a leucine-binding protein from *Escherichia coli. J. Biol. Chem.* 243: *5921-5928* (1968).

PÉNZES, L. Intestinal absorption of glycine, L-alanine and L-leucine in the old rat. *Exper. Geront.* 9: *245-252* (1974).

PÉNZES, L. Further data on the age-dependent intestinal absorption of dibasic amino acids. *Exper. Geront.* 9: *259-262* (1974).

PÉNZES, L. & M. BOROSS. Intestinal absorption of some heterocyclic and aromatic amino acids from the aging gut. *Exper. Geront.* 9: *253-258* (1974).

SEGAL, S., C. REA, & I. SMITH. Separate transport systems for sugars and amino acids in developing rat kidney cortex. *Proc. Nat. Acad. Sci.* 68: *372-376* (1971).

SIPPEL, T.O. Energy metabolism in the lens during aging. *Invest. Ophth.* 4: *502-513* (1965).

SIPPEL, T.O. The effect of aging on amino acid transport in the rat lens. In: Biochemistry of the Eye. Symposium, Tutzing Castle, 1966. Karger, Basel/New York. pp. 277-285 (1968).

YATVIN, M.B., G.B. GERBER & J. DEROO. Effect of age and strain on uptake of α-aminoisobutyrate. *Arch. Inter. Physiol. Biochem.* 82: *251-257* (1974).

Keywords:

Amino acids
Transport
Bovine lens
Epithelium
Fiber cells
Aging
Differentiation

Authors' address:

Department of Ophthalmology
Albert Einstein College of Medicine
of Yeshiva University
1300 Morris Park Avenue
Bronx, New York 10461, USA

CHOLESTEROL, CHOLESTEROL ESTER, AND SPHINGOMYELIN COMPLEXED TO PROTEIN OF NORMAL HUMAN LENS AND SENILE CATARACTS*

Y. OBARA, E. COTLIER, R. LINDBERG.& J. HORN

(Chicago, Illinois)

ABSTRACT

The protein fractions of the lens after urea or guanidine digestion contain lipids. Cholesterol, cholesterol ester, sphingomyelin, and phosphatidyl ethanolamine were un- covered in the urea-insoluble protein fractions of human lens. Marked increases of cholesterol were found in the guanidine-soluble and guanidine-insoluble fractions of senile cataracts. Cholesterol esters increased three-fold in the guanidine-insoluble frac- tions of cataracts. Copolymerization of oxidized lipids with protein is the most likely mechanism for protein aggregation and insolubilization in senile cataracts.

INTRODUCTION

Recently, TAO & COTLIER (1975) found that in senile human cataracts, a fast-moving ceramide fraction (A fraction) and its sphinganine and 4-sphin- genine bases were increased up to 450% as compared to age-matched lenses. This finding, indicative of lipid storage in senile cataracts, was further con- firmed and amplified by our studies on lens sphingomyelin fractions in human lenses and cataracts (OBARA and associates, in press). We found significant increases in three sphingomyelin fractions (A, B, and D) of human cataracts as compared to age-matched controls. Furthermore, pro- nounced shifts in the distribution of fatty acids in each sphingomyelin fraction were found in the cataracts (OBARA and associates, in press). The possible association and complexing of lens lipids to insoluble protein has been suggested by COTLIER (1975) as the cause of nuclear sclerosis but has not been investigated previously. The present study was undertaken to de- termine whether lipids are complexed to various protein subfractions of human lenses and senile cataracts.

MATERIALS AND METHODS

Lenses

Autopsy human eyes were obtained from the Eye Bank of the University of Illinois within 72 hours of death. The globes were sectioned at the equator immediately upon receiving the eyes. The lenses were then dissected from the zonules with blunt scissors. Each lens was transferred to a Petri dish, the

---

* Supported by U.S. Public Health Service Grant PHS EY 703-05 capsule incised and removed with fine tweezers. The decapsulated lenses were then individually frozen at $-20\,°C$, lyophilized, and weighed. Surgically removed cataracts were decapsulated, lyophilized, and weighed as the normal autopsy lenses. The cataracts with various degrees of cortical and nuclear opacities corresponded to groups II and III of Pirie's classification (PIRIE, 1968). Pairs of normal autopsy lenses and cataracts were matched for age and processed simultaneously.

Protein subfractions and lipid extractions

Decapsulated, lyophilized clear lenses and cataracts were weighed, homogenized in 20 volumes of water under N_2, and spund down at 2500 rpm at room temperature. The water-insoluble fractions were then subjected to further digestion with 7M urea, 6M guanidine HCl-50 m molar dithiothreitol, and 2N methanolic KOH as shown in Fig. 1. At various stages of fractionation, the lipids were extracted with chloroform: methanol (2 : 1 v/v) under N_2, with constant swirling motion provided by magnetic stirring. The water

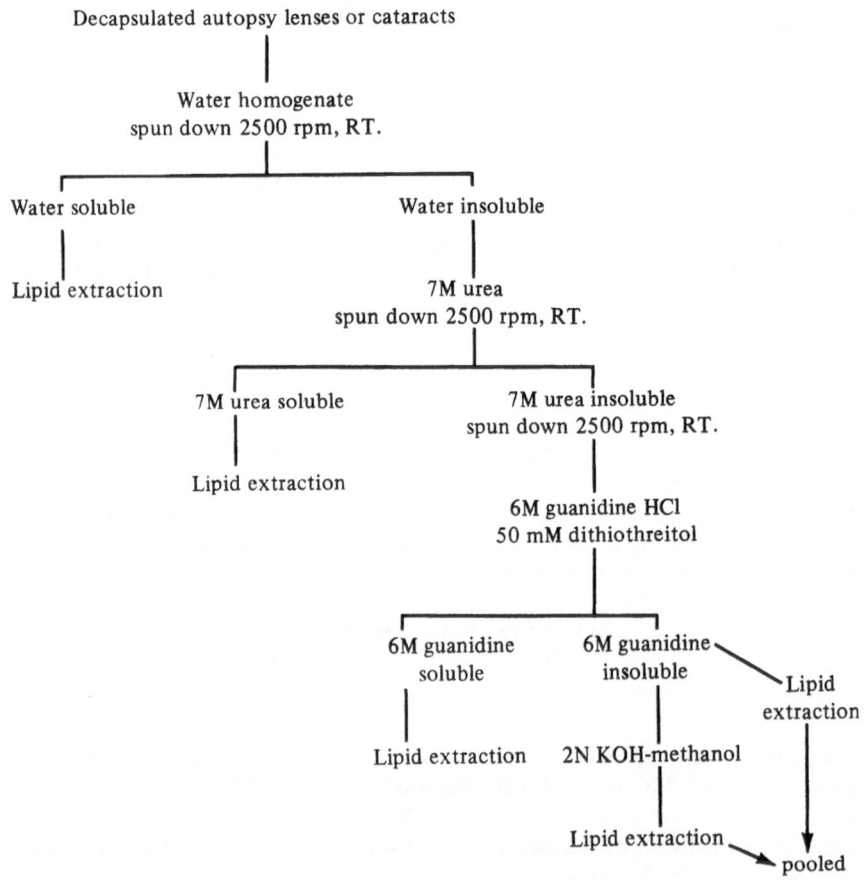

Fig. 1. Procedure for separation of lens proteins and lipid extraction from each one.

194

and guanidine fractions were lipid extracted at 4 °C, whereas the urea fractions were extracted at room temperature. After centrifugation (2500 rpm, RT) for 20 minutes, the residue was subjected to chloroform : methanol (1 : 2 v/v) extraction. The collected extracts were pooled and dried under N_2. The dry lipids were then redissolved in 5.0 ml of chloroform : methanol (1 : 2 v/v), 0.2 ml of water added, and centrifuged. The upper phase was removed by aspiration and the lower phase washed four times with 2.0 ml of chloroform : methanol : water (3 : 48 : 47, v/v/v) and five times with 2.0 ml of chloroform : methanol : 0.1% NaCl (3 : 48 : 47, v/v/v) as described by FOLCH, LEES, & SLOAN-STANLEY (1957). The lower phase was then dried under N_2 and weighed.

Lipid extraction of decapsulated lenses (not digested)

Decapsulated entire lenses were lyophilized, homogenized in 20 volumes of chloroform : methanol 2 : 1, and lipid was extracted as the protein subfractions. Then the neutral lipid fraction was separated by silicic acid column chromatography as described before (TAO & COTLIER, 1975).

Chromatography

Dry lipids from entire lenses and each protein fraction were dissolved in chloroform : methanol (2 : 1 v/v) and spotted on silica gel Q_4 plates (from Quantum Industries, Fairfield, New Jersey and from Analtech, Inc., Newark, Delaware). Lipid fractions were separated by the two-solvent, one-dimensional method of KELLEY (1966). The first solvent was petroleum ether : ethyl ether : acetic acid (70 : 30 : 1 v/v/v), and the second solvent was petroleum ether : ethyl ether : acetic acid (30 : 70 : 1 v/v/v). Standards were run simultaneously, and the chromatograms were visualized by the ammonium molybdate-perchoric acid spray (AMPA) or by iodine vapors.

Cholesterol determinations

Cholesterol spots (free and esterified) were scraped from the thin-layer chromatography silica gel plates, transferred to scintered glass funnels, and eluted with 20 ml of ethyl ether. The samples were then evaporated to dryness under N_2, and cholesterol was determined according to COURCHAINE, MILLER & STEIN (1959). In the decapsulated lenses, total cholesterol was determined directly from the neutral lipid fraction.

Protein determinations

Protein concentrations were determined according to LOWRY et al. (1951).

RESULTS

Lipid extraction of decapsulated entire lenses and cataracts

The one-dimensional, two-solvent system used here allowed separation of all lens lipids in a single procedure. Lipids found in the intact decapsulated

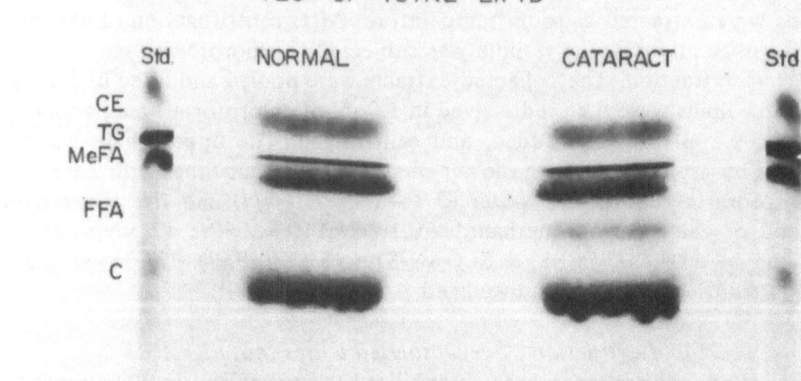

Fig. 2. Thin-layer chromatography of lipids in normal lenses and age-matched senile cataracts. CE signifies cholesterol esters; TG, triglycerides; MeFA, esterified fatty acids; FFA, free fatty acids; C, cholesterol; MG. monoglyceride; PL, phospholipids.

lenses (not digested) were in order of faster to slower migration : cholesterol esters, triglycerides, esters of fatty acids, cholesterol, monoglycerides, unknown spot, and phospholipids (Fig. 2). The spots corresponding to cholesterol, phospholipids, triglycerides, cholesterol esters, or esterified fatty acids did not differ significantly between normal lenses and cataracts (Fig. 2). However, increased levels of a) free fatty acids, b) monoglycerides, and c) unknown spot were found in the cataracts. Determinations of total cholesterol (free and esterified) in decapsulated lenses are shown in Table 1. In agreement with the findings by FELDMAN (1968), no significant differences were found in cholesterol content between age-matched clear lenses and cataracts.

Lipids in protein-digested fractions

In the water-soluble fraction, the spots corresponding to cholesterol and triglycerides did not differ in intensity (Fig. 3); however, the free fatty acids, 1,3-diglyceride, 1,2-dyglyceride, and unknown spot stained more darkly than those of normal lenses. In the 7M urea-soluble fraction, increases in cholesterol levels, 1,3-diglyceride, 1,2-dyglyceride, free fatty acids, cholesterol ester, and the unknown spot were found in cataracts as compared to normal lenses (Fig. 3). In the 6M guanidine-soluble fraction, a major cholesterol spot was detected only in the cataract group (Fig. 4). Free cholesterol determinations in the water-soluble, 7M urea-soluble, and 6M guanidine-soluble and insoluble fractions are shown in Table 2.

196

Table 1. Total cholesterol (free and esterified) in lens and cataracts

IDENT. #	NORMAL LENS			CATARACTS		
Lenses	Age, Sex	µg/lens	µg/mg (dry)	Age, Sex	µg/lens	µg/mg (dry)
1	60, M	844	17.7	56, F	965	19.8
2	49, F	1210	15.2	48, F	881	21.2
3	82, M	1470	21.9	74, F	1230	19.8
4	78, F	1190	17.1	75, F	1030	17.5
5	67, F	1020	17.3	62, F	935	14.1
6	60, F	1140	20.0	56, F	1090	20.1
7	67, F	1000	18.4	68, M	1320	21.3
8	67, F	808	16.6	69, F	833	15.0
Mean ± S.D.	66 ± 9.2	1090 ± 215	18.0 ± 2.1	64 ± 9.6	1040 ± 170	18.6 ± 2.8
Pooled lenses						
1	68, F; 68, F; 70, F	902	17.3	64, F; 68, F; 69, F	974	18.2
2	68, F; 58, F; 75, M	988	18.1	57, F; 73, F; 75, M	1150	20.6

M, males; F, females

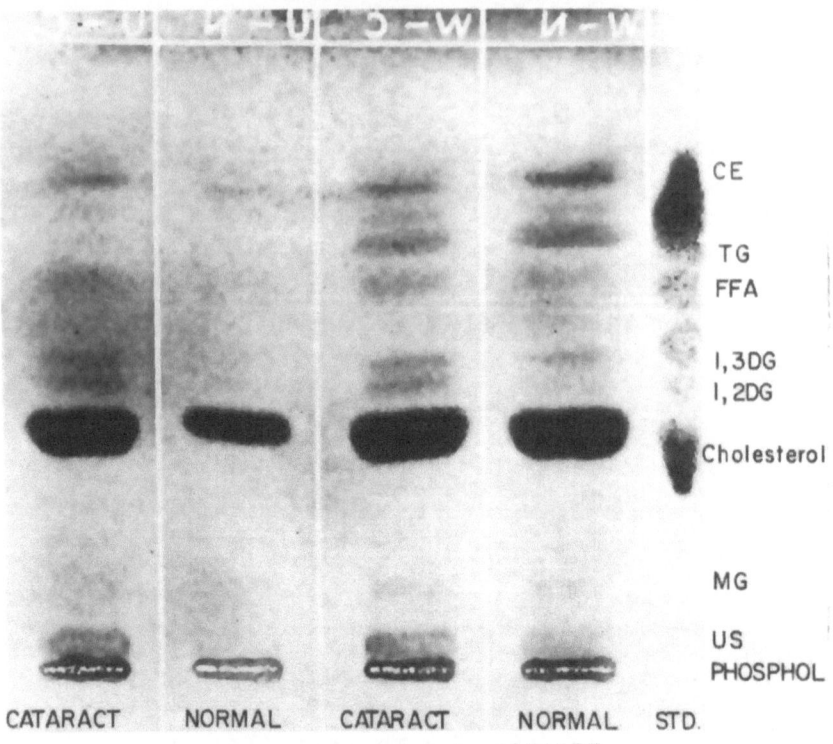

Fig. 3. Thin-layer chromatography of lipids in 7M urea-soluble and water-soluble fractions of normal lenses and age-matched cataracts. In addition to abbreviations specified for Fig. 2, 1,3 DG signifies 1,3 diglyceride; 1,2 DG, 1,2 diglyceride; and U.S., unidentified spot.

Table 2. Cholesterol (free) in various lens fractions*

| | in μg/mg protein | | μg/lens | |
	NORMAL	CATARACT	NORMAL	CATARACT
Water soluble	7.89	11.01	583	428
7M urea soluble	17.33	26.55	410	868
6M guanidine soluble	4.46	7.39	130	243
6M guanidine insoluble	0.76	1.66	40	93
Total, above fractions			1163	1632
7M urea insoluble (addition of 6M guanidine soluble + insoluble fractions)	5.52	9.05	170	336

* Two normal lenses (Average age to 5 years) and two senile cataracts (Average age 72.5 years).

198

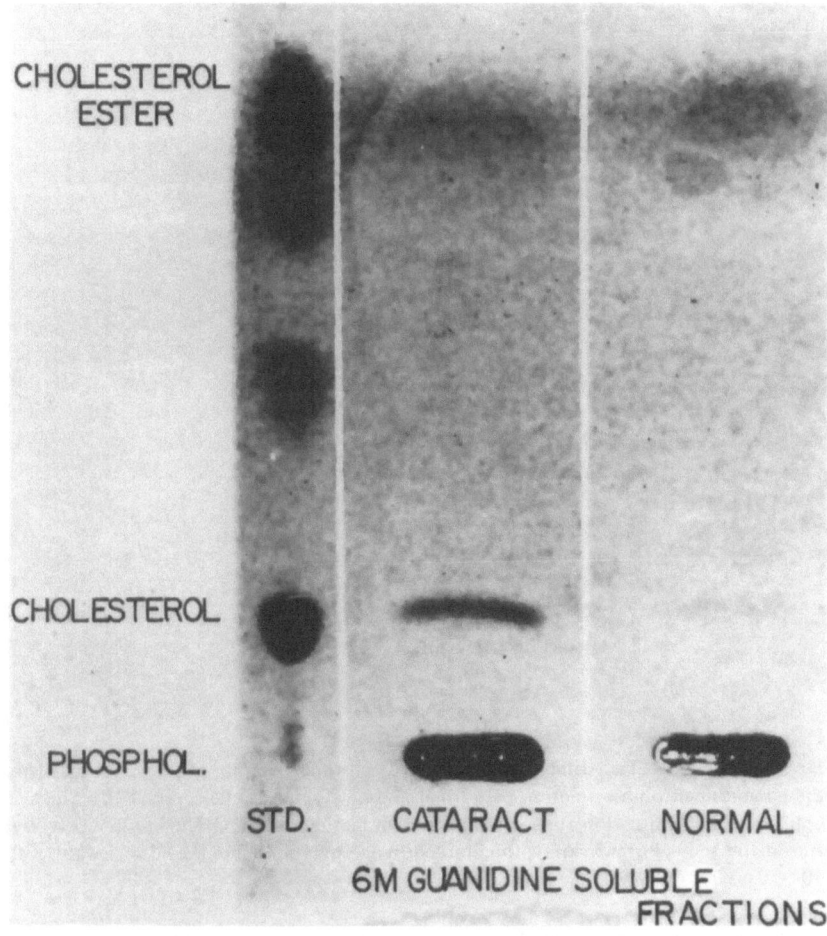

CHOLESTEROL ESTER

CHOLESTEROL

PHOSPHOL.

STD.   CATARACT   NORMAL

6M GUANIDINE SOLUBLE
FRACTIONS

Fig. 4. Thin-layer chromatography of lipids in the 6M guanidine-soluble fractions of normal lenses and cataracts.

Table 3. Cholesterol esters in various lens fractions*

	in μg/mg protein		μg/lens	
	NORMAL	CATARACT	NORMAL	CATARACT
6M guanidine soluble	6.56	6.34	194	209
6M guanidine insoluble	0.35	1.10	23	62
7M urea insoluble (addition of 6M guanidine soluble + insoluble fractions)	6.91	7.44	217	271

* Same material as in table 2.

199

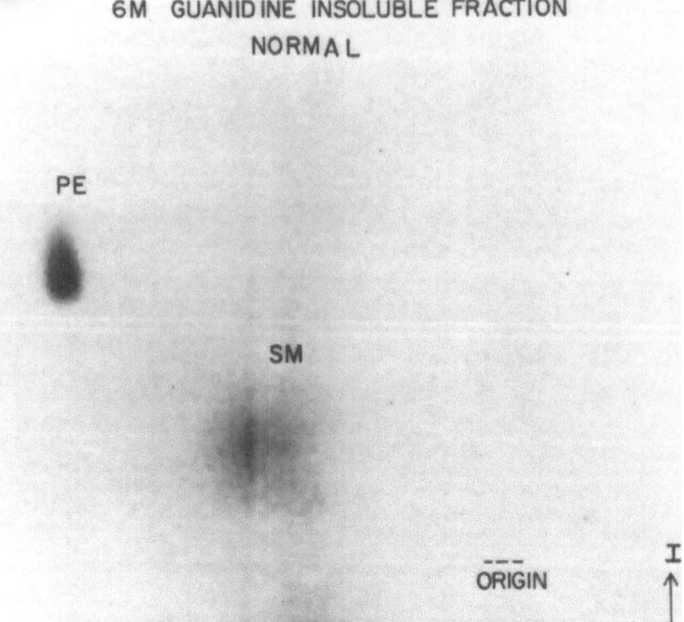

Fig. 5. A and B) Two-dimensional thin-layer chromatography of phospholipids from the guanidine-insoluble fraction of normal lenses (A) and senile cataract (B). Silica gel G plates. First dimension run with chloroform-methanol-NH$_4$OH, 65 : 25 : 5 (v/v/v), and in the second dimension with chloroform-acetone-methanol-acetic acid-water, 30 : 40 : 10 : 10 : 5 (v/v/v/v/v).

The free cholesterol levels were increased in cataracts of the urea-soluble, guanidine-soluble, and guanidine-insoluble fractions when expressed on a μg/mg protein or μg/lens basis (Table 2). Thus free cholesterol is stored or complexed to the proteins in the urea-soluble, guanidine-soluble, and guanidine-insoluble protein fraction of cataracts as in clear lenses expressed on a protein or per lens basis (Table 2). Cholesterol esters were three times higher in the guanidine-insoluble fraction of cataracts as compared to clear lenses (Table 3). Phospholipids from the guanidine-insoluble fraction of clear lenses and cataracts were further separated by two-dimensional thin-layer chromatography. Sphingomyelin and phosphatidyl ethanolamine were identified (Fig. 5A and B). A marked increase in the levels of sphingomyelin was found in the senile cataracts (Fig. 5B) as compared to the normal lenses (Fig. 5A).

DISCUSSION

The increase of free cholesterol and sphingomyelins in the urea and guanidine-insoluble fractions of senile cataracts opens new avenues regarding

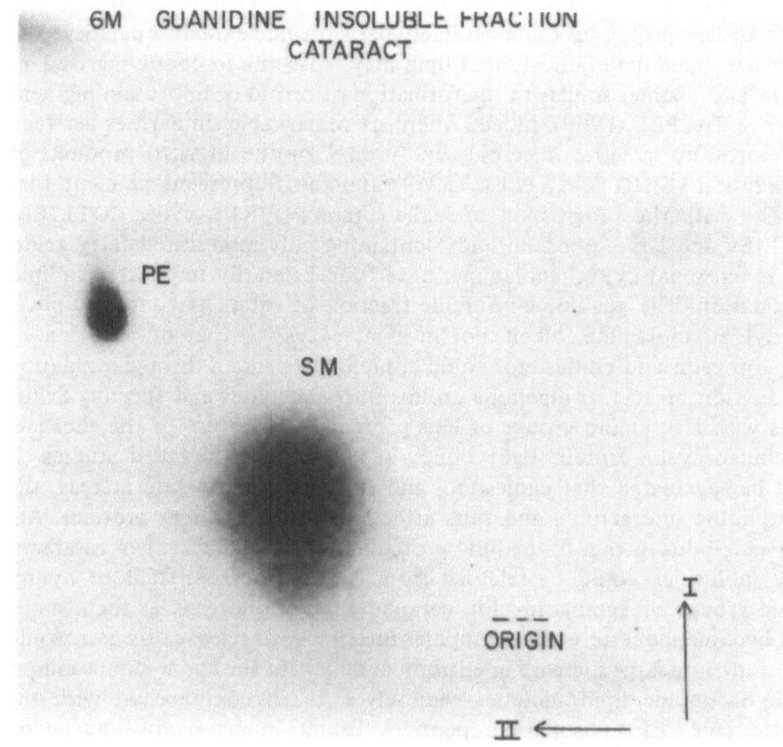

the chemical abnormalities associated with nuclear cataracts. It is known that a majority of the urea-insoluble or guanidine-insoluble protein of cataracts is found in the nucleus (DILLEY & PIRIE, 1974). It appears then that the formation of tight complexes among cholesterol, sphingomyelin, ceramides, and protein may be a major chemical anomaly of nuclear senile cataract.

The question as to whether cholesterol is increased in senile cataract has led to innumerable studies which have been summarized by SALIT (SALIT & O'BRIEN, 1935; SALIT, 1941). A major fault with these studies is the lack of age-matched controls and inadequate extraction conditions. BROEKHUYSE (1973) has documented the progressive increase of cholesterol with age in humans. Age-matched cataracts and clear lenses are mandatory in such studies. Furthermore, as shown here, chloroform: methanol extractions of homogenized entire cataracts are inadequate. Obviously, cholesterol is not completely accessible to the solvents unless tight protein-lipid bonds or the anomalous protein, themselves, are first broken down. This explains the failure of FELDMAN (1968), who matched cataracts with clear lenses, to find increased cholesterol in the former. In a series of studies (to be published), we found that the high cholesterol levels occur in the various protein fractions (urea-soluble, guanidine-soluble, guanidine-insoluble) of cataracts even after prolonged dialysis. This indicates tight binding of lipid to protein, probably of a covalent nature.

HARDING (1973) and DILLEY & PIRIE (1974) have invoked cross-linking of lens protein as the most likely basis for nuclear lens opacities. The results presented here indicate that lipid may cross-link or copolymerize lens protein in a manner similar to the formation of ceroid or lipofuscin pigment (CHIO & TAPPEL, 1969). Indeed, there are remarkable similarities between the fluorescent spectra of ceroid, lipofuscine, or the in vitro products of peroxidation (CHIO & TAPPEL, 1969) and the fluorescent pigment that increases with the progression of senile cataract (PIRIE, 1968; COTLIER, 1975). By and large, phospholipids containing polyunsaturated fatty acids, such as phosphatidyl ethanolamine, have been primarily implicated in lipid peroxidation. The guanidine-insoluble fraction of cataracts contained phosphatidyl ethanolamine, albeit not in great excess to that of clear lenses. Sphingomyelin and cholesterol could complex to protein through oxidation or reduction of acid or alcoholic groups into aldehydes and forming Schiff bonds with free amino groups of lens proteins. The nature of the cholesterol-sphingomyelin-protein tight bonds in lens requires detailed studies. It could be speculated that cholesterol and sphingomyelin would increase the hydrophobic interactions and thus affect the folding of lens proteins. Another possibility is that in the lipid protein complex(es) of nuclear cataracts, water molecules could be released from the hydrocarbon tails of hydrophobic groups of sphingomyelin, ceramides, or cholesterol, as these molecules become sequestered in a nonpolar interior. This release of water would also result in a large increase in entropy and explain the stable bonds among the hydrophobic lipid moieties themselves, or in combination with the 'tryptic core' of hydrophobic peptides found in cataractous nuclei by DILLEY & PIRIE (1974). Furthermore, closely packed hydrocarbon tails and sterol rings would shorten the distances between atoms to the van der Waals contact distance which would also favor clustering of sphingomyelins, cholesterol, and hydrophobic peptides.

The remarkable similarities in chemical composition between the hydrophobic urea-insoluble lipid protein complex and those of lens fiber membranes (or other mammalian cell membranes) cannot be ignored. In the normal lens, it is likely the former represents aged lens membranes that had been pushed toward the center of the lens nucleus. In the cataractous lenses, abnormalities in synthesis or degradation in the cholesterol and/or sphingomyelin moieties of fiber membranes may copolymerize or cross-link the proteins or the membranes or even the less rigid globular proteins of the fiber interior.

REFERENCES

BROEKHUYSE, R.M. The Human Lens – In Relation to Cataract, Ciba Foundation Symposium 19 (new series). Amsterdam, Elsevier, pp. 135-149 (1973).

CHIO, K.S. & A.L. TAPPEL. Inactivation of ribonuclease and other enzymes by peroxidizing lipids and by malonaldehyde. *Biochemistry* 8: *2821-2832* (1969).

COTLIER, E. The lens. In Moses, R. (ed.): Adler's Physiology of the Eye. St. Louis, C.V. Mosby Co. (1975).

COURCHAINE, T., W.H. MILLER, & D.B. STEIN, Jr. Rapid semimicroprocedure for estimating free and total cholesterol. *Clin. Chem.* 5: *609* (1959).

DILLEY, K.J. & A. PIRIE. Changes to the proteins of human lens nucleus in cataract. *Exp. Eye Res.* 19: *59-72* (1974).

FELDMAN, G.L. Lipids of the human lens. In Dardenne, M.V. & J. Nordmann (eds.): Biochemistry of the Eye, Symposium. Basel, New York, S. Karger, pp. 348-358 (1968).

FOLCH, J., M. LEES & G.H. SLOAN-STANLEY. A simple method for the isolation and purification of total lipids from animal tissues. *J. Biol. Chem.* 226: *497-509* (1957).

HARDING, J.J. Disulfide cross-linked protein of high molecular weight in human cataractous lens. *Exp. Eye Res.* 17: *337-383* (1973).

KELLEY, T.F. Separation with uni-dimensional TLC of all neutral lipid classes. *J. Chromatog.* 22: *457* (1966).

OBARA, Y., E. COTLIER, J.O. KIM, K. LUECK & R.V. TAO. Sphingomyelin species stored in human senile cataract. *Invest. Ophthalmol.* (in press).

PIRIE, A. Color and solubility of the proteins of human cataracts. *Invest. Ophthalmol.* 7: *634-650* (1968).

SALIT, P.W. Total lipid and cholesterol content of cataractous and sclerosed human lenses. *Am. J. Ophthalmol.* 24: *191-195* (1941).

SALIT, P.W. & C.S. O'BRIEN. Cholesterol content of cataractous human lenses. *Arch. Ophthalmol.* 13: *227-237* (1935).

TAO, R.V. & E. COTLIER. Ceramides of human normal and cataractous lens. *Biochim. Biophys. Acta* 409: *329-341* (1975).

LOWRY, O.H., N.J. ROSEBROUGH, A.L. FARR, & R.J. RANDALL. Protein measurement with the Folin phenol reagent. *J. Biol. Chem.* 193: *265-275* (1951).

Authors' address:

Biochemical Laboratories
Department of Ophthalmology
University of Illinois and Ear Infirmary
Chicago, Illinois 60612, USA

Requests for reprints to be addressed to

Prof. E. Cotlier
1855 W. Taylor Street
Department of Ophthalmology
University of Illinois
Chicago, Illinois 60612, USA

STUDIES ON THE MODE OF ACTION OF 1-HYDROXY-PYRIDO-(3,2a)-5-PHENOXAZONE-3-CARBOXYLIC ACID IN BOVINE LENSES

INGE KORTE, O. HOCKWIN, F. WINKLER & P. RABE

(Bonn, W. Germany)

The effect of 1-hydroxy-pyrido-(3,2a)-5-phenoxazone-3-carboxylic acid (Catalin®)* on the carbohydrate metabolism in bovine lenses has recently been investigated and reported by KORTE et al. (1975a). In vitro experiments showed that addition of 0.6×10^{-4} M or 1.8×10^{-4} M Catalin respectively to the incubation medium effects the carbohydrate breakdown, thereby impairing the energy supply of lens metabolism. Other studies revealed that Catalin reacted with the reduced coenzymes NADH and NADPH and disturbed the optical enzyme test in which these coenzymes were used as parameters (KORTE et al., 1975b). Continuing these studies we determined the gas exchange of intact lenses as well as that of lens homogenates after addition of Catalin to the medium.

We also applied some well known enzyme inhibitors in order to get better insight into the mode of action of Catalin.

MATERIALS AND METHODS

Measurements of gas exchange

Gas exchange of a 10% calf lens homogenate or intact bovine lenses respectively by consumption of O_2 and formation of CO_2 was measured using a Warburg apparatus (Fa. B. Braun, Melsungen, T VL 166). The incubation medium consisted of 96% 0.154 M NaCl, 2% 0.154 M KCl, 2% 0.110 M $CaCl_2$ and 20% 0.155 M $NaHCO_3$. Calf lenses were homogenized in this solution and 8 ml of the homogenate, containing 10^{-4} M Catalin were filled into each vessel.

Bovine lenses were incubated as intact organs with an appropiate amount of the Ringer solution, containing 10^{-4} M Catalin, so that 8 ml including the lens volume were filled into each vessel. For the controls, no Catalin was added.

0.2 ml of a 1 M glucose solution (36 mg) served as energy source and were filled into the side arms, allowing 10 min for saturation of the medium with air and attaining a temperature of 37 °C. Potassium cyanide (KCN),

* We are indebted for the providing of the compound and for the support of the study to Senju Pharmaceutical Co. Lt.: Takeda Chemical Ind. Lt. Japan, via M. Woelm, Eschwege, Germany.

Table I. Gas exchange of lens homogenates within 1 h in dependence on Catalin concentration. $\bar{x}$, n = 6 to 42. Underlined figures differ from the controls on a 5% level.

Molarity of added Catalin	$\mu l\ CO_2$ per 100 g lens wet weight	$\mu l\ O_2$ per 100 g lens wet weight	$RQ = CO_2/O_2$
0	1662	364	4.5
10^{-6}	1643	364	4.2
10^{-5}	<u>1650</u>	459	3.6
10^{-4}	<u>1801</u>	<u>686</u>	2.6
10^{-3}	<u>1819</u>	624	2.9

mono iodine acetic acid (JAA) and malonic acid (MA) were used as enzyme inhibitors in a final concentration of 10^{-3}M in the medium. Readings of the pressure differences in the vessels were made at 5, 10, 15, 30, 45 and 60 minutes after glucose addition. Then the amount of glucose was consumed and the experiments were stopped. The 60 minutes readings were used exclusively for the calculation of CO_2 formation and O_2 consumption. Before and after the experiments the pH values were between 7.2 and 7.4.

Determination of glutathione and ascorbic acid

Glutathione was determined according to ELLMANN (1958) and ascorbic acid according to MOHR (1956) with the methods modified for lenses by HOCKWIN et al. (1974).

RESULTS

All data are presented as mean values. Analysis of variance and comparison of the mean values were carried out according to Student-t-test. μl gas are referred to 100 g lens fresh weight or to whole lenses respectively.

1. Influence of Catalin on the gas exchange of lens homogenates

Determination of suitable Catalin concentrations

Before starting the experiments we tested the concentrations of Catalin which actually influence the gas exchange of lens homogenates. Addition of 10^{-6} to 10^{-3}M Catalin revealed that a 10^{-4}M Catalin containing medium affected the formation of carbon dioxide and the consumption of oxygen significantly (Table 1). Therefore all following experiments were performed with a 10^{-4}M Catalin medium.

Interaction between enzyme inhibitors and Catalin

To get better insight into the mode of action of Catalin certain enzyme inhibitors were added besides Catalin to the lens homogenate, such as: potassium cyanide (KCN), which is known to inhibit i.a. the respiration of the lens to one third (HOCKWIN et al., 1956); mono iodine acetic acid, (JAA) which reacts i.a. with the SH-groups of the triose phosphate dehydrogenase and completely blocks lens metabolism (HOCKWIN et al., 1956); and malonic acid (MA) which inhibits normal respiration by blocking the oxidation of succinic acid in the citric acid cycle and moreover largely blocks the formation of oxaloacetic acid (WEBB, 1966). Succinic acid is present in the lens in a concentration of 8.5 to 17 μM (MANDEL et al., 1954).

The data obtained are presented in Table 2, Part a) of the table shows the effect of enzyme inhibitors on untreated lens homogenates. Formation of CO_2 is reduced by KCN and slightly increased by JAA and MA. The consumption of oxygen is reduced by each of the three inhibitors. Part b) of the table shows the influence of Catalin on the effects of the enzyme inhibitors. The oxygen consumption and the CO_2 formation of poisoned lens homogenates was increased by Catalin to a higher degree than that of the controls, reaching that of Catalin-treated homogenates. This Catalin influence on the effect of the three poisons was significant on a 5% level. As regards the reverse effect, i.e. the influence of the inhibitors on the Catalin action, the table shows that the CO_2-formation of Catalin-treated lens homogenates was reduced by KCN and increased by JAA and MA. The

Table II. Interaction between Catalin effect and effect of enzyme inhibitors on the gas exchange of lens homogenates after 1 h incubation $\bar{x}$, n = 12 to 24

Added substance	μl CO_2 per 100 g lens	μl O_2 per 100 g lens	RQ
a) O	1662	364	4.5
KCN	1362	128	10.6
JAA	2076	289	7.2
MA	1985	244	8.1
Catalin	1801	686	2.6
b) KCN + Catalin	1525	647	2.4
JAA + Catalin	2244	783	2.8
MA + Catalin	2079	811	2.6

⌙‾‾‾⌞ significant difference on a 5% level
⌙‑‑‑‑⌞ no significant difference

Table III. Content of glutathione and ascorbic acid in lens homogenates after 1 h incubation with and without Catalin. $\bar{x}$, n = 3

Added Catalin	mg glutathione per 100 g lens wet weight	mg ascorbic acid per 100 g lens wet weight
0	128	24
10^{-4} M	66	2.3

Table IV. Oxygen consumption of intact bovine lenses after 1 h incubation with and without Catalin. $\bar{x}$, n = 10. Underlined figure differs significantly from the control on a 5% level.

Added Catalin	$\mu l\ O_2$ per lens $\cdot$	g lens wet weight
0	2.55	2.36
10^{-4} M	5.94	2.36

O_2-consumption of such homogenate was not changed by KCN but was significantly increased by JAA and MA.

Influence of Catalin on the content of glutathione
and ascorbic acid in lens homogenates

To elucidate the process which might be influenced by Catalin in the lens homogenate we determined the content of glutathione and ascorbic acid in a lens homogenate before and after one hour incubation with and without Catalin. Table 3 shows that the glutathione content was reduced by 50% and the content in ascorbic acid was reduced by as much as 90% after Catalin addition. In the non-treated controls, these two substances were only slightly decreased.

2. Influence of Catalin on the gas exchange of intact lenses

Intact lenses are less suitable for investigations in the Warburg apparatus. It seemed to be important, however, to find out whether the gas exchange of intact lenses might be different from that of lens homogenates under the influence of Catalin. For this purpose we incubated intact bovine lenses for one hour in the Warburg apparatus and determined the oxygen consumption under the conditions employed for homogenates. Table 4 shows that the oxygen consumption of intact bovine lenses was nearly doubled by Catalin. The μl are referred to whole lenses. The average weight of the lenses was about 2.3 g, which corresponds to an age of 4 years. Formation of CO_2 was not determined.

In another series we determined the interaction of enzyme inhibitors and Catalin with regard to the oxygen consumption of the intact lens. The lenses weighed between 2.0 and 2.3 g, which corresponds to an age of 2 to 4 years. The μl are again referred to the whole lens.

Table 5, part a) shows the influence of enzyme inhibitors on the O_2-consumption of intact lenses. It was reduced by KCN and by JAA, and, on the other hand, was increased even by malonic acid. Part b) shows the effect of Catalin on poisoned lenses. Catalin reduced the KCN effect, though not significantly; it compensated the effect of JAA and raised the O_2-consumption to the level of Catalin-treated lenses.

There was no influence on the unexpected effect of malonic acid. Part c) of Table 5 shows the reverse influence of the enzyme inhibitors on the Catalin

208

effect. The Catalin effect was significantly reduced by KCN, JAA had no influence at all and malonic acid increased the O_2-consumption significantly and to a higher degree than Catalin alone.

DISCUSSION

The experiments were performed in order to elucidate further the mode of action of Catalin®. Certain interactions of the gas exchange of normal lenses or their homogenate, as well as that of poisoned lenses or their homogenate, with the influence of Catalin were found. The phenoxazone-compound increased the O_2-consumption of lenses and lens homogenates and also increased the CO_2-production of lens homogenates. In the case of poisoned lenses or lens homogenates respectively, the effect of the enzyme inhibitor could be influenced.

There is a suggestion that the influence of Catalin extends to other O_2-consuming processes in the lens besides respiration. If only the citric acid cycle and the respiration were affected changes in RQ (CO_2/O_2) would never occur. The RQ, however, decreased from 4.5 (controls) to 2.6 after addition of 10^{-4} M Catalin (Table 1); this is caused mainly by increased O_2-consumption without the corresponding increase in CO_2-formation. Although there is also a small augmentation of CO_2, this might be due to increased glycolysis with a higher rate of lactic acid production. In this case oxygen consumption must have taken place within another process of lens metabolism. One may assume an increased oxidation of glutathione and ascorbic acid, and Table 3 shows clearly that they decrease considerably in

Table V. Interaction between Catalin effect and effect of enzyme inhibitors on the O_2 consumption of intact bovine lenses, $\bar{x}$, n = 8 to 38, after 1 h incubation

Added substance	μ L O_2 consumption per lens	lens wet weight
a) O	2.96	2.25
KCN	*	2.18
JAA	*	2.02
MA	10.16	2.01
b) KCN + Catalin	3.00	2.23
JAA + Catalin	6.43	2.30
MA + Catalin	8.18	2.22
c) Catalin	5.19	2.27
Catalin + KCN	2.37	2.27
Catalin + JAA	9.00	2.34
Catalin + MA	7.37	2.16

⌐___⌐ significant differences on a 5% level

⌐-------⌐ no significant difference

* no O_2 consumption was detectable

In contrast to table III are the experiments of b and c from different series, as can be seen by the $\bar{x}$ of the lens wet weight

the presence of Catalin in lens homogenates. This is in good agreement with the results of KORTE et al. (1975b), who found that Catalin reacts with the hydrogen of the reduced coenzymes NADH en NADPH. Thus there is no NADPH available for the reduction of GSSG formed by autoxidation.

Experiments with enzyme inhibitors also indicate that Catalin not only influences the respiration, but the RQ-values also show considerable changes. Each of the three blockers inhibits O_2-consumption (Table 2a). KCN, the well known respiration blocker, inhibits CO_2-production in an order of magnitude corresponding to the decrease in O_2-consumption, which clearly indicates an exclusive effect on respiration. Simultaneous addition of Catalin and KCN resulted in considerably increased O_2-consumption, approximating the values found for the O_2-consumption of homogenates treated with Catalin alone. This is demonstrated in Table 2b, where the values for O_2-consumption of Catalin-treated homogenates are compared to those treated with Catalin + KCN. However, there is no corresponding change in CO_2. Regarding the RQ-values, it may be assumed that interaction between Catalin and JAA or MA respectively are similar to those found with Catalin and KCN.

The increase in CO_2-production, already observed with Catalin alone, which was approximately the same in poisoned lenses with additional Catalin treatment, need not necessarily be due to respiration, but might be caused by increased formation of lactic acid which releases CO_2 from the $NaHCO_3$ of the medium. This assumption, however, could not entirely be verified in the present study. Although lenses incubated with Catalin (KORTE et al., 1975a) did not show any increase of lactic acid, it is possible that the latter has been released into the medium; analyses on this problem, however, have not yet been performed.

In general, Catalin-induced changes of the O_2-consumption of whole bovine lenses are similar to those found for homogenates.

Glutathione and ascorbic acid decrease with Catalin treatment. It is to be assumed that Catalin exerts its influence on other redox-systems, too, as is evident from the ratio NAD/NADH or NADP/NADPH reported by KORTE et al., (1975b).

Measurements on the gas exchange of lenses and lens homogenates indicate disturbances in metabolism which may cause the previously observed changes (KORTE et al., 1975 a,b). Unfortunately the method of measurement for the gas exchange does not allow a detailed determination of the Catalin effect.

With regard to its importance in lens metabolism, further studies on the problem are requisite.

SUMMARY

The influence of Catalin on the gas exchange of lens homogenates and intact bovine lenses was studied. The consumption of oxygen was increased by addition of the substance to the medium. The reduced oxygen consumption due to enzyme inhibitors came to an almost normal level by Catalin addition. Concentrations of glutathione and ascorbic acid were reduced in the lens homogenate after Catalin treatment.

REFERENCES

ELLMANN, G.L. Tissue sulfhydryl groups. *Arch. Biochem. Biophys.* 82: *70-77* (1958).

HOCKWIN, O., KLEIFELD, O. & ARENS, P. Einfluss des Kalium-cyanid und der Monojodessigsäure auf den Stoffwechselablauf der Linse. *Albrecht von Graefes Arch. Ophthal.* 158: *47-53* (1956).

HOCKWIN, O., WINKLER, F. & KORTE, I. Veränderungen im Glutathion- und Ascorbinsäuregehalt von Rinderlinsen in Abhängigkeit vom Lebensalter. *Albrecht v. Graefes Arch. Ophthal.* 192: *215-225* (1974). '

KINSEY, V.E., WACHTL, C., CONSTANT, M.A. & CAMACHO, E. Studies on the crystalline lens. VI. Mitotic activity in the epithelia of lenses cultured in various media. *Amer. J. Ophthal.* 40, II: *216-223* (1955).

KORTE, I., HOCKWIN, O., TULLIUS, H., DIEDERICH, D., STEIDTEL, C.U. & SCHOLL, W. Studies on the influence of 1-hydroxy-pyrido-(3,2a)-5-phenoxazone-3-carboxylic acid on the carbohydrate metabolism of the lens. *Ophthal. Res.* 7: *282-291* (1975a).

KORTE, I., HOCKWIN, O., TULLIUS, H. & DIEDERICH, D. Effect of 1-hydroxy-pyrido-(3,2a)-5-phenoxazone-3-carboxylic acid on the reduced coenzymes NADH and NADPH. *Ophthal. Res.* 7: *440-446* (1975b).

MANDEL, P. & KLETHI, J. Sur l'acide succinique et la succino-dehydrase du cristallin. *C.R. Soc. Biol.* 148: *577-579* (1954).

MOHR, H. Zitat in: Strohecker, K. & Henning, H. Vitaminbestimmungsmethoden, Merck AG., Darmstadt. Weinheim, Bergst. Verlag Chemie (1963).

WEBB, J.L. Enzyme and Metabolic Inhibitors II. *1-244* Academic Press, New York, London (1966).

Authors' address:

Section Biochemistry of the Eye
Institute of Experimental Ophthalmology
University of Bonn
Bonn, W. Germany

211

SODIUM AND POTASSIUM IN THE NORMAL HUMAN LENS IN RELATION WITH AGE

JEAN KLETHI

(Strasbourg, France)

SUMMARY

Sodium and potassium were estimated by three different procedures on bovine lenses. While sodium content was independent from the technique used, potassium showed highest values with the mineralisation technique. Until 5 h post-mortem no changes in sodium and potassium could be noticed on bovine lenses. In selected normal post-mortem (1-5 h) human lenses of different ages sodium and potassium concentrations were measured. There were no changes in these cations in relation with age. A slight rise of sodium was noticed when 1-2 h and 4-5 h post-mortem lenses were compared.

INTRODUCTION

Several papers dealing with the determination of sodium and potassium in human cataractous lenses have appeared the last years (ANDREE, 1970; VAN HEYNINGEN, 1972; MARAINI & MANGILI, 1973; MARAINI & TORCOLI, 1974; DUNCAN & BUSHELL, 1975). However, values concerning normal human lenses are scarce because of the lack of material. These values still represent fundamental references which are not included in certain comparative studies of lenses at different cataractous stages. In this work we attempted to have more information concerning the variations with age of the two cations in normal human lenses. All efforts were made to obtain post-mortem lenses as quickly as possible. The lenses were selected by slit lamp examination. Only clear lenses were used in this analysis. In a preliminary study on bovine lenses we tested the influence of the possible post-mortem variations on the respective sodium and potassium contents. In addition we tried three different lens extraction techniques for flame photometry.

MATERIALS AND METHODS

Study on bovine lenses

Concerning the results of Table I, the lenses were removed at the slaughter house immediately after death and brought to the laboratory on ice. Analysis started within 20 min after removal of the lenses. Lenses of same fresh weights were collected and divided into 4 groups of 6 lenses each. The first group served for lens water determinations. In the next two groups each lens was homogenized in a Potter with 3 volumes of bidistilled water or TCA 10% for the calf lenses, 6 volumes of bidistilled water or TCA 10% for the

Table I. Sodium and potassium content of bovine lenses (mequiv./kg lens water ±S.E.)

Extraction procedure	Calf		Ox	
	Na^+	K^+	Na^+	K^+
Bidist. H_2O	23.5 ±2.3	97.6 ±4.4	29.7 ±2.8	99.7 ±3.6
TCA 10%	22.2 ±3.3	119.5 ±7.6	28.7 ±2.1	108.0 ±1.1
Mineralisation in HNO_3	21.9 ±3.7	125.8 ±12.8	28.7 ±0.8	122.2 ±3.5

Table II. Influence of different post-mortem stages on the sodium and potassium content of bovine lenses (mequiv./kg lens water ±S.E.)

Lens removal time	Calf		Ox	
	Na^+	K^+	Na^+	K^+
5 min after slaughter	21.9 ±1.8	128.5 ±5.8	29.0 ±4.6	128.9 ±3.6
1 h post-mortem	22.3 ±1.7	133.3 ±2.2	34.4 ±4.9	132.1 ±1.2
3 h post-mortem	18.4 ±1.0	127.7 ±4.3	30.6 ±4.5	133.1 ±3.1
5 h post-mortem	22.6 ±1.5	125.6 ±5.4	32.1 ±5.1	130.2 ±4.2

ox lenses. After centrifugation at 100,000 x g for 30 min the supernatant were diluted to 1 : 200 with bidistilled water. Sodium and potassium were determined by an Eppendorf flame emission photometer. The lenses of the fourth group were mineralised in the presence of successive amounts of concentrated nitric acid until clarification. The mineralisate was taken up in bidistilled water and diluted for flame photometry.

To study the influence of the different post-mortem stages on the content of sodium and potassium we removed the lenses according to the specifications indicated in Table II.

Study on human lenses

The lenses, obtained within 1-5 h after death (Table III), were removed, cleaned, rinsed, blotted on filter paper without ash, weighed and put in an oven at 105 °C for 24 h. Lens water was determined. The dry lenses were mineralised and sodium and potassium estimated as indicated above.

In all instances care was taken to avoid the cation shift phenomenon.

RESULTS AND DISCUSSION

In order to choose among the different techniques, we tested three procedures on bovine lenses. We compared the results after different extraction techniques such as homogeneisation with bidistilled water, with TCA 10% or by mineralisation with nitric acid. Table I summarizes the values obtained for sodium and potassium in calf and ox lenses. The data for sodium are nearly identical for all three extraction methods used. This can be explained if one considers that sodium is mostly localized extracellularly. The usual rise of sodium in function of age is noticed (about 20%). In contrast, the potassium contents behave differently. Here the mineralisation technique gives the highest values. In this case, potassium being intracellular, can be trapped, especially in the nuclear region, into the insoluble fraction, either in water or in TCA 10%. Using the mineralisation technique this can be avoided. The data obtained are in good agreement with those of MEROLA, KERN & KINOSHITA (1960), AVIRAM, SCHALITT, KASSEM & GROEN (1966) and PATERSON (1969).

To justify to what extent post-mortem lenses can be used as parameters

Table III.   Sodium and potassium content of normal human lenses at different ages

Age in years	Post-mortem time	Fresh weight mg	Dry weight mg	% H_2O	mequiv./kg lens water	
					Na^+	K^+
19	1 h 30	170.6	54.8	67.9	29.8	97.1
		177.9	54.5	69.4	20.7	94.2
41	4 h	189.3	61.7	67.4	14.7	102.9
		190.5	62.3	67.3	14.6	109.8
44	1 h 30	235.2	74.0	68.5	27.9	101.0
		232.1	73.1	68.5	23.6	102.6
45	1 h	178.8	56.3	68.5	20.2	91.8
		184.8	55.7	69.9	20.1	81.3
50	5 h	203.1	59.2	70.9	28.9	92.1
		197.8	59.5	69.9	26.4	87.9
51	4 h	215.4	68.0	68.4	29.9	92.3
		217.2	67.8	68.9	30.5	89.2
63	1 h 45	200.0	62.6	68.7	27.5	71.3
		200.2	61.8	68.5	27.1	92.7
65	2 h	207.8	70.1	66.3	27.2	98.0
		208.3	64.8	68.9	26.1	115.0
66	1 h	219.4	69.7	69.5	18.0	94.3
		230.0	71.0	69.1	18.1	94.3
67	2 h	253.4	80.2	68.4	23.2	102.1
		250.3	78.8	68.5	26.2	100.9
68	1 h 30	212.1	65.5	69.1	19.0	103.6
		221.3	68.1	69.1	20.7	103.2
68	5 h	259.7	81.2	68.7	24.7	108.5
		259.3	82.2	68.3	24.2	102.5
74	2 h	248.4	76.0	69.4	17.7	105.4
		243.5	75.4	69.0	20.2	113.0
78	4 h	213.5	66.7	69.6	21.1	105.4
		219.1	66.7	69.6	18.9	98.0

for the *in vivo* situation, we studied the influence of the post-mortem time on the content of sodium and potassium in bovine lenses. We assumed that the best representative values for sodium and potassium *in vivo* are reflected in lenses which are removed immediately after slaughter of the animal. Since we obtained human lenses between 1-5 h post-mortem we measured consequently sodium and potassium within this time span on bovine lenses. Table II summarizes our results which led to the conclusion that for sodium and potassium there are no significant alterations within 5 h after death. As judged from these results it is to be expected that studies on human lenses would behave similarly.

After these preliminary studies we analysed normal human lenses of different ages. Of the 28 lenses most were obtained within 1-2 h after death. As shown in Table III the variation for sodium as well as for potassium do not allow us to establish any correlation between age and content of sodium and potassium. In contrast to bovine lenses, the effect of the post-mortem time seems to influence the sodium content of the human lenses. As shown in Table III. except for the first two (19, 41 years), a rise of sodium is noticed for similar aged human lenses when the post-mortem time increases. If we separate the post-mortem lenses into two groups, which is possible since the lens age is equally represented, we can evaluate a mean for the first group (1-2 h post-mortem) of 22,6 meq and 25,5 meq for the second (4-5 h post-mortem). This corresponds to an increase of about 11%. On the contrary, potassium seems less susceptible to changes. Here also no correlation with age seems to exist. Highest values can be found at 68 years as well as at 41 years.

CONCLUSION

At first sight there is no difference in sodium and potassium content between human lenses of 40 years and those of 68. It seems that human lenses are more exposed to variations than bovine lenses. This might be due to the great variability of the individual antecedents which exist in a human population as well as to the smaller human lens Na^+ K^+ ATPase activity compared to that of the bovine lens as we found elsewhere. The present work was done with whole lenses; a study in various dissected areas from the lens would give more information regarding the variations of sodium and potassium concentrations in function of age of the human lens.

ACKNOWLEDGEMENTS

This work was in part supported by a grant from the Centre National de la Recherche Scientifique. I wish to thank Professor Nordmann for providing and selecting the human lens material. The skilful technical assistance of Mrs. M. Bakish is gratefully acknowledged.

REFERENCES

ANDRE, G. Natriumakkumulation in Kataraktlinsen. *Ber. Deut. Ophthalmol. Ges.* 70: *354-358* (1970).

216

AVIRAM, A., SCHALITT, M., KASSEM, N. & GROEN, J.J. Glucose utilization, gluta-thion, potassium and sodium content of isolated bovine lens. *Clin. Chim. Acta* 14: *442-449* (1966).

DUNCAN, G. & BUSHELL, A.R. Ion analysis of human cataractous lenses. *Exp. Eye Res.* 20: *223-230* (1975).

MARAINI, G. & MANGILI, R. Differences in proteins and in the water balance of the lens in nuclear and cortical type of senile cataract. In The human lens in relation to cataract, Ciba Symposium, Elsevier, Amsterdam (1973).

MARAINI, G. & TORCOLI, D. Electrolyte changes in the lens in senile cataract. *Ophthal. Res.* 6: *197-205* (1974).

MEROLA, L.O., KERN, H.L. & KINOSHITA, J.H. The effect of Ca on the cations of calf lens. *Arch. Ophthalmol.* (Chicago) 63: *830-835* (1960).

PATERSON, C.A. Distribution of sodium and potassium in ox lenses. *Exp. Eye Res.* 8: *442-446* (1969).

VAN HEYNINGEN, R. The human lens I, II, III. *Exp. Eye Res.* 13: *136-160* (1972).

Keywords:

Sodium and potassium
Human lens
Bovine lens
Aging

Author's address:

Institut de Chimie Biologique
Faculté de Médecine
11 rue Humann
67085 Strasbourg Cedex, France

CELL VOLUME REGULATION IN THE LENS*

JOHN W. PATTERSON

(Farmington, Conn.)

ABSTRACT

Rat lenses incubated in media with different osmolarities change in volume as water shifts across cell membranes to achieve osmotic balance. This process, however, is accompanied by another which tends to counteract the volume change. This effect can not be explained by changes in the leak or pump of the usual pump-leak model. Instead it appears to relate to permeability changes to sodium and potassium that are volume dependent. This volume regulating mechanism is well established for other types of cells and this work suggests that it is also active in the lens.

The lens is involved in the refraction of light and this in turn is dependent on the shape and refractive index of the organ. It would not be surprising, therefore, if volume regulating mechanisms that have been demonstrated for other cells were also active in the lens. In mammals this process has been studied most extensively in red blood cells. Cells from cats (SHA'AFI & PASCOE, 1972) dogs (PARKER & HOFFMAN, 1975), man (POZNANSKY & SOLOMON, 1972) and ducks (KREGENOW, 1971, 1971, 1974) all have volume regulating mechanisms. Duck red cells have been studied extensively and, unlike cat and dog erythrocytes, have a high potassium content that makes them similar to the cells of other organs including the lens.

Interest in this process was initiated with the finding that lenses incubated in hypotonic media failed to swell and that lenses incubated in a 185 mOsm medium for periods up to 24 hours behaved in a manner comparable with duck red cells (PATTERSON & FOURNIER, 1976).

This paper presents additional data supporting this observation with an emphasis on changes at different osmolarities and with a suggestion as to the relationship of lens volume regulation to the development of cataracts that are associated with lens swelling.

MATERIAL & METHODS

Lenses were obtained from male Sprague-Dawley rats weighing 80-100 gms. The lenses were removed from the enucleated eye with a posterior approach under a dissecting microscope. The media used had final mM concentrations as follows: KH_2PO_4-0.5, Na_2HPO_4-0.8, $MgSO_4$-1.0, $CaCl_2$-1.5, $NaHCO_3$-

* This research was supported in part by research grant EY-00902 from the National Eye Institute, National Institutes of Health, Bethesda, Maryland.

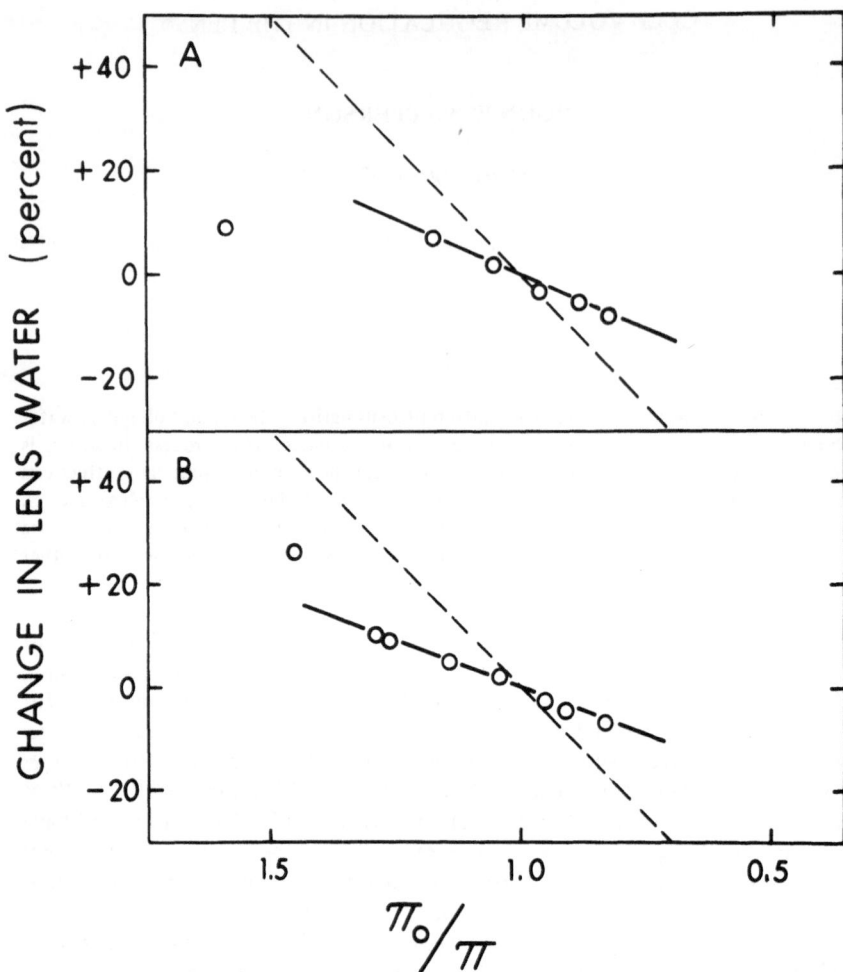

Fig. 1. The percent change in lens water plotted against the ratio of the initial osmolarity to the new osmolarity. The dotted lines indicate the theoretical relationship. Part A is experimental data for rat lenses (see Figure 3) and Part B is data from KINOSHITA, MEROLA & HAYMAN (1965) for rabbit lens.

11.0, KCl-6.0, glucose-6.7, and NaCl as required to establish the desired osmolarity. Phenol red was incorporated at a concentration of 2 mg per 100 ml. Dry weights were obtained by drying to constant weight in a 95 ° oven. For comparative purposes all values were adjusted to reflect levels for a lens with a dry weight equal to 10 mg. Sodium concentrations were corrected for extracellular content by using an extracellular space equal to 6 percent. Sodium and potassium concentrations were determined by using a Perkins-Elmer atomic absorption spectrophotometer.

RESULTS

Volume changes in cells that are incubated in dilute solutions with varying osmolarities are described by the equation

$$\Delta V = V_o \, (\pi_o/\pi) - 100$$

where V_o and V equal the initial and new volumes for cell water and π_o and π equal the initial and new osmolarities of the incubating media. If the volume is adjusted to 100 then ΔV equals the percent change in lens water. In Fig. 1 this theoretical relationship is shown with a dotted line.

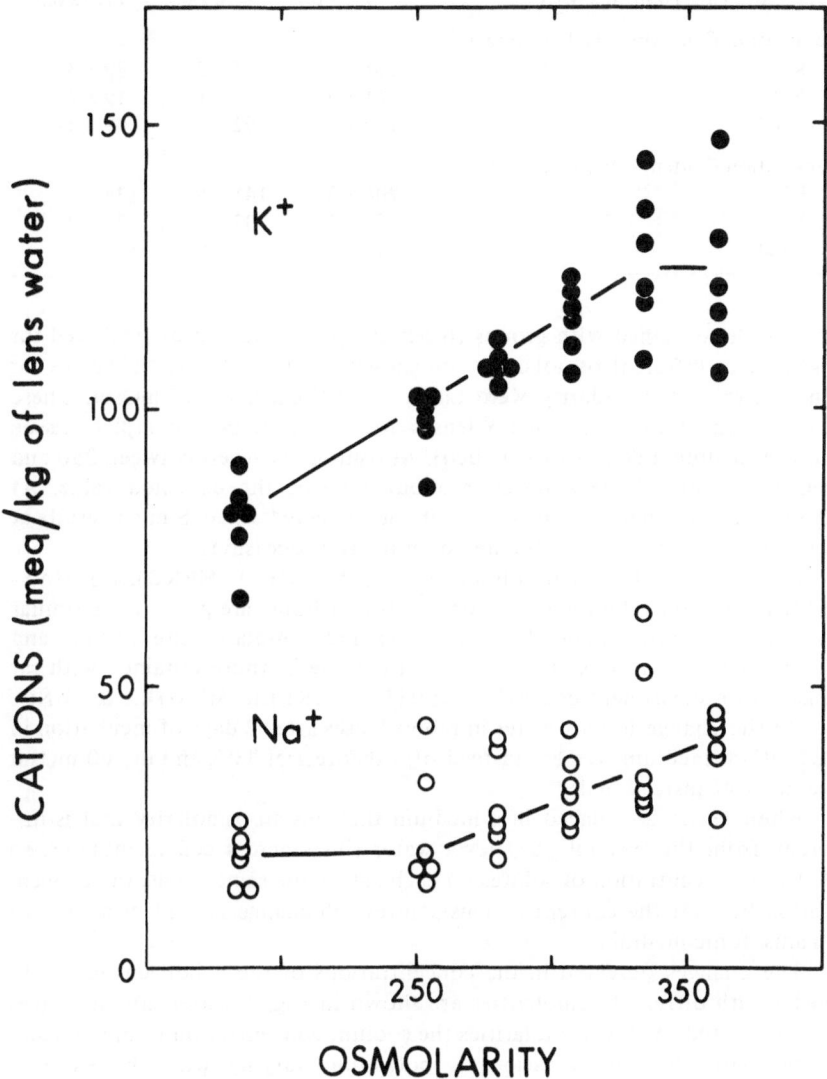

Fig. 2. Changes in cation concentration with osmolarity.

Table 1. Effect of High Glucose and Hypotonic Media on Rat Lenses (mean ± S.E.)

	Fresh Lenses	High Glucose Medium	Hypotonic Medium
Lenses (number)	6	5	6
Osmolarity (mOsm)	300	304	185
Incubation time (hours)	0	24	24
Glucose Conc. (mM)	5.5	60.0	6.7
Lens Water (mg/10 mg dry wt.)	17.0 ± 0.4	18.8 ± 0.1	17.4 ± 0.5
Lens Cation Conc. (meq/kg lens water)			
K^+	121 ± 3	75 ± 2	80 ± 3
Na^+	21 ± 3	17 ± 1	19 ± 2
Total	142 ± 3	92 ± 3	99 ± 3
Lens Cation Content (meq/kg dry wt.)			
K^+	206 ± 3	141 ± 5	139 ± 7
Na^+	36 ± 5	32 ± 2	34 ± 3
Total	242 ± 5	173 ± 6	171 ± 8

The results obtained with groups (6 lenses each) of rat lenses incubated for 24 hours at different osmolarities are shown in Figure 1A. Initial values for lens water and osmolarity were taken as 15.9 mg and 295 mOsm. These were obtained by incubating 9 lenses for 24 hours in a complete tissue culture medium (TC199 from Gibco). At osmolarity levels between 250 and 360 the change in lens water is about 40% of the expected value. At 185 mOsm the change is only 16% of the expected value. Similar results at this osmolarity have been obtained on numerous occasions.

In Figure 1B the results obtained by KINOSHITA, MEROLA & HAY-MAN (1965) on rabbit lenses incubated for 21 hours are plotted in a similar manner. The initial values for lens water and osmolarity are 117 mg and 292 mOsm. The results are essentially the same as those obtained with rat lenses. In a subsequent paper (KINOSHITA, BARBER, MEROLA & TUNG, 1969) the change in lens water in rabbit lenses after 2 days of incubation in 222 mOsm medium was 8% instead of a theoretical 33%, and in 360 mOsm medium 6% instead of 19%.

When lenses are placed in a medium that has an osmolarity that is different from the physiological level water shifts across cell membranes so that the concentration of solutes on each side is the same. Thus, the concentration but not the content of lens solutes will change as the lens adjusts to an anisotonic medium.

The changes observed in the concentrations of the major lens cation in media with different osmolarities are shown in Fig. 2. Three circumstances may be noted. At low osmolarities the sodium concentration is minimal and stable with the concentration of potassium varying with the external osmolarity. At somewhat higher osmolarities sodium and potassium concentrations increase as the osmolarity increases. At still higher osmolarities the potassium concentration levels off and the concentration of sodium varies with the external osmolarity. The critical osmolarity at which these changes occur is variable and relates to the composition of the medium. In these experiments the medium consisted of glucose and a salt mixture. It may be noted in Table I that a fresh lens at about a 300 mOsm level has an intracellular concentration of sodium that is at the minimal level.

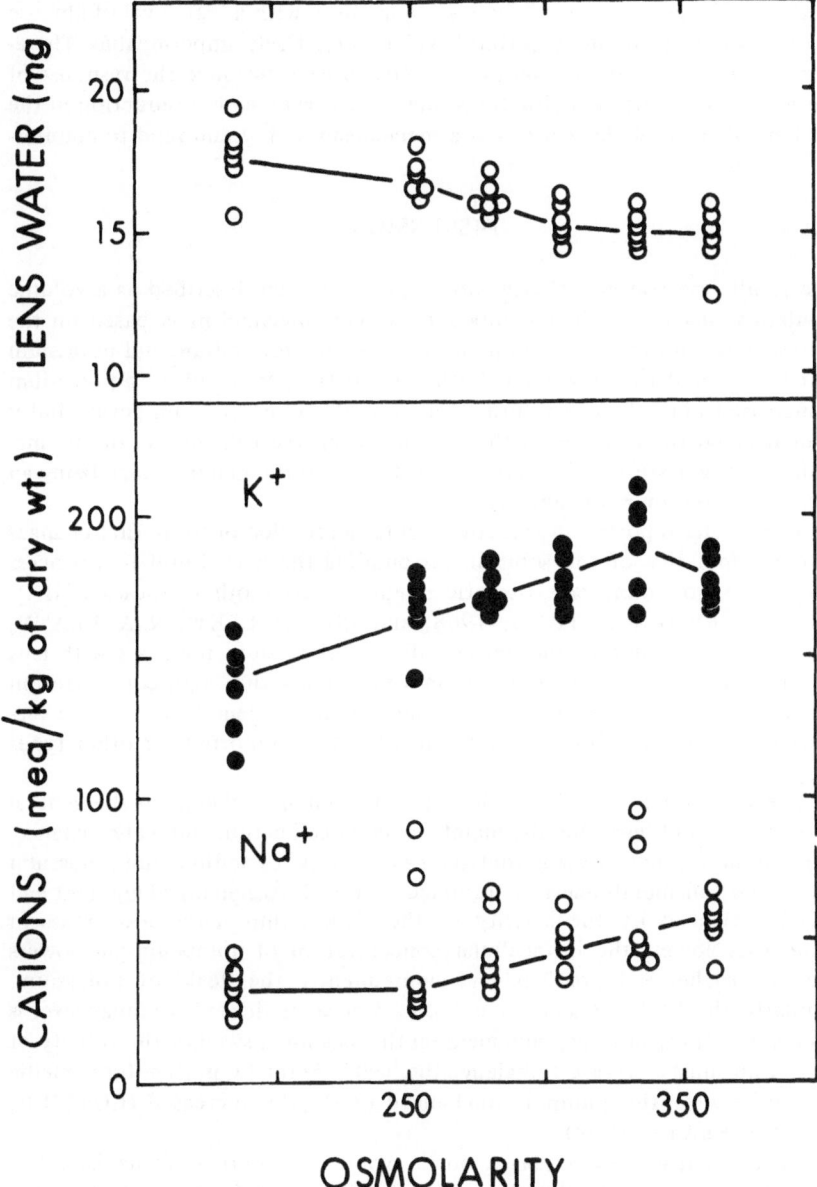

Fig. 3. Changes in cation content with osmolarity. The upper plot shows the change in lens water with osmolarity.

The changes observed in the content of the major lens cations at different osmolarities are shown in Figure 3. Changes in cation content do occur with changes in osmolarity. Thus the shift in water accompanying osmotic equilibration must be associated with an additional process.

The changes in lens cation concentration and content that are observed in a hypotonic medium are similar to those observed in lenses incubated in an isotonic medium with a high concentration of glucose. This is demonstrated in Table I. Lenses incubated in a medium with a high level of glucose are known to accumulate sorbitol which is relatively impermeable. Therefore, there is a resultant osmotic swelling. In each instance the response of the lens to two different situations that induce swelling is a reduction in the content of intracellular cations — a mechanism that would tend to counteract swelling.

DISCUSSION

The results are consistent with those that have been described as a volume regulating mechanism in red blood cells. This mechanism is based on the existence of an inherent membrane permeability for sodium and potassium which is related to cell volume. With swelling the permeability to potassium is increased until the cell returns to its initial volume. Sodium permeability is unaffected or decreases with swelling. When the cell shrinks the permeability changes are in the opposite direction with the major change being an increase in sodium permeability.

The results reported in this study on rat lenses demonstrate that changes in the osmolarity of the solution surrounding the lens stimulate a process that tends to counteract osmotic swelling. From other studies (KINOSHITA, MEROLA & TUNG, 1968; and COTLIER, KWAN & BEATY, 1968) it is known that the permeability of potassium increases with lens swelling in hypotonic medium and in a medium with a high concentration of sugar. Therefore, it may be concluded that the lens has a volume regulating mechanism similar to that which has been reported for other types of cells.

The acceptance of this conclusion will result in a change in the general view that is held regarding the maintenance of cell cation and water balance. The commonly held view is that the passive 'leak' of sodium and potassium across the cell membrane is determined by the electrochemical gradient and this is balanced by the activity of the Na-K pump. Thus, a decrease in osmolarity lowers the intracellular concentration of potassium and lowers the electrochemical gradient and consequently the 'leak' of potassium. Similarly the 'leak' of sodium is reduced because the extracellular level is decreased. Thus, in hypotonic medium the lens must swell or the activity of the pump must decrease to balance the 'leak'. Actually, in hypotonic media the activity of the pump is unchanged or slightly increased (COTLIER, KWAN & BEATY, 1968).

An alternative view is based on the volume regulating mechanism. The pump-leak model is modified so that the dominant factor controlling the leak is the permeability of the membrane at any given volume rather than the electrochemical gradient. The effects of the latter are secondary and probably account for the fact that complete volume regulation is not attained. The activity of the pump is determined by the concentrations of extracellular potassium and intracellular sodium and the availability of energy (SACHS, KNAUF & DUNHAM, 1975). Therefore, the pump is not affected by changes in osmolarity if the concentration of extracellular potassium is constant. The pump, however, is responsible for the influx of potassium which accounts for about 80% of the actively transported solutes that accumulate in the lens. Thus the observed volume of the lens, under ordinary circumstances, is the volume at which the permeability of potassium permits a rate of efflux that equals the rate at which it is being pumped into the lens. The data obtained on rabbit lenses by COTLIER, KWAN & BEATY (1968) are consistent with this interpretation. Their findings are summarized in modified form in Table II.

The data in Figures 2 and 3 may be considered against this interpretive background. At low osmolarities the cells swell and the efflux of potassium exceeds the rate at which it is being pumped. Therefore, the potassium along with anions and water are lost until the imbalance is corrected. At osmolarities above the physiological level and at lower osmolarities in a medium consisting of a salt mixture and glucose the lens shrinks and the permeability of potassium decreases; however, the permeability and concentration of sodium increase. The latter stimulates the pump so that the content of potassium and water increase until the volume equals that at which the potassium permeability will permit efflux to equal influx. At higher osmolarities the pump is saturated and increases in volume to attain a balance are dependent on the accumulation of sodium as its permeability varies with volume. All of these effects are modulated by changes in the electrochemical gradient.

In a hypotonic medium the cation content of the lens is decreased. This must be accompanied by a decrease in anions and in water. Glutamate and aspartate are major anions in the lens and amino acids are known to decrease when lenses are incubated in a hypotonic medium or in a medium with a high level of glucose (KINOSHITA, BARBER, MEROLA & TUNG, 1969). These effects are prevented if swelling is prevented. Thus it is possible that the volume regulating mechanism results in a loss of glutamic acid so that it is not avialable as a substrate for glutathione synthesis or for

Table 2. Relative Influx (pump) and Efflux (leak) of ^{86}Rb at Different Osmolarities during the First 4 Hours of Incubation (COTLIER, KWAN BEATY, 1968)

Osmolarity	Influx	Efflux
238	112	262
270	103	175
300	100	100
333	94	51
366	99	50

amino acid transport by glutamyltranpeptidase as suggested by RATHBUN & WICKER (1973).

The time required for the development of nuclear sugar cataracts is known to correlate inversely with lens swelling (PATTERSON & BUNTING, 1966). Therefore, the effects of the volume regulating mechanism that are observed with hypotonic swelling can be expected to occur under cataractogenic conditions. The permeability of potassium is known to increase with swelling (KINOSHITA, MEROLA & TUNG, 1968). Therefore, the potassium concentration will decrease and glutamate and aspartate may well be lost. It is known that cataracts may be delayed or prevented with dietary supplements consisting of unessential amino acids including aspartate and glutamate (PATTERSON, 1960).

ACKNOWLEDGEMENT

The author is grateful for the technical assistance provided by Janis Langston in the performance of this work.

REFERENCES

COTLIER, E., B. KWAN & C. BEATY. The Lens as an Osmometer and the Effects of Medium Osmolarity on Water Transport, [86]Rb Efflux and [86]Rb Transport by the Lens. *Biochim. Biophys. Acta* 150: *705* (1968).

KINOSHITA, J.H., L.O. MEROLA & S. HAYMAN. Osmotic Effects on Amino Acid-concentrating Mechanism in the Rabbit Lens. *J. Biol. Chem.* 240: *310* (1965).

KINOSHITA, J.H., L.O. MEROLA & B. TUNG. Changes in Cation Permeability in Galactose Exposed Rabbit Lenses. *Exp. Eye Res.* 7: *80* (1968).

KINOSHITA, J.H., G.W. BARBER, L.O. MEROLA & B. TUNG. Changes in the Levels of Free Amino Acids and Myo-inositol in Galactose-exposed Lens. *Invest. Ophthal.* 8: *625* (1969).

KREGENOW, F.M. The Response of Duck Erythrocytes to Nonkemolytic Hypotonic Media, Evidence for a Volume Controlling Mechanism. *J. Gen. Physiol.* 58: *372* (1971).

KREGENOW, F.M. The Response of Duck Erythrocytes to Hypertonic Media. *J. Gen. Physiol.* 58: *396* (1971).

KREGENOW, F.M. Functional Separation of the Na-K Exchange Pump from Volume Controlling Mechanism in Enlarged Duck Red Cells. *J. Gen. Physiol.* 64: *393* (1974).

PARKER, J.C. & J.F. HOFFMAN. Interdependence of Cation Permeability, Cell Volume, and Metabolism in Dog Red Blood Cells. *Fed. Proc.* 24: *589* (1965).

PATTERSON, J.W. Effects of Galactosemia. *Anat. Rec.* 138: 395 (1960).

PATTERSON, J.W. & K.W. BUNTING. Sugar Cataracts, Polyol Levels and Lens Swelling. *Docum. Ophthal.* 20: *64* (1966).

PATTERSON, J.W. & D.J. FOURNIER. The effect of Tonicity on Lens Volume. *Invest. Ophthal.* (Accepted for Publication 1976).

POZNANSKY, M. & A.K. SOLOMON. Regulation of Human Red Cell Volume by Linked Cation Fluxes. *J. Membrane Biol.* 10: *259* (1972).

RATHBUN, W.B. & K. WICKER. Bovine Lens γ glutamyl Transpeptidase. *Exp. Eye Res.* 15: *161* (1973).

SACKS, J.R., P.A. KNAUF & P.B. DUNHAM. Transport through Red Cell Membranes.

In the Red Blood Cell. D. Mac. N. Surgenor, Editor. Academic Press Inc., N.Y. (1975).

SHA'AFI, R.I. & E. PASCOE. Further Studies of Sodium Transport in Feline Red Cells. *J. Gen. Physiol.* 61: *709* (1973).

Keywords:

lens
osmotic swelling
hypotonic medium
volume regulation
hypertonic medium
cataract

Author's address:

Dept. of Physiology
University of Connecticut
Farmington, Connecticut
U.S.A.

DIFFERENCES IN THE CALCIUM BINDING CAPACITY
OF NORMAL AND CATARACTOUS LENSES

GEORGE DUNCAN & RUTH VAN HEYNINGEN

(Oxford, England)

ABSTRACT

Fresh bovine lenses, and human post mortem and senile cataracts (Group III PIRIE, 1968), bind [45] calcium when frozen and thawed and incubated at 4°C in isotonic sodium-free buffer containing [45] calcium. The calcium-binding properties of bovine and post mortem human lenses are similar, and differ from those of the senile cataractous lens.

There appears to be a higher density of calcium binding sites in Group III cataracts and only these lenses bind calcium in the presence of EGTA.

INTRODUCTION

It has long been appreciated that the calcium concentration of cataractous lenses is extremely variable (ADAMS, 1929; MACKAY, STEWART & ROBERTSON, 1932) but recently DUNCAN & BUSHELL (1975) have demonstrated a correlation between the sodium and calcium content of cataractous lenses. They showed that cataracts with low sodium values in the range 20-30 mM had low calcium levels, and that cataracts with sodium concentrations of 80 mM or more had high calcium levels. DUNCAN & BUSHELL (1976) attempted to reproduce this pattern of ion-distribution in the cataractous lenses by using bovine lenses that had had their membrane permeability barriers destroyed by freezing and thawing. When these lenses were incubated in a medium of similar composition to that of the bovine aqueous humour, they found that the calcium concentration of the lens did indeed increase as the sodium concentration of the lens increased, although they were not able to reproduce the high calcium levels (> 5 mM/kg lens water) found in many cataracts.

A possible explanation for this discrepancy is that there are differences between the binding sites of bovine and human lenses, and/or between the sites of normal human and cataractous lenses. In this communication we present data that argue in favour of the latter possibility.

MATERIALS

Bovine eyes were obtained from the slaughterhouse within a few hours of death, while post mortem eyes were received approximately 48 hr after death. $^{45}CaCl_2$ in aqueous solution (1.34 mCi/ml) was obtained from

Radiochemicals, Amersham, Bucks., U.K. and EGTA (ethyleneglycolbis-N, N-Tetraacetic Acid) was from Sigma, U.S.A.

METHODS

Lenses were removed from the eyes and stored frozen in pre-weighed polythene pots until required. Cataractous lenses (Group III PIRIE, 1968) were placed in pre-weighed pots immediately after the operation.

When required, the lenses were thawed at room temperature and a one-third segment (approximately) was dissected out and reweighed. It was then homogenised in 10 ml ice-cold trichloroacetic acid (4%) and the homogenate centrifuged at 5000 g for 15 min. The sediment was dried overnight at 60 °C and the difference between the wet weight of the segment and the dry weight of the precipitate gave the weight of water in the segment. The supernatant was analysed for sodium and calcium by conventional flame photometric techniques (DUNCAN & BUSHELL, 1975). Only lenses with a sodium value in the segment of greater than 80 mM/kg water (Group C, DUNCAN & BUSHELL, 1975) were used.

The remaining two-thirds of the lens was placed in buffer containing 100 mM Tris (Sigma) adjusted to pH 7.3 with 6 M HCl, 1 mM $CaCl_2$ and 5 μCi/ml $^{45}CaCl_2$. The ratio of the buffer volume to lens volume always exceeded 50 to 1. The lenses were incubated for 24 hr at 4 °C with occasional gentle shaking, removed from the solution, blotted and weighed. There were then homogenised in 4% trichloroacetic acid and the weight of water determined as above. The radioactivity in 1 ml samples of the supernatant, and 100 μl samples of the bathing solutions, was assayed in a Beckman liquid scintillation counter. The specific activity ratio (R), where

$$R = \frac{cts/min/kg \text{ lens water}}{cts/min/kg \text{ bathing solution}}$$

was determined for each lens.

RESULTS AND DISCUSSION

The abnormally high initial value for sodium (and probably calcium) in the human post-mortem lens (Table I) is due to the fact that the lens remains in the eye for many hours after death (VAN HEYNINGEN, 1972). The values for sodium and calcium in the bovine lens are normal (DUNCAN & BUSHELL, 1975) and the senile cataracts were selected for their high concentrations of sodium, and therefore calcium (DUNCAN & BUSHELL, 1976).

The specific activity ratio (R) gives some estimate of the extent of calcium binding in the lens, and previous investigations (DUNCAN & BUSHELL, 1976) have shown that the bovine lens incubated in an isotonic salt solution can sequester calcium. Further studies (DUNCAN, 1976) have demonstrated that sodium ions can to some extent compete for the calcium sites, and so we have carried out the present study in a sodium-free buffer. The data presented in Table I show a consistent difference between the R values attained in fresh bovine and post-mortem human lenses, but the

230

Table I. Effect of EGTA on the uptake of ^{45}Ca by part of a frozen-thawed lens incubated at 4°C.

Type of lens	No. of Expts.	Initial Conc. of ion in one-third of lens (mM/kg water)		Specific activity ratio (R) in $\frac{2}{3}$ portions after incubation	
		Na^+	Ca^{++}	no EGTA	plus 1mM EGTA
human, post mortem	5	71± 2	3.2±0.6	2.6,2.4,2.2	0.83,0.82
human, senile cataract	5	135±13	14.2±4.0	8.2,5.7,4.8	2.7,2.4
bovine	6	22± 1	0.55±0.06	1.7,1.7,1.7,1.6	0.84,0.82

human lenses were all about 65 years old. The initial ion concentrations are expressed as the mean ± S.D.

differences are much less than those between human post-mortem and senile cataractous lenses. This indicates that the high calcium levels attained in Group III (or Group C) cataracts are not simply due to calcium ions adsorbing on to sites present in the normal lens, but that they adsorb on to additional sites created during cataract formation. These sites could arise as a result of the considerable amount of protein unfolding that is now believed to occur in cataract (HARDING & DILLEY, 1976).

The fact that, in the presence of EGTA, R attains a value of about 0.83 in the normal bovine and human lens (Table I) indicates that near equilibrium is reached between the free calcium in the lens and that in the medium. It also shows that normal bovine and post-mortem human lenses do not bind calcium in the presence of EGTA. The high ratios achieved in Group III lenses under the same circumstances indicate that the additional binding sites in these lenses have a higher affinity than EGTA for calcium ions.

ACKNOWLEDGEMENTS

We acknowledge many stimulating discussions with Dr. Keith J. Dilley and Dr. John J. Harding and we thank Miss Joy Rosser for excellent technical assistance. G.D. wishes to thank the Royal National Institute for the Blind for support, and Mr. Anthony J. Bron, Margaret Ogilvie's Reader in Ophthalmology, for the hospitality and facilities of the laboratory. We thank the Medical Research Council for a Grant to purchase the Scintillation Counter.

REFERENCES

ADAMS, D.R. The role of calcium in senile cataract. *Biochem. J.* 23: *902-912* (1929).
DUNCAN, G. The concentration and state of calcium in the lens. Colloq. d'INSERM, 1976 (in press).
DUNCAN, G. & BUSHELL, A.R. Ion analyses of human cataractous lenses. *Exp. Eye Res.* 20: *223-230* (1975).
DUNCAN, G. & BUSHELL, A.R. The bovine lens as an ion-exchanger: a comparison with ion levels in human cataractous lenses. *Exp. Eye Res.* 1976 (in press).

231

HARDING, J.J. & DILLEY, K.J. Structural proteins of the mammalian lens: A review with emphasis on changes in development, aging and cataract. *Exp. Eye Res.* 22: *1-73* (1976).

MACKAY, G., STEWART, C.P. & ROBERTSON, J.D. A note on the inorganic consti- tuents of normal and cataractous human lenses. *Brit. J. Ophthalmol.* 16: *193-198* (1932).

PIRIE, A. Color and solubility of the proteins of the lens. *Invest. Ophthalmol.* 7: *634-642* (1968).

VAN HEYNINGEN, R. The human lens III. Some observations on the post-mortem lens. *Exp. Eye Res.* 13: *155-160* (1972).

Keywords:

Lens
Cataractous lens
Human lens
Senile cataract
Calcium binding

Authors' address:

Oxford University
Nuffield Laboratory of Ophthalmology
Walton Street
Oxford, ox2 6AW, England

INTRACELLULAR MARKERS IN THE CRYSTALLINE
LENS OF THE RAT

J.L. RAE & T.R. STACEY

(Galveston, Texas)

INTRODUCTION

STRETTON & KRAVITZ (1968) reported the usefulness of Procion dyes for marking cells in the nervous system. Because of their ionic nature, these dyes can be injected by iontophoresis from the tip of a microelectrode which has impaled the cell to be marked. The most used of these dye markers is procion yellow which, because it is highly fluorescent, can be located in histologic sections by fluorescence microscopy. More recently, CHRISTENSEN (1973) has reported the use of Procion brown as a marker for cells in the lamprey spinal cord. This dye, because it contains chromium, is electron dense and can be localized by electron microscopy.
RAE (1973, 1974) and RAE & BLANKENSHIP (1973) described the use of Procion dyes to mark cells in the crystallin lens of the frog. These studies had the disadvantage that they were performed on an animal in which experimental cataracts are not easily produced. In addition, the histologic studies were done using low resolution paraffin embedding procedures. To rectify these shortcomings, the present studies were undertaken using Sprague-Dawley rats and the high resolution histology associated with Epon embedding and glass and diamond knife sectioning techniques.

MATERIAL & METHODS

All studies were done on 80-120 gm. female Sprague-Dawley rats. The animals were anesthetized by a single intraperitoneal injection of 25% Urethan (25 mg. per Kg.). The eyes were enucleated and the posterior portion of the globe dissected away. The remaining globe, with the lens attached, was pinned into a Sylgárd (Dow-Corning) lined chamber filled with a Hepes buffered (pH 7.4) mammalian Ringer's solution at room temperature, and illuminated from below by a fiber-optic illuminator. The lens was impaled with a glass microelectrode filled with either a 50-50 mixture of 6% Procion scarlet and 6% Procion yellow, or with a 4% solution of electron dense Procion rubine, using previously described techniques (RAE, 1974). The electrodes were selected to have resistances in the 20-30 megohm range when filled with the appropriate solution. The negatively charged dyes were injected into the cells iontophoretically by passing 300, 2.5 to 50 nA negative current pulses (.1 sec. duration, 1 per sec.) through the current injection circuit of a W.P.I. M4 electrometer to which the microelectrode was connected. To prevent the dye from precipitating in the electrode tip, every third current pulse was reversed in polarity.

Movement of the dye during injection was observed directly through a Wild M5 dissecting microscope (62.5x), to allow detection of microelectrode tip breakage with subsequent dye leakage, or to detect excessive lens dimpling at the electrode tip. After removal of the electrode, the globe was left in the Ringer's solution for thirty minutes to allow the injected dye time to diffuse. The globe was then immersed for ten minutes in a 10% Formaldehyde solution in .1 M phosphate buffer (pH 7.4), after which, the lens was removed and reimmersed in the fixative overnight. After fixation, the lenses were cut initially in a plane perpendicular to the injected fibers and were then cut into approximately 1 mm. cubes containing the injected fibers. Tissues to be used for fluorescence microscopy were then dehydrated in ethanol and embedded in Epon. Tissues for electron microscopy were post-fixed for ninety minutes in 1% osmium tetroxide buffered to pH 7.4 in .1 M phosphate buffer and subsequently stained for one hour enbloc in 2% Mg uranyl acetate. Dehydration in ethanol and embedding in Epon followed. For fluorescence microscopy, 1 micron sections were cut with glass knives on a sorvall MT 1 ultramicrotome and mounted unstained, but coverslipped, on glass slides. Silver to silver-gold sections were cut for electron microscopy using a Sorvall MT2 ultramicrotome and a diamond knife. The sections for electron microscopy were stained for twenty minutes in a saturated uranyl acetate solution in 50% ethanol and ten minutes in a modified Reynolds' lead citrate solution (REYNOLDS, 1963), and were viewed and photographed with a Phillip's 200 electron microscope. Sections for non-fluorescence light microscopy were stained for thirty seconds to one minute with a 50-50 mixture of 1% methylene blue-1% Na Borate and 1% Azure II.

RESULTS

Figure 1 shows typical light micrographs from a Procion rubine injected rat lens. Three separate penetrations (Figure 1a, 1b — arrows) with known spacing were made, so that localization of injected cells would be unequivocal. This was necessary because cells of the posterior cortex exhibited such staining heterogenity that some non-injected cells stained as darkly as the injected cells. It can be seen that multiple cells were always injected. Ten to 15 cells in the same column in which the microelectrode tip was located, as well as 3 to 5 columns of adjacent cells, were usually involved. Occasionally, one or more cells within a column of injected cells appeared not to have dye in them. Such a result is shown in Figure 1c (arrow). However, serial sectioning back in the direction of the injection site showed that dye could be found in these cells at locations closer to the injection site.

Figure 2a shows electron micrographs of the same injected cells seen in Figure 1. Each of these injected cells shows a cell to cell 'tight junction' both on its top and bottom surface. Such junctions are also seen laterally between adjacent columns of cells. Figure 2b is an intermediate magnification of such a junction (arrow), whereas Figure 2c shows a junction at very high magnification. The junctions were found to be of the seven-layered type described by others as gap junctions (GILULA, 1974).

Figure 3 (a and b) depicts a cell injection obtained with a mixture of

234

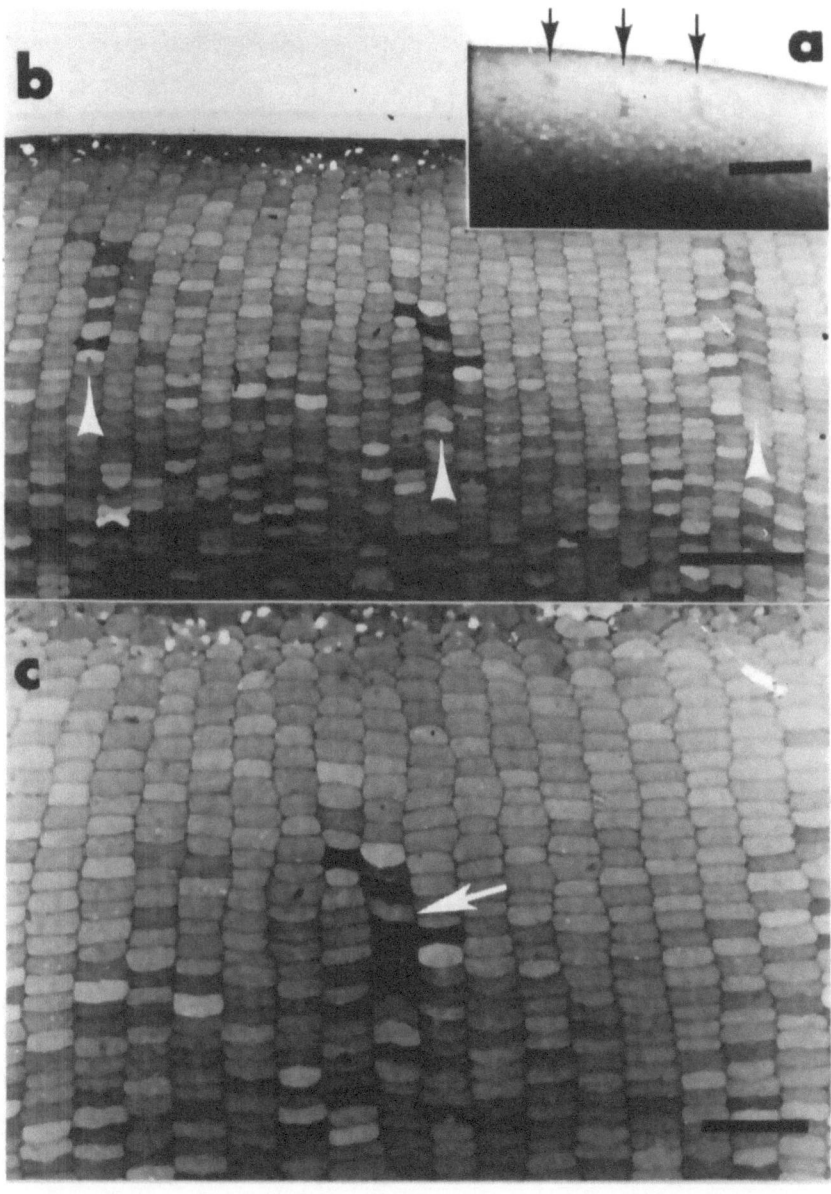

Fig. 1. Light micrographs of lens fibers from the posterior cortex of the rat lens which have been injected with Procion rubine through the tip of a glass microelectrode. Three injected fiber columns (1a, black arrows, bar = 10μ) are shown at two different magnifications (1b, white arrows, bar = 40μ). In 1c (bar = 20μ), one cell in the column (arrow) appears not to be dye filled (see text). Epon, cross section.

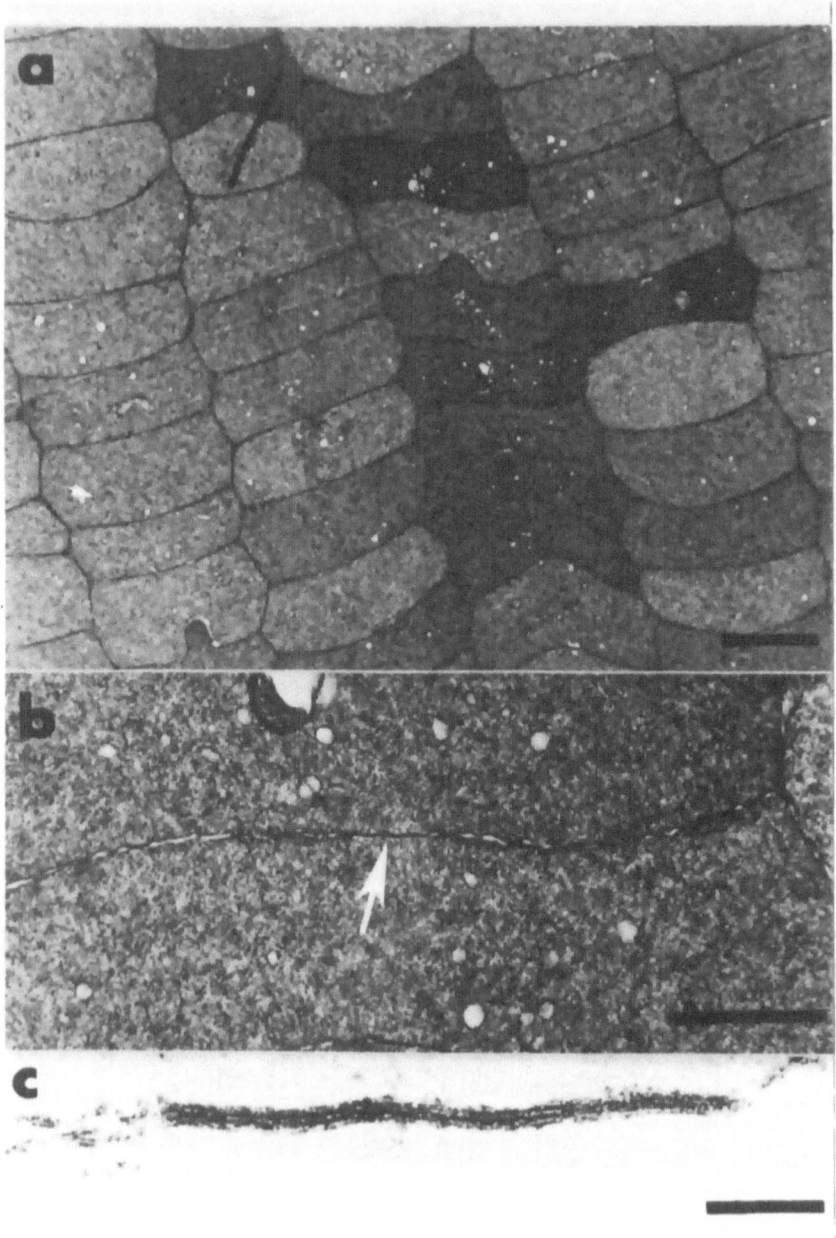

Fig. 2. Electron micrographs of same cells shown in Figure 1c. Electron dense dye, Procion rubine, can be seen within the injected cells (2a, bar = 5μ). Numerous cell to cell junctions occur between the cells (2b, arrow, bar – 1μ) on dorsal, ventral, and lateral surfaces. At high magnification (2c, bar – .1μ), many of these are seven-layered gap junctions. Epon, cross section.

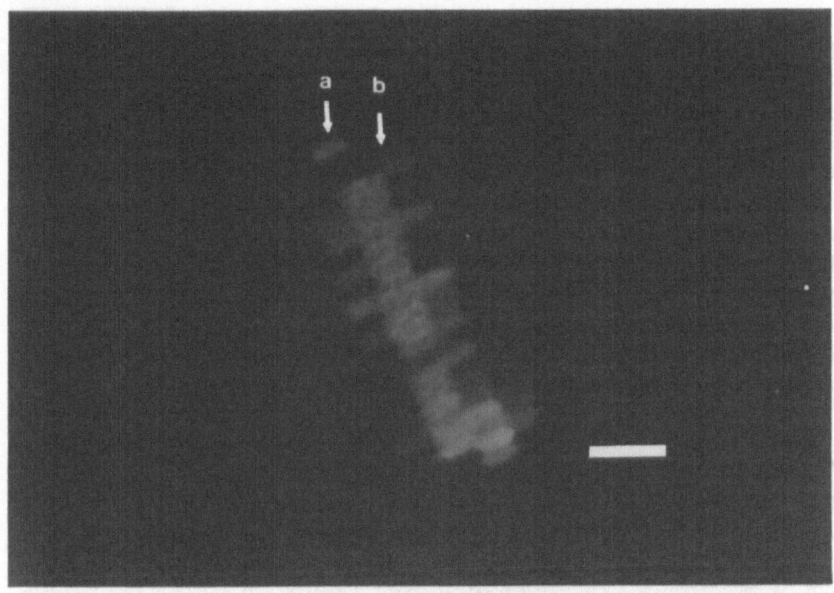

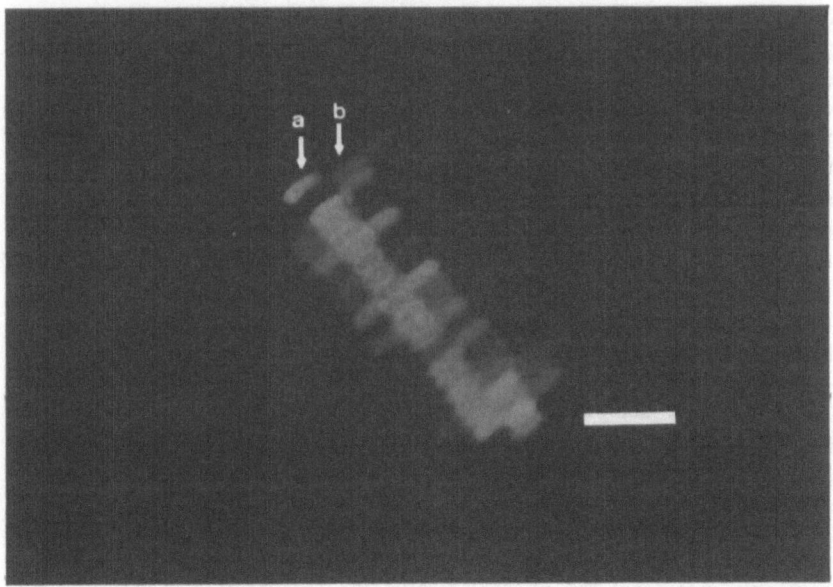

Fig. 3. Fluorescent light micrographs of lens cells injected with a 50-50 mixture of 6% Procion scarlet and 6% Procion yellow. In 3a (bar = 20μ), a section cut about 1 mm. from the injection site, cell a appears completely isolated from the rest of the cell columns (cell b). In 3b (bar = 20μ), a section cut about .75 mm. from the injection site, cell a appears to have almost joined cell b and the rest of the injected columns.

237

Procion scarlet and Procion yellow dyes in the microelectrode. These dyes diffuse in cells more readily than Procion rubine (STRETTON & KRAVITZ, 1968). Again, it can be appreciated that the dye does not remain within a single cell. Rather, it moves approximately 11 to 15 cells up and down a single column as well as 9 to 11 columns laterally. The dye appears to move more readily up and down columns than it does between columns. It can also be appreciated that the concentration of the dye falls off progressively as one moves laterally from the injection site, a pattern consistent with diffusion. It is interesting to note that the isolated cell a (Figure 3a — arrow) was found to be attached to cell b (arrow) when serial sectioning was done in the direction of the injection site (Figure 3b). Note also that there is no dye evident in the extracellular space around the cells lying between the isolated cell a and the column of injected cells.

DISCUSSION

The results presented are similar to those reported previously for the frog lens (RAE, 1974). Dye injected from a microelectrode, which because of its tip size is presumably in a single cell of the lens, does not stay within that cell. Rather, it moves readily both up and down a cell column and laterally between columns. The lateral diffusion is much more substantial when a highly diffusive dye such as Procion yellow is used. Before a microelectrode penetrates the lens, a significant amount of dimpling of the capsule is observed. With the electrode tapers used here, no such dimpling could be observed after the tip penetrated. However, one cannot be certain that 'creeping' of the tissue past the electrode did not occur from some time following penetration. This would have resulted in a number of cells in the same column being penetrated sequentially as the tissue returned to its orginal position. Such creeping would amount to depth 'jitter of the electrode tip. Such depth jitter, however, could not explain the lateral movement of the dye, since virtually no lateral jitter occurs with our experimental preparation. In short, there is no way that the electrode tip could have physically penetrated every cell in which dye is found. Therefore, the dye must have moved either from cell to cell through specialized junctions which we have demonstrated, or alternatively it might have entered from the extracellular space. We do not favor penetration from the extracellular space for the following reasons:
1. When the tip of a microelectrode breaks upon penetration, dye is indiscriminately released in the region around the tip. Thereafter, by the use of the dissecting microscope, diffuse coloration can be seen in the lens for some distance from the microelectrode tip. This coloration is presumably due to movement of dye in the extracellular space. In the studies reported here, no diffuse coloration was seen in the extracellular space.
2. No dye was ever seen in the extracellular space with either fluorescence microscopy or electron microscopy.
3. Previous studies on the frog lens, using pressure injection techniques, have suggested that dye does not move from the extracellular space across cell membranes in the lens.
4. Since electric current easily moves from one cell to another in the rat

lens (RAE, unpublished observations), it would be anticipated that small molecular weight dyes would also move.

These studies support previous suggestions that in the crystalline lens, adjacent fibers are not functionally independent of one another. Rather, their cytoplasm is joined through low resistance junctions. These junctions apparently allow the passage of small molecular weight substances from one cell to another, thus facilitating the movement of metabolites and ions throughout the lens.

SUMMARY

When either fluorescent or electron dense dyes are iontophoresed into lens fibers through glass capillary microelectrodes, the dye substances move readily from one cell to another. More highly diffusive dyes such as Procion yellow move much more readily than dyes such as Procion rubine which contain heavy metals. Gap junctions can be demonstrated between the cells where the movement occurs. No evidence was found for leakage of the dye into the extracellular space. It is concluded that movement of the dye substances must occur from one cell to another through low resistance cell to cell junctions.

ACKNOWLEDGMENT

These studies were supported by a research grant from the U.S.P.H.S. National Eye Institute (EY-01207).

REFERENCES

CHRISTENSEN, B.N. Procion Brown: An Intracellular Dye for Light and Electron Microscopy. *Science* 182: *1255-1256* (1973).

GILULA, N.B. Junctions Between Cells. in Cell Communication, Cox, R.P., Editor. New York, John Wiley & Sons, Inc., p. 1 (1974).

RAE, J.L. & J.E. BLANKENSHIP. Bioelectric Measurements in the Frog Lens. *Exp. Eye Res.* 15: *209* (1973).

RAE, J.L. Discussion of paper, Socolar, S.J., Cell Coupling in Epithelia. *Exp. Eye Res.* 15: *697* (1973).

RAE, J.L. The Movement of Procion Dye in the Crystalline Lens. *Invest. Ophthal.* 13: *147* (1974).

REYNOLDS, E.S. The Use of Lead Citrate at High pH as an Electron Opaque Stain in Electron Microscopy. *J. Cell Biol.* 17: *208* (1963).

STRETTON, A.O.W. & E.A. KRAVITZ. Neuronal Geometry: Determination with a Technique of Intracellular Dye Injection. *Science* 162: *132* (1968).

Keywords: Authors' address:

Crystalline lens   Departments of Ophthalmology and Physiology and Biophysics
Intracellular markers   University of Texas Medical Branch
Iontophoresis   Galveston, Texas, USA

LENS FLUORESCENCE IN AGING AND CATARACT FORMATION

SIDNEY LERMAN, M.D.

(Atlanta, Georgia)

ABSTRACT

The phenomenon of lens fluorescence in aging and cataract formation is reviewed and two specific fluorogens are demonstrated in the normal aging lens. Evidence is presented regarding the role of UV radiation (above 290 nm) in the generation of at least one fluorogen by means of a free radical induced photodegradation reaction involving protein bound tryptophan in the lens (particularly in the nucleus). The fluorogens can serve as aging parameters and are associated with the development of two other aging parameters; the increase in insoluble protein and decline in SH with age. A mechanism is proposed to account for lenticular aging and nuclear (brown) cataract formation as related to the effects of prolonged exposure of the lens to UV radiation above 290 nm.

Lenticular fluorescence was first described well over 100 years ago (REGNAUD, 1858) and has long been utilized by ophthalmic surgeons as an aid in estimating the amount of lens matter remaining in the eye following an extracapsular cataract extraction. Since 1858 sporadic reports have appeared in the literature regarding the nature, origin and function of this phenomenon in which the fluorescence was attributed to a variety of substances including melanin, lipofuscins, pteridines, flavinoids and other pigments. Aside from the controversy regarding the origin and composition of the lens pigment or pigments responsible for lenticular fluorescence, there has also been a considerable amount of speculation regarding the function of this material. WALLS & JUDD (1933) suggested that the yellow pigmentation in the lens might serve as an intraocular filter for blue light which is the wave length of the visible spectrum subject to the greatest dispersion, and WALD (1952) proposed that the lens pigments served to correct for chromatic aberration in the lens.

The last decade has seen a significant resurgence of interest in lens pigments and fluorescence and a considerable amount of confusion relating to this area has now been clarified. This can probably be attributed to the utilization and better understanding of more refined chemical techniques which enable research workers to study fluorescence, fluorescence life time, and phosphorescence in biological compounds and in the whole lens as well (CHEN, 1967; KURZEL et al., 1973a,b; and LERMAN et al., 1975, 1976a,b). The results of these investigations now suggest that a significant amount of lenticular fluorescence and corresponding lens pigmentation derives from one or two possible mechanisms; the most likely mechanism is one in which the lens fluorogen(s) develop by means of a photooxidation process induced by prolonged exposure of the lens to ultraviolet light above 295 nm (between 295 and 380 nm). The action of the ultraviolet light would be on one or more of the aromatic amino acid residues in the lens proteins resulting in the generation of a specific fluorogen(s) tightly bound to at least one peptide within the protein (LERMAN et al., 1970; LERMAN, 1972). Tryptophan is the most likely candidate proposed for this role and a significant amount of evidence has recently accumulated in favor of this hypothesis. A second and much less likely possibility is the development of a free radical induced lipofuscin in a manner somewhat analogous to the aging lipofuscin pigments generated in the internal organs of the body by means of ionizing radiation (TAPPEL, 1973). It is well known that the lipofuscin pigments accumulate in animal tissues particularly in the brain and heart as a function of age. They are considered to be due to lipid peroxidation and the presence of these lipofuscin pigments, which represent chromophoric molecular damage sites, is proposed as evidence of unconfined free radical reactions. Although some research workers have suggested a similar mechanism to explain the presence of the lens pigments (COTLIER & LUECK, 1975), it is generally believed by most workers in this area that the fluorescent pigment(s) in the lens derive from one or more aromatic amino acids. It is also generally agreed that the lens fluorogen(s) are responsible to a significant degree for the increasing yellow coloration of the lens core with age and that their function is to serve as a protective filter with respect to the underlying vitreous and retina (WEALE, 1973; WOLBARSHT, 1976). Thus the increasing accumulation of the lens pigments results in the absorption of ultraviolet light between 300 and 380 nm within the lens thereby preventing this form of radiation from reaching the vitreous and retina. BALAZS, 1960 and TOTH et al., 1962 have presented evidence that exposure of the vitreous to ultraviolet light results in shrinkage of the vitreous gel and denaturation of the collagen network. There is also some evidence that UV absorbing material can be generated in the vitreous exposed to UV at wavelengths shorter than 320 nm (BALAZS et al., 1959). Aside from potential damage resulting from UV light above 300 nm the possibility of retinal damage by UV radiation at 315 nm has also been suggested (ZIGMAN 1971). However, the latter possibility is less likely since there is evidence that exposure of the vitreous to ultraviolet radiation over 300 nm results in the formation of UV absorbant material (BALAZS et al., 1959) and even in specific fluorescent compounds (LERMAN, unpublished data) and the normal aging vitreous also shows a small but significant accumulation of these fluorogens. Aside from its protective function the lens pigment may also play a second role; both the cone and rod pigments have secondary absorption maxima at 325 and 350 nm, respectively (DARTNELL, 1957), thus UV radiation in this region could result in some visual stimulation and possibly produce color confusion. There is evidence that this indeed occurs in aphakic patients (TAN, 1971).

Prior to considering lenticular fluorescence it is important to note that most proteins are endowed with an intrinsic ultraviolet fluorescence because they contain aromatic amino acids (particularly phenylalanine, tyrosine and tryptophan). Of these three aromatic amino acids, phenylalanine has the lowest fluorescence quantum yield as compared with tyrosine and tryptophan (approximately 1/10 to 1/20 of the latter two). Protein fluorescence spectra are thus generally considered with respect to tyrosine and tryptophan. In those proteins where no tryptophan is present (for example, insulin or ribonuclease) it is possible to demonstrate intrinsic tyrosine fluorescence only (Teale, 1960), however, the presence of even one tryptophan residue in a protein (for example, horse serum albumin which has 17 tyrosines and 1 tryptophan) will result in an intrinsic fluorescence essentially that of tryptophan alone. Thus in most proteins containing at least one tryptophan residue, tyrosine appears to have a very low quantum efficiency so that the emission from this residue is markedly overshadowed by tryptophan fluorescence. There are several mechanisms for quenching tyrosine fluorescence in proteins; for example tyrosine-tyrosine energy transfer (WEBER, 1960) and it has been postulated that a non-fluorescent tyrosine could serve as an energy sink for dissipation of excitation energy of other residues, e.g., tryptophan. It is also evident that changes in the secondary and tertiary structure of a protein will result in increased tyrosine fluorescence; TEALE (1961) has demonstrated that urea and detergents markedly increase tyrosine fluorescence of serum albumins. Thus in most tyrosine containing proteins there is a significant quenching of tyrosine fluorescence by a variety of mechanisms including tyrosine-tyrosine energy transfer and the quantum yield of tyrosine fluorescence from proteins such as insulin (which contain no tryptophan) is significantly lower than for pure tyrosine in water. However, tryptophan fluorescence in protein appears to have quantum yields which in some cases are equivalent to those of the free amino acid (TEALE, 1960) and it has also been shown that the tryptophan emission maxima in proteins can vary from 332 to 342 nm depending on the protein. It should be noted that free tryptophan has a characteristic fluorescence emission at approximately 350-360 nm but this shifts to the blue side of the spectrum when tryptophan emission is measured in a protein. In lens proteins and in most other proteins the fluorescence emission of protein bound tryptophan is 332 nm which represents a significant blue shift. KONEV et al. (1965) have proposed that the fluorescence emission of a protein bound tryptophan arises from the singlet state of the indole moiety. There is also some evidence that energy transfer from tryptophan to ionized tyrosine is a pathway for deactivation of the the tryptophan excited state (EDELHOCH et al., 1963, 1967 and COWGILL, 1963). Such energy transfer could occur since ionized tyrosine which has an absorption max of 295 nm (as compared to 278 in the unionized state) overlaps the initial portion of the tryptophan emission band in proteins.

Mammalian lens proteins in general have a considerably higher content of tyrosine as compared to tryptophan (Table 1) but the presence of the tryptophan residues in the proteins results in an intrinsic protein fluorescence due to tryptophan alone (Figure 1). However, it is possible to demonstrate the presence of tyrosine fluorescence in such proteins if one subjects them to ultraviolet radiation for a period of time sufficient to photo-oxidize a significant amount of the tryptophan. This results in the generation of a fluorogen derived as a photo-degradation product from the protein bound tryptophan with an emission maximum shifted significantly towards the red thus unmasking the tyrosine fluorescence emission.

Table I. Amino acid composition of dogfish lens proteins*

Amino acid	α-crys-tallin	β-crys-tallin	γ-crys-tallin	Insoluble Fraction
Lysine	7	7	3.4	4
Histidine	4	5	3.4	3.5
Arginine	11	12	20	14
Aspartic acid	15	14	17	17
Threonine	5	5	3	3.5
Serine	10	10	9	9
Glutamic acid	18	22	15	18
Proline	15	7	10	8
Glycine	8	13.5	12	14
Alanine	5	5	1.3	3.5
Valine	8	4	5	6
Methionine	4	4.3	7	7.4
Isoleucine	7	4.4	5	5.3
Leucine	9	5	2	4.5
Tyrosine	5	10	17	12
Phenylalanine	9	8	9.5	9
Tryptophan	2	3.5	2	3

* Expressed as residues per 20,000 g protein.

FRANCOIS et al. (1961) demonstrated the presence of a fluorescent peptide in primate lenses which could be activated by UV light. The presence of specific fluorescent proteins in the human lens (and other mammalian lenses) has been demonstrated by several investigators (PIRIE, 1968, 1971, 1972; LERMAN et al., 1970, 1971; LERMAN, 1972; VAN HEYNINGEN, 1971, 1973a,b; SATOH et al., 1973; ZIGMAN et al., 1973; DILLEY & PIRIE, 1974; SPECTOR et al., 1975; AUGUSTEYN, 1974, 1975). In addition to the fluorescence due to tryptophan these proteins demonstrate a fluorescence spectrum with an activation wavelength at approximately 340 to 360 nm and an emission at 420 to 440 nm. This type of fluorescence has been shown to be present both in the soluble and insoluble fractions of the human lens, and it increases with age, particularly in the insoluble lens protein fraction. It is generally agreed that this fluorogen (activation 340 to to 360 nm; emission 420 to 440 nm) is tightly bound to at least one or more of the lens proteins and increases in concentration as the lens ages. It is also generally accepted that the increasing yellow coloration of the lens core is due (at least in part) to the presence of one or more fluorogens associated with specific protein fractions of the ocular lens (LERMAN, PIRIE VAN HEYNINGEN, SATOH, SPECTOR, AUGUSTEYN). It has been postulated that this fluorogen could derive from one or more of the aromatic amino acids in the soluble lens proteins by means of a photo-oxidation reaction in which the process would be initiated by prolonged exposure of the lens to ultraviolet light above 295 nm (LERMAN, 1972a,b). While the cornea filters out almost all of the ultraviolet light below 295 nm, the lens is constantly exposed to the longer ultraviolet radiation. It is therefore conceivable that the initiating process in the formation of this fluorogen could be prolonged exposure of the lens to long ultraviolet radiation throughout life; the process being initiated by UV-induced free radical formation.

Ultraviolet light and ionizing radiation are capable of generating free radicals (HENRICKSEN, 1967; BOAG, 1968; COPELAND, 1972). It is accepted by many investigators that aging itself must be due at least in part to

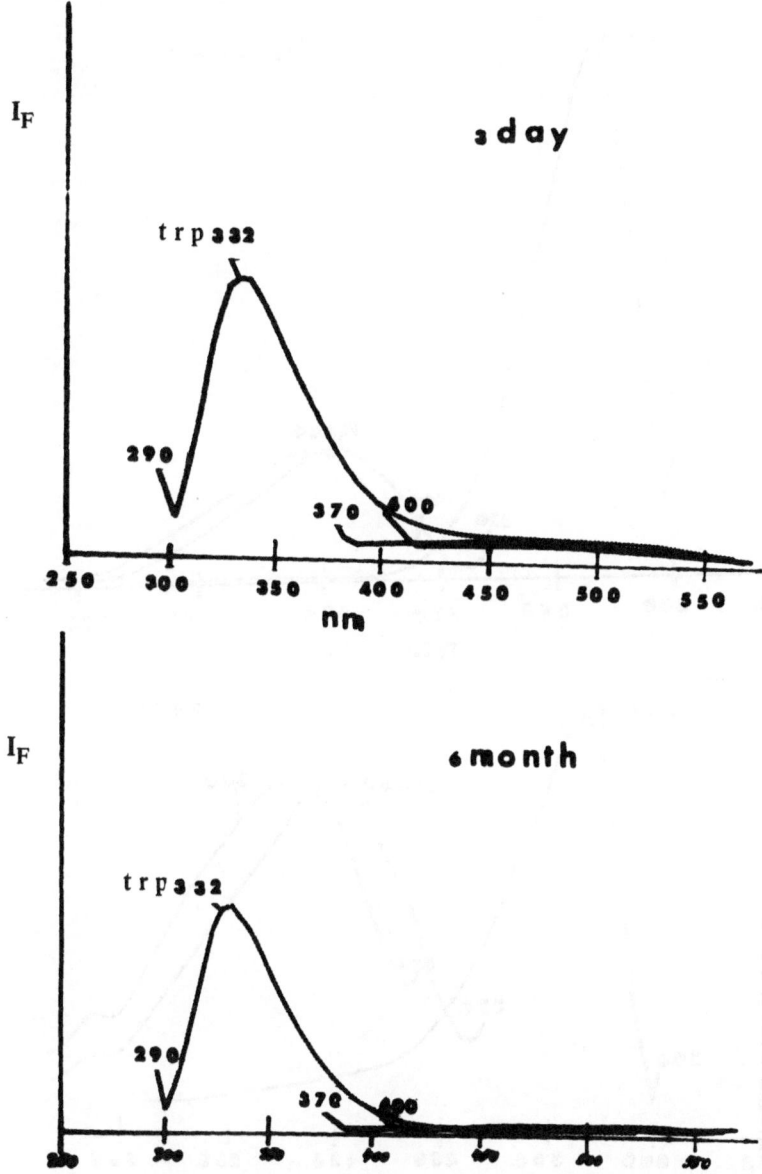

Fig. 1. Fluorescence spectra on 3 day and 6 month old human lenses. Only intrinsic tryptophan (trp 332) fluorescence present (290 nm activation; 332 nm emission). No detectable fluorogen (444 nm emission) even with instrument sensitivity increased from 10^{-6} to 10^{-8} gain. (10^{-6} gain).

damage caused by radical reactions within tissues. An important effect of the induction of a free radical state in a compound by ultraviolet light (or other physical agents) is the fact that the resulting free radicals have considerably altered physical chemical properties leading to an alteration in their function (RUSSELL, 1968). It has also been shown that proteins can

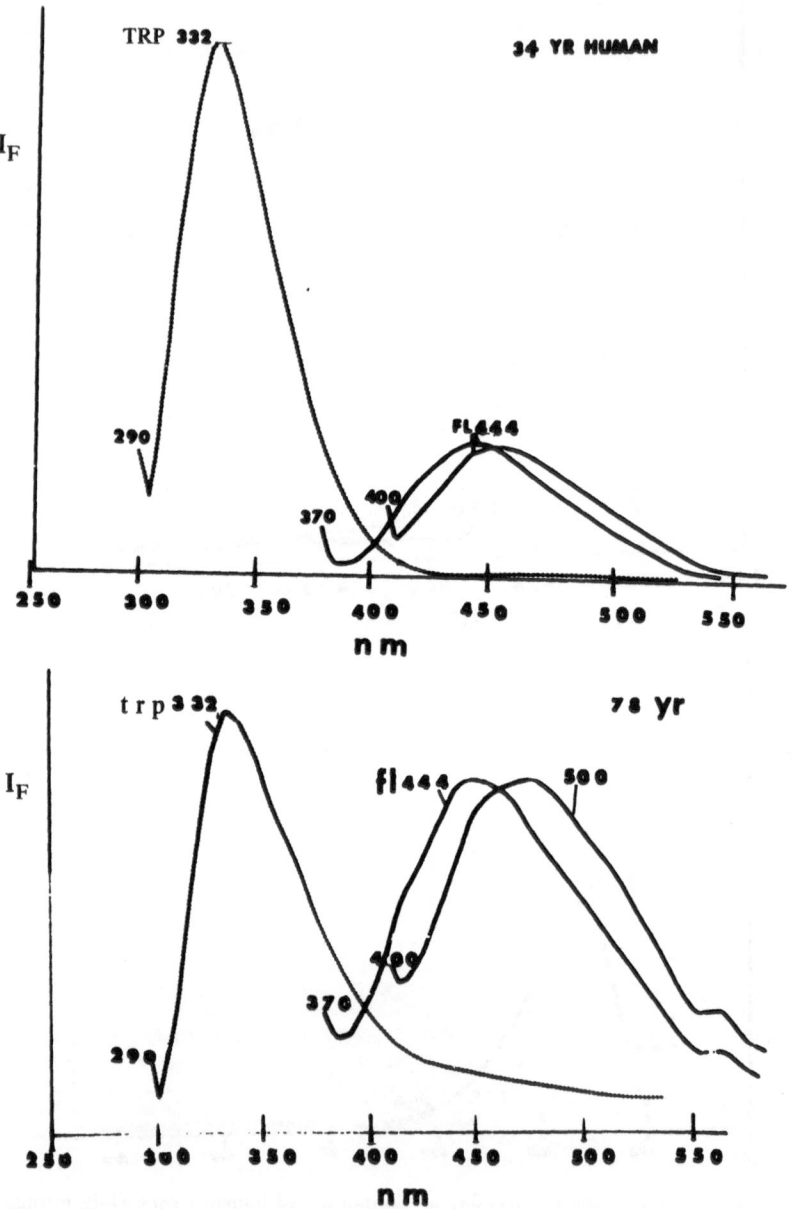

Fig. 2. Fluorescence spectra of normal 34 and 78 year human lenses. Intrinsic tryptophan (trp 332) and fluorogen (fl 444) fluorescence present; latter markedly increased in 78 year as compared with 34 year lens. (10^{-7} gain).

be significantly altered by radical reactions (ZIRLIN, 1969; MEYBECK, 1969; SHIELDS, 1970) with the aromatic amino acid residues in the proteins being particularly susceptible. Thus prolonged exposure of the ocular lens to long UV radiation could result in free radical formation and the generation of one or more fluorogens in increasing concentrations.

The proposal of protein tryptophan depletion via oxidation, resulting in protein pigmentation (KURZEL et al., 1973a) correlates with our findings regarding the inverse relationship between tryptophan fluorescence intensity and fluorogen emission intensity in the whole lens (LERMAN et al., 1976a,b; BORKMAN et al., 1976). Previous studies in our Laboratory have demonstrated an in vitro and in vivo induction and acceleration of the fluorogen in the ocular lens of the mouse, rat and human species (LERMAN, 1975; LERMAN et al., 1976a,b). Studies on normal human lenses ranging in age from 6 months fetal material to 90 years of age have demonstrated that this fluorogen is not present to any significant extent within the first year of life but then becomes manifest and increases in emission intensity with age as shown in Figure 2. This progressive increase in the fluorogen is paralleled by a similar increase in the relative concentration of the insoluble fraction with age (Figure 3). A similar relationship exists in the rat

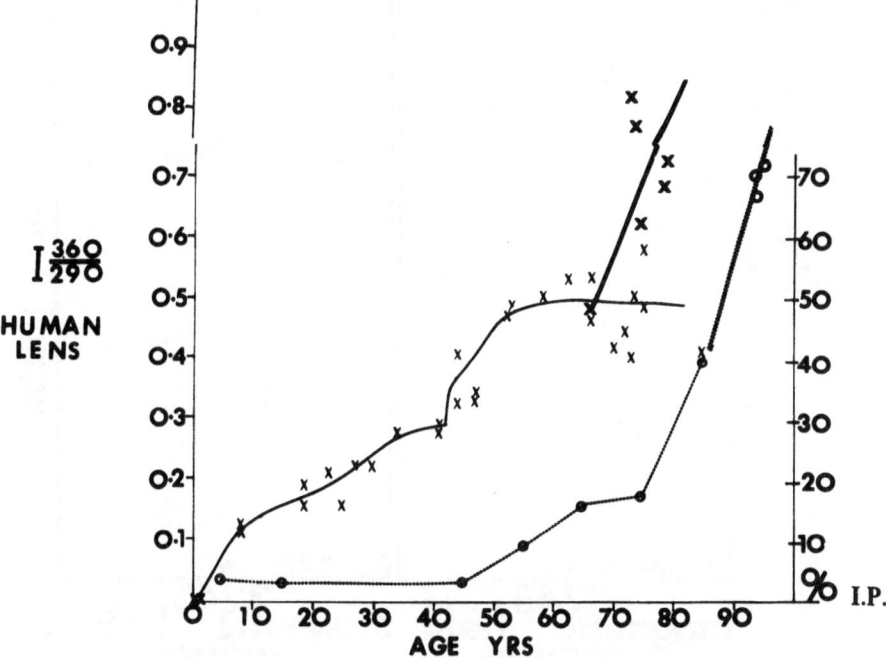

Fig. 3. $I\frac{360}{290}$ ratios in normal human lenses (solid line) and in nuclear cataracts (heavy solin line) compared with relative percent of insoluble lens protein (% I.P.) in comparably aged lenses. $I\frac{360}{290}$ ratio refers to emission intensity of the fluorogen activated at 360 nm over the emission intensity of the intrinsic protein bound tryptophan activated at 290 nm.

and mouse lens. In vitro studies with lens incubates (mouse, rat and human lenses) have demonstrated that this fluorogen can be induced and/or markedly accelerated in lens incubation systems in which the lenses are exposed to 3-amino-triazole (AT) and ultraviolet radiation (LERMAN et al., 1976a,b). AT is a catalase (peroxidase) inhibitor, thus more glutathione is being used up by the lens and a significant decrease in the concentration of glutathione in lenses incubated with AT has been demonstrated (BHUYAN et al., 1973, 1974, 1975; KUCK, 1974). The resultant depletion of an important free radical scavenger in the lens increases its sensitivity to UV radiation, thereby accelerating the photo-induced fluorogen formation.

Action spectra performed on 4 to 6 hour in vitro lens incubation systems (exposed to UV and AT) have demonstrated that tryptophan depletion

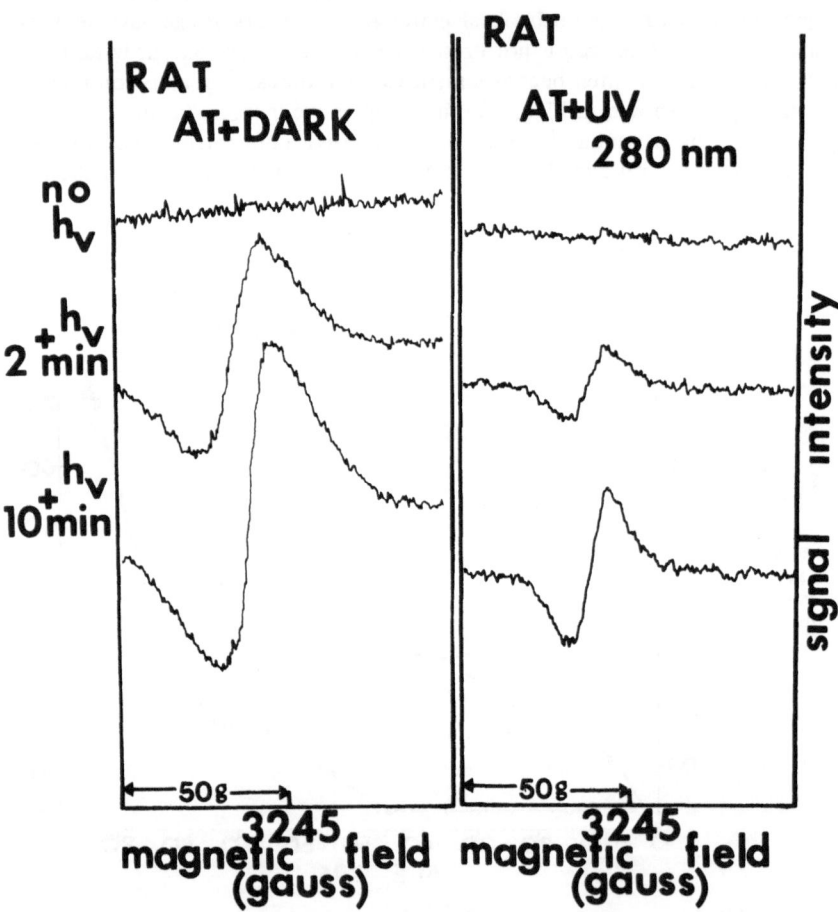

Fig. 4. EPR spectra of normal rat (a) and human (b) lenses showing growth of tryptophan free radical after 2 and 10 minute exposure to UV light compared with marked decrease in signal intensity in contralateral lenses which had previously been incubated in a culture medium containing 3-aminotriazole (AT) and exposed to UV light (280 or 300 nm) for 6 hrs. EPR spectroscopy performed at 75 milliwatts power, 77 °K, 500 g sweep at 2.5 minutes, 0.1 time constant.

occurs specifically with the generation of the fluorogen (BORKMAN et al., 1976). A plot of the rate of fluorogen production (normalized to constant photon flux) versus irradiation wavelength showed relatively little action at 360, 340 and 320 nm but the action increased sharply at 300 nm and remained constant at 290 and 280 nm. This indicates that the fluorogen is generated photo-chemically with tryptophan as the prime UV light absorbing species and this conclusion is supported by the observation that the photo-chemical production of fluorogen is accompanied by a decrease in tryptophan fluorescence. Similar results have been obtained with mouse lenses and young human lenses (BORKMAN et al., 1976).

Furthermore, EPR spectra on whole rat and mouse lenses and on the nuclear core from human lenses demonstrate that a significant tryptophan free radical can be demonstrated in the normal rat and human lens (Figure 4) after 10 minutes irradiation with ultraviolet light, but a marked decrease in the signal is noted in those lenses which had been previously exposed to UV plus AT for at least 4-6 hours (Figure 4).

There is also a direct relationship between the signal intensity of the UV induced tryptophan free radical and the age of the human lens. The highest intensity is seen in the young lens and the signal decreases significantly with

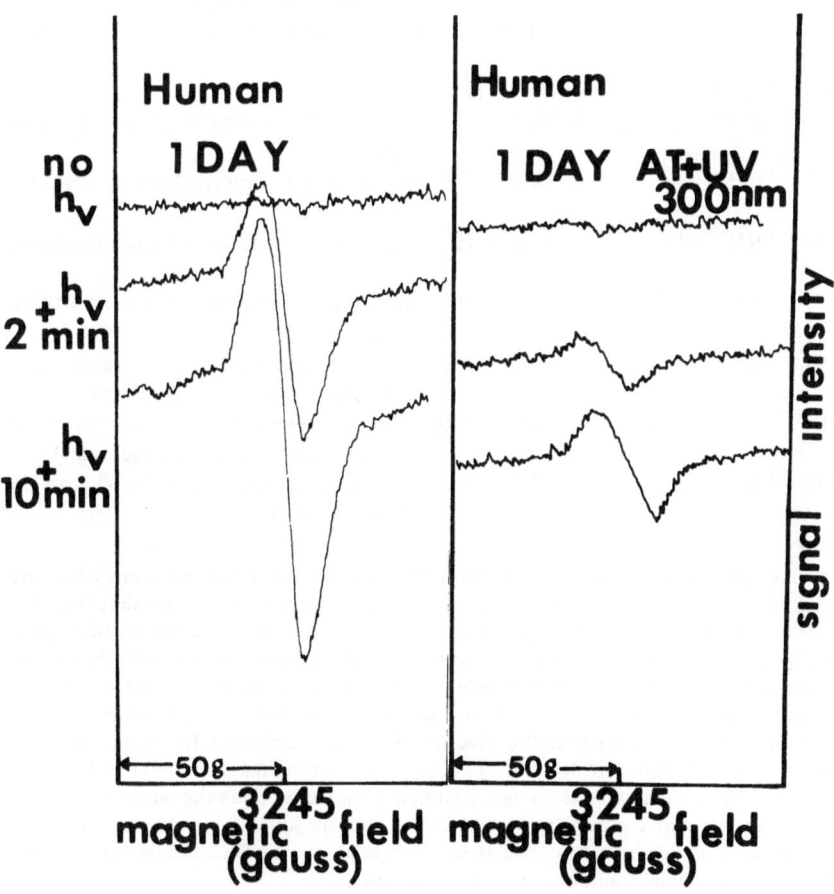

age, particularly after the fifth or sixth decade (LERMAN et al., 1976c; LERMAN & BORKMAN, 1976). This correlates with the evidence previously cited that tryptophan depletion is associated with fluorogen generation as aging proceeds (the fluorogen being generated as a UV induced photo-degradation product of tryptophan). The specific site of the UV induced action thus appears to be on one or more protein bound tryptophan residues in which a photo-chemical degradation occurs. That is, tryptophan is elevated to an excited state by absorbing UV energy (over a wavelength range between 280 to 315 nm) and its energy must be dissipated. This can occur by one or more routes as demonstrated by FEITELSON (1971) in the following manner. Since the indole ring of tryptophan is the portion subject to photo-chemical attack one can utilize FEITELSON's scheme in which RH denotes the indole chromophore.

1) $RH + h\nu_{abs} \longrightarrow {}^1RH^*$ (denotes the excited singlet state of indole)***

2) ${}^1RH^* \longrightarrow RH + h\nu_{fl}$ (dissipation of energy by fluorescing at a higher wavelength)

3) ${}^1RH^* \longrightarrow {}^3RH^*$ (intersystem crossing to form the triplet state)

4) ${}^3RH^* \longrightarrow RH + h\nu_p$ (phosphorence)

5) ${}^3RH^* \longrightarrow RH$ (intersystem crossing to the ground state)

6) ${}^1RH^* \longrightarrow RH$ (radiationless deactivation by internal conversion)

7) ${}^1RH^* + H^+ \longrightarrow RH^+ + H$ (hydrogen abstraction from the singlet state)

8) ${}^3RH^* + H^+ \longrightarrow RH^+ + H$ (hydrogen abstraction from the triplet state)

9) ${}^1RH^* \longrightarrow RH^+ + e^-aq$ (electron ejection from singlet state – formation of solvated electron)

10) ${}^3RH^* \longrightarrow RH^+ + e^-aq$ (electron ejection from triplet state – formation of solvated electron)

11) ${}^1RH^* + Q \longrightarrow RH + Q$ (fluorescence quenching by Q; can be O_2 or H^+ etc)

*** A molecule is defined as a singlet if it has an even number of electrons which are all arranged in pairs with opposite spins. The term spins denotes the fact that electrons have a magnetic moment and can point up or point down (this property is called spin). A triplet is a molecule in which one pair (of its even number of electrons) have parallel spins. A molecule with an odd number of electrons must have one electron with an unpaired spin. This molecule is called a radical. The magnetic properties of this odd electron can be measured in the Electron Spin (paramagnetic) Resonance Spectrometer. This technique involves the application of a strong magnetic field to the compound being studied and the energy absorbed is measured when the odd electrons flip their spins so that they are now pointing in opposite directions. One measures the amplitude of the energy peaks and their location at specific field strenghts to identify the nature and relative amount of the radical present.

The foregoing scheme suggests a number of possibilities regarding the nature of the excited state and specific mechanisms involved in the photo-degradation of tryptophan when this molecule absorbs ultraviolet light. However, studies on the photoinactivation of proteins by several investigators (KONEV & VOLOTOVSKII, 1966; FEITELSON, 1971) have demonstrated that the primary processes are due mainly to the singlet excited state of tryptophan. The singlet state can dissipate energy by several routes. It can undergo photochemical reaction either directly or by intersystem crossing to the triplet state. WEITER & FINCH (1975) have demonstrated the tryptophan triplet in UV exposed human lens material (as well as the tryptophan free radical). This excited triplet state may be dissipated by a photochemical reaction which ultimately generates fluorogens, by intersystem crossing to the ground singlet state as suggested by KURZEL et al. (1973) or by other routes. Thus the effect of UV light (of specific wavelength) on the lens is to generate the excited singlet state of tryptophan either directly or via intersystem crossing to the triplet state. The photo-chemical degradation is initiated by the photo-ionization of the excited tryptophan molecule and results in cleavage of the indole ring at the C^2-C^3 position. Laser flash photolysis experiments on aqueous tryptophan have recently shown that UV degradation of aqueous tryptophan occurs via such a photo-ionization mechanism (BRYANT et al., 1975).

Previous experiments in our Laboratory have indicated that the UV-induced fluorogen is one that is tightly bound to the lens protein and has a molecular weight of approximately 300 (LERMAN, 1962; LERMAN et al., 1976c). It is postulated that the photo-chemical degradation of tryptophan could result in the generation of a condensation product of anthranilic acid resulting in the formation of a tricyclic compound (m.w. $<$ 300, e.g. phenoxazine or β carbolene) with fluorescence and UV spectra identical to those previously reported (LERMAN, 1972a,b).

Aside from an increase in the yellow color of the lens core as it ages, the mechanism whereby this fluorogen is induced could result in a process of polymerization and insolubilization of the previously soluble lens protein fractions (LERMAN, 1972a,b; ÁUGUSTEYN, 1974, 1975; PIRIE, 1972; SATOH et al., 1973; WEITER & FINCH, 1975). ORD and CD studies on alpha and gamma crystallin derived from several species (LI & SPECTOR, 1967; JONES & LERMAN, 1971) have indicated that these proteins contain no alpha helical structure and are mainly in the beta configuration with some degree of random coil also present. More recent reports utilizing Lasar Raman Spectroscopy have confirmed that the lens proteins are mainly in an anti-parallel beta-pleated configuration both in protein extracts and in the whole lens (YU & EAST, 1975: SCHACHER & SOLIN, 1975). This type of protein configuration would be amenable with the proposed mechanism involving the polymerization and insolubilization of lens proteins with age based on the photo-degradation of tryptophan as well as disulfide bond formation. Furthermore, Raman spectroscopy does not reveal any changes in the secondary structure of the proteins in lenses exposed to UV and AT for varying periods of time (LERMAN et al., 1976c) although there appears to be an increase in SS bonds with a corresponding fall in SH bonds in the nuclear portion of such lenses. There is a significant increase in SS formation in ultraviolet exposed lenses both in vitro and in vivo with a concomitant decline in SH levels as measured by means of Raman spectroscopy and similar results have been noted in the aging lens. These observations regarding SH and SS levels correlate with previous reports regarding a decrease in SH and an increase in SS with aging and following exposure of the lens to ionizing radiation (KINOSHITA & MEROLA, 1958; LERMAN et al., 1966, 1967; LERMAN, 1967, 1972b; CLARK et al., 1969; FORBES & HAMLIN, 1969).

Table II. Age-related changes in the concentration of lens proteins

	Normal Human Lenses	
Age (years)	Soluble protein as % of total	Insoluble protein as % of total
0 to 9	96.7	3.3
10 to 19	97.1	2.9
40 to 49	96.7	3.3
50 to 59	90.9	9.1
60 to 69	84.3	15.7
70 to 79	82.6	17.4
80 to 89	60.1	39.9
Brunescent and nigricant cataract		
75 to 90	29.0	71.0
	Rat Lenses	
At birth	95	5
35 days	88	12
42 to 45 days	87	13
70 days	80	20
365 days	64	36
3 years	43	57

Table III. Age-related changes in the concentration of α-, β- and γ-crystallins*

Species and age	α-crys-tallin (%)	β-crys-tallin (%)	γ-crys-tallin (%)
Human			
10 to 19 years	37	38	25
60 to 69 years	55	33.6	11.4
80 to 89 years	57.6	33.7	8.7
Rat			
5 to 6 weeks	20	20	60
6 months	38	42	20
11 months	41	46	13

* Concentration expressed as percentage of total soluble proteins.

CONCLUSIONS

The preceding discussion has demonstrated that fluorescence spectroscopy can be utilized to measure an aging parameter in the lens, and that the major fluorescent compound appears to be derived from tryptophan on the basis of prolonged exposure of the lens to ultraviolet light above 295 nm. This fluorogen which has an activation peak at 340 to 360 nm and an emission peak at 420 to 440 nm is definitely age related as is the increase in the water insoluble proteins (Tables II and III) and the decline in SH and concomitant increase in the level of SS bonds (Table IV-VI). The age related increase in fluorogen concentration enhances the yellowing of the lens core and accompanies polymerization of the soluble protein precursors into the insoluble protein fraction. There is also a progressive fall in SH levels (with age or UV exposure) and an increase in SS bonds without any significant alteration in the secondary configuration of the lens proteins which remain mainly in the anti-parallel beta-pleated configuration. It is postulated that ultraviolet radiation above 295 nm plays a significant role in lenticular aging, particu-

Table IV. Sulfhydryl values for soluble protein fractions (μmoles/g protein)

Material	Soluble fractions		
	α-crys-tallin	β-crys-tallin	γ-crys-tallin
Human			
Normal (0-10 years)	35	40	128
Normal (60-69)	58	47	76
Cataractous (80-89)	47	42	78
Rat			
5 weeks			
6 months	25	34	154
11 months			78
5 week old rat			53
exposed to 1,500 r			40

Table V. SH and SS content of protein fractions in the rat lens*

Protein Fractions	SH	SS
	moles/20,000 gm.	protein
α-crystallin (old)	0.43	0.32
β-crystallin (old)	0.74	0.77
γ-crystallin (young, 3-5 wks)	3.17	1.85
γ-crystallin (1 yr. old)	1.03	2.88
Insoluble protein (1 yr. old)	1.04	2.68

* Average of five determinations.

Table VI.   Rat lens glutathione*.

	Av. Lens Wt.	Whole Lens (mg%)	Cortex (mg%)	Nucleus (mg%)
Young Rat	25.3 mg	156 ± 7	277 ± 33	71.7 ± 7.7
Old Rat	53.0 mg	114 ± 5	204 ± 23	36.8 ± 6.3

*Courtesy J.F. KUCK Jr.

larly nuclear sclerosis and its extreme state characterized by the brunescent cataract. Preliminary experiments in our Laboratory also indicate that a second fluorescence activation and emission peak develops in the lens as it ages (approximately 420-435 activation and 500-520 nm emission) and becomes particularly pronounced (an increase of 2-3 fold) in the brunescent cataract (Figure 5). It is still not clearly defined whether this second fluorescence emission peak is characteristic of a separate fluorogen species or derives from the previously discussed fluorogen (320-340 nm activation, 420-440 nm emission). In contrast with the aging changes and the nuclear and brunescent cataract formation, lenticular fluorescence does not appear to play a role in cortical cataracts. Fluorescence and EPR spectra performed on a variety of cortical cataracts do not demonstrate any change in the level of the fluorogen or the intensity of the tryptophan free radical compared to a normal lens of the same age. The fluorescence spectra do, however, show a marked degree of light scattering in comparison with spectra obtained from normal and/or nuclear cataracts. While the nuclear cataract appears to be an accelerated form of the normal aging process of the lens in which the visual reduction is mainly due to the increased coloration of the lens and perhaps to protein polymerization forming less soluble high molecular weight aggregates and in which at least the secondary protein configuration remains relatively unchanged, it is likely that the cortical opacities are derived by means of a different mechanism. In the latter case it is postulated that localized alterations in protein configuration could play a significant role in the pathogenesis of these opacities.

It is interesting to note that avian lenses differ significantly from mammialian lenses with respect to several aging parameters. These include a difference in the lens protein fractions in the birds as compared to those found in the mammalian lens particularly with respect to the absence of gamma crystallin and a relative lack of the water insolbule protein fraction in the avian lens as it ages. An increase in the size of the lens nucleus and nuclear sclerosis which are concomitant of the aging process in the mammalian lens does not occur in the bird lens. We have also been unable to demonstrate fluorogens similar to those present in the mammalian lens in a variety of avian lenses including lenses derived from young chickens and from pigeons of various age groups. Furthermore, in vitro lens incubation experiments similar to the ones previously described were also performed and no fluorogen could be generated in such incubations. Aside from the relative lack of the so-called insoluble protein fraction in avian lenses, Raman spectroscopy indicates that at least some bird lenses contain a significant amount of alpha helical configuration in contrast with mammalian

254

lenses in which the lens proteins are mainly in the beta-pleated configuration (YU, 1976, personal communication). Thus, the inability to demonstrate a fluorogen in certain avian lenses as well as inability to generate such a fluorogen in incubation systems identical to those utilized for the mammalian lenses correlates with the observation that there is a significant difference with respect to certain aging parameters in the bird as compared to the mammalian lens (particularly the lens fluorogens, the insoluble proteins, and protein configuration).

Aside from the direct damage by ultraviolet radiation to the ocular lens there is also the possibility of lenticular damage by means of photosensitized reactions involving such drugs as the phentothiazines (chlorpromazine) and particularly the psoralens.

It is generally accepted that the most likely mechanism involving the photosensitization reaction of psoralens and other photosensitizing mole-

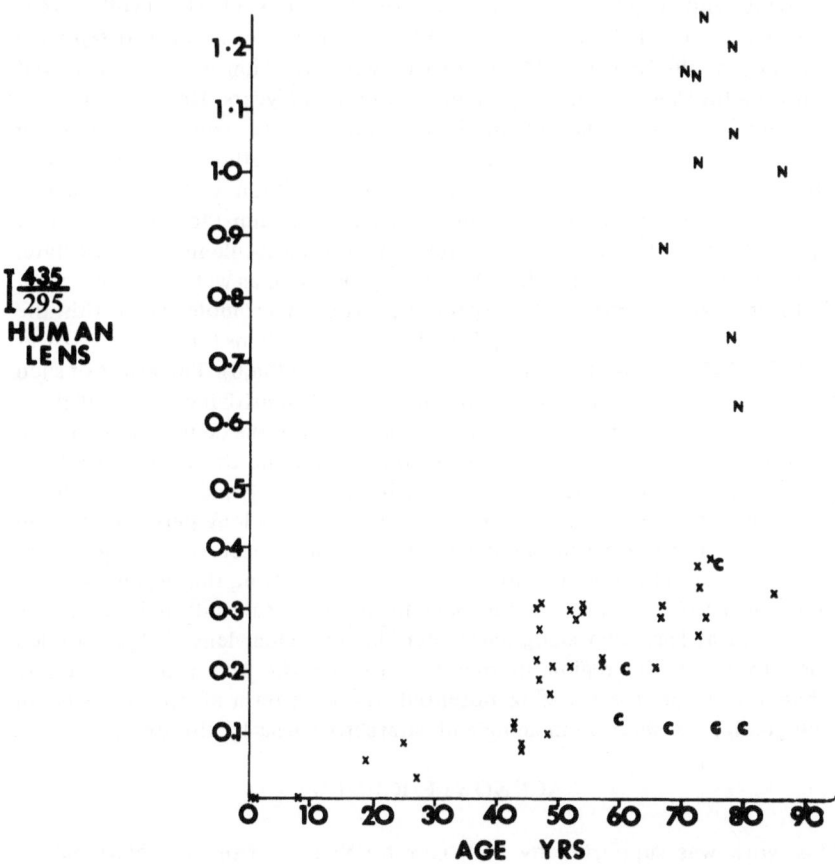

Fig. 5. $I\frac{435}{295}$ ratios of normal human lenses (x), cortical cataracts (c) and nuclear cataracts (N). Ratio refers to the emission intensity of the fluorogen activated at 435 nm over the emission intensity of intrinsic protein bound tryptophan activated at 295 nm.

255

cules, upon exposure to UV radiation above 310-320 nm involves internal electronic transition of the metastable triplet state resulting in the formation of free radicals (FOWLKS, 1959; OGINSKY et al., 1959; PATHAK, 1962; PATHAK et al. 1961, 1965, 1967). Such free radicals had been noted in human lens following radiation with UV light between 290 and 320 nm (WEITER & FINCH, 1975; LERMAN et al., 1968, 1976c). The psoralens have also been shown to form loose complexes with the pyrimidine basis of DNA and RNA (WALTER et al., 1973) and exposure to longer wave UV radiation (300-400 nm) results in a photo-oxidation reaction with the eventual occurrence of intrastrand cross linkages between the nucleic acids.

Since 1947 when the psoralens were introduced as a method for treating vitiligo (EL MOFTY, 1948) and more recently for treating psoriasis, there has been sporadic interest as to the potential relationship between psoralens and cataract formation. Although some reports have appeared in the literature regarding the experimental production of cataracts in animals given psoralens and exposed to UV radiation (CLOUD et al., 1960, 1961; CLARK, 1961; FREEMAN, 1966), FITZPATRICK et al. (1966) reported that they could find no evidence of cataract formation in patients treated with 8-methoxy-psoralen for periods as long as 12 years. However, the current therapy of psoriasis utilizing the psoralens in doses ranging up to 80 mg per day could be a potential hazard to the lens. 8-methoxy-psoralen has an ultraviolet absorption peak of approximately 248 nm and 305 nm and a fluorescence emission peak at approximately 510 nm (activation max at approximately 320 nm). This data refers to the molecule in its native state. There is also some evidence that 8-methoxy psoralen as well as certain other photosensitizing agents bind to specific areas of macromolecules within the body tissues such as DNA, and probably certain proteins (DALL'ACQUA et al., 1970, 1974; BEN-HUR & ELKIND, 1972a,b, 1973a,b). The result of such binding is an enhanced potentiation of the photosensitizing action of these drugs. Thus the danger of the psoralens with respect to the ocular lens is at least two-fold. The drug can and probably does enter the ocular lens from the general circulation (albeit in very small quantities) and could exert its photosensitizing effect as it slowly accumulates over a long period of time in addition to the normal ultraviolet induced changes occurring in the ocular lens as it ages. This could result in a cumulative action; that is, an enhancement and acceleration of the photochemical processes resulting in the development of at least two aging parameters in the ocular lens. If the psoralen binds to a specific region in one or more of the lens proteins thereby enhancing its photosensitizing potential, the long term effect would be an even greater acceleration in aging and cataractogenesis by this drug.

ACKNOWLEDGEMENT

This work was supported by PHS Grant EY01575 from the National Institutes of Health.

REFERENCES

AUGUSTEYN, R.C. Distribution of fluorescence in the human cataractous lens. *Ophth. Res. 7: 217-224* (1975).

AUGUSTEYN, R.C. Human lens albuminoid. *Jap. J. Ophth.* 18: *127-134* (1974).

BALAZS, E.A. Physiology of the vitreous body. In: Proceedings of the Second Conference of the Retinal Foundation. (C.L. Schepens, ed.). C.V. Mosby, St. Louis, p. 29-47 (1960).

BALAZS, E.A., LAURENT, T.C., HOWE, A.F. & VARGO, L. Irradiation of mucopolysaccharides with ultraviolet light and electrons. *Radiat. Res.* 11: *149-164* (1959).

BEN-HUR, E. & ELKIND, M.M. Damage and repair of DNA in 5-bromodeoxyuridine-labeled Chinese hamster cells exposed to fluorescent light. *Biophys. J.* 12: *636-647* (1972a).

BEN-HUR, E. & ELKIND, M.M. Survival response of asynchronous and synchronous Chinese hamster cells exposed to fluorescent light following 5-bromodeoxyuridine incorporation. *Mutation Res.* 14: *237-245* (1972b).

BEN-HUR, E. & ELKIND, M.M. DNA cross-linking in Chinese hamster cells exposed to near ultraviolet light in the presence of 4,5',8-trimethylpsoralen. *Biochim. Biophys. Acta.* 331: *181-193* (1973a).

BEN-HUR, E. & ELKIND, M.M. Psoralen plus near ultraviolet light inactivation of cultured chinese hamster cells and its relation to DNA links. *Mutation Res.* 18: *315-324* (1973b).

BHUYAN, D.K. & BHUYAN, K.C. Regulation of hydrogen peroxide levels in eye humors. *IRCS Med. Sci.* 3: *415* (1975).

BHUYAN, K.C., BHUYAN, D.K. & KATZIN, H.M. Amizol induced cataract and inhibition of lens catalase in rabbit. *Ophth. Res.* 5: *236-247* (1973).

BHUYAN, K.C., BHUYAN, D.K. & TURTZ, A. Aminotriazole-effect on the ocular tissue in rabbit. *IRCS Med. Sci.* 2: *1594* (1974).

BOAG, J.W. Overlapping effects of ultraviolet and ionizing radiations. *Brit. J. Radiol.* 41: *879-881* (1968).

BORKMAN, R.F., DALRYMPLE, A. & LERMAN, S. Ultraviolet action spectrum for production of a fluorogen in the ocular lens. (abstract) ARVO annual meeting (1976).

BRYANT, F.D., SANTUS, R. & GROSSWEINER, L.I. Laser flash photolysis of aqueous tryptophan. *J. Phys. Chem.* 79: *2711-2716* (1975).

CHEN, R.F. Extrinsic and Intrinsic Fluorescence in the Study of Protein Structure: A Review in Fluorescence, Theory, Instrumentation, and Practice. (George C. Guilbault, ed.). Marcel Dekker Inc., New York, pp. 443-499 (1967).

CLARK, J.H. (1961). Photosensitization by 8-methoxypsoralen. *J. Invest. Derm.* 37: *171-174* (1961).

CLARK, R., ZIGMAN, S. & LERMAN, S. Studies on the structural proteins of the human lens. *Exp. Eye Res.* 8: *172-182* (1969).

CLOUD, T.M., HAKIM, R. & GRIFFIN, A.C. Photosensitization of the eye with methoxsalen. *Arch. Ophthal.* 64: *346-351* (1960).

CLOUD, T.M., HAKIM, R. & GRIFFIN, A.C. Photosensitization of the eye with methoxsalen. II. Chronic effects. *Arch. Ophthal.* 66: *689-694* (1961).

COPELAND, E.S. Electron spin resonance studies in radiation biology. In: Biological Application of Electron Spin Resonance. (H.M. Swartz, J.R. Bolton & D.C. Borg, eds.). Wiley-Interscience, New York, p. 449 (1972).

COTLIER, E. & LUECK, K. Lipid fluorescent pigments of human lens and senile cataract. A ceroid pigment theory. (abstract) ARVO annual meeting, p. 84 (1975).

COWGILL, R.W. Fluorescence and the structure of proteins. II. Fluorescence of peptides containing tryptophan or tyrosine. *Biochim. Biophys. Acta.* 75: *272-273* (1963).

DALL'ACQUA, F., MARCIANI, S. & RODIGHIERO, G. Inter-strand cross-linkages occurring in the photoreaction between psoralen and DNA. *FEBS letters* 9: *121-123* (1970).

DALL'ACQUA, F., MARCIANI, S., VEDALDI, D. & RODIGHIERO, G. Studies on the photoreactions (365 nm) between DNA and some methylpsoralens. *Biochim. Biophys. Acta.*, 353: *267-273* (1974).

DARTNALL, H.J.A. The Visual Pigments. Methuen & Co., Ltd., London, New York (1957).

DILLEY, K.J. & PIRIE, A. Changes to the proteins of the human lens nucleus in cataract. *Exp. Eye Res.* 19: *59-72* (1974).

EDELHOCH, H., BRAND, L. & WILCHEK, M. Fluorescence studies with tryptophyl peptides. *Biochemistry* 6: *547-559* (1967).

EDELHOCH, H., BRAND, L. & WILCHEK, M. *Israel J. Chem.* 1: *216* (1963).

EL MOFTY, A.M. Preliminary clinical report on treatment of leucodermia with Ammi majus Linn. *J. Roy. Egyptian M.A.*, 31: *651-665* (1948).

FEITELSON, J. The formation of hydrated electrons from the excited state of indole derivatives. *Photochem. & Photobiol.* 13: *87-96* (1971).

FITZPATRICK, T.B., ARNDT, K.A., EL MOFTY, A.M. & PATHAK, M.A. Hydroquinone and psoralens in the therapy of hypermelanosis and vitiligo. *Arch. Derm.* 93: *589-600* (1966).

FORBES, W.F. & HAMLIN, C.R. Determination of SH and SS groups in proteins – the age dependence of SH and SS contents in the soluble protein fractions of the eye lens. *Exp. Geront.* 4: *151-158* (1969).

FOWLKS, W.L. The mechanism of the photodynamic effect. *J. Invest. Derm.* 32: *233-247* (1959).

FRANCOIS, J., RABAEY, M. & RECOULES, N. A fluorescent substance of low molecular weight in the lens of primates. *Arch. Ophth.* 65: *118-126* (1961).

FREEMAN, R.G. Morphologic changes resulting from photosensitization of the eye with 8-methoxypsoralen – a comparison with ultraviolet injury. *Texas Reports on Biol. and Med.* 24: *588-596* (1966).

HENRICKSEN, T. Effect of oxygen on radiation-induced free radicals in proteins. *Radiation Res.*, 32: *892-904* (1967).

JONES, H.A. & LERMAN, S. Optical rotatory dispersion and circular dichroism on ocular lens proteins. *Can. J. Biochem.* 49: *426-430* (1971).

KINOSHITA, J.H. & MEROLA, L. The distribution of glutathione and protein sulfhydryl groups in calf and cattle lenses. *Amer. J. Ophth.* 46: *36-42* (1958).

KONEV, S.V. & VOLOTOVSKII, I.D. Investigation of the role of singlet and triplet excited states of tryptophan in the photoinactivation of trypsin. *Biofizika* 11, (5): *791-795* (1966).

KONEV, S.V., BOBROVICH, V.P. & CHERNITSKII, E.A. Boliarizatsionnye spektry fluorestsentsii belkov po ipuskaniiu i vozmozhnost' mezhtriptofanovoi migratsil energil. *Biofizika* 10: *42-47* (1965).

KUCK, J.F. Effect of long wave ultraviolet light on the lens in vitro with 3'aminotriazole (abstract). ARVO annual meeting. p. 84 (1974).

KURZEL, R., WOLBARSHT, M.L., YAMANASHI, B.S., STATON, G.W. & BORKMAN, R.F. Tryptophan excited states and cataracts in the human lens. *Nature* 241: *132-133* (1973a).

KURZEL, R., WOLBARSHT, M.L. & YAMANASHI, B.S. Spectral studies on normal and cataractous intact human lenses. *Exp. Eye Res.* 17: *65-71* (1973b).

LERMAN, S., FORBES, W.F., ZIGMAN, S. & KIRMAN, J. A study on gamma crystalline derived from the rat and dogfish lens. Biochem. of the Eye, Symp. XX, International Congress of Ophthalmology. Munich, 1966. Karger/Basel/New York, pp. 292-300 (1966).

LERMAN, S. The structural proteins of the ocular lens. *Survey Ophth.* 12: *112-129* (1967).

LERMAN, S., FORBES, W.F. & ZIGMAN, S. The effect of aging irradiation on the thiol content of the soluble lens proteins. *Invest. Ophth.* 6: *552-553* (1967).

258

LERMAN, S., TAN, A.T., LOUIS, D. & HOLLANDER, M. Anomalous absorptivity of lens proteins due to a fluorogen. *Ophth. Res.* 1: *338-343* (1970).

LERMAN, S., LOUIS, D. & HOLLANDER, M. Characterization of a fluorogen in the ocular lens. *Can. J. Ophth.* 6: *148-152* (1971).

LERMAN, S. Lens proteins and fluorescence. *Israel J. Med. Sci.* 8: *1583-1589* (1972a).

LERMAN, S. Lens Proteins in Aging and Cataract Formation. In: Contemporary Ophthalmology. (J. Bellows, ed.), p. 476-493 (1972b).

LERMAN, S., KUCK, J.F., BORKMAN, R. & SAKER, E. Fluorescence spectroscopy of the aging human lens. (abstract). ARVO annual meeting p. 84 (1975).

LERMAN, S. & BORKMAN, R.F. Spectroscopic evaluations on the normal lens and cortical and nuclear cataracts. *Ophth. Res.*, 8: *558-561* (1976).

LERMAN, S., KUCK, J.F., BORKMAN, R. & SAKER, E. Induction of an aging parameter (fluorogen) in the ocular lens. *Ann. Ophth. 8:* 558-561 (1976a).

LERMAN, S., KUCK, J.F., BORKMAN, R. & SAKER, E. Induction, acceleration, and prevention (in vitro) of an aging parameter in the ocular lens. *Ophth. Res.*, in press (1976b).

LERMAN, S., BORKMAN, R.F., YU, N.T., KUCK, J.F. & SAKER, E. Spectroscopic studies on normal and ultraviolet accelerated aging in the lens. (abstract). ARVO annual meeting (1976c).

LI, L.K. & SPECTOR, A. The optical rotary dispersion and circular dichroism of calf lens alpha-crystallin. *J. Biol. Chem.* 242: *3234-3236* (1967).

MEYBECK, A. & WINDLE, J.J. Electron paramagnetic resonance study of x-ray and gamma-ray irradiated peptides in the solid state. *Radiation Res.* 40: *263-275* (1969).

OGINSKY, E.L., GREEN, G.S., GRIFFITH, D.G. & FOWLKS, W.L. Lethal photosensitization of bacteria with 8-methoxypsoralen to long wave length ultraviolet radiation. *J. Bact.* 78: *821-833* (1959).

PATHAK, M.A., ALLEN, B., INGRAM, D.J.E. & FELLMAN, J.H. Photosensitization and the effect of ultraviolet radiation on the production of unpaired electrons in the presence of furocoumarins (psoralens). *Biochim. Biophys. Acta.* 54: *506-515* (1961).

PATHAK, M.A., DANIELS, F. & FITZPATRICK, T.B. The presently known distribution of furocoumarins (psoralens) in plants. *J. Invest. Derm.* 39: *225-239* (1962).

PATHAK, M.A. & STRATTON, K. Proceedings of the Fourth International Photobiological Congress. Pergamon Press, Oxford, pp. 419-440 (1965).

PATHAK, M.A., WORDEN, L.R. & KAUFMAN, K.D. Effect of structural alterations on the photosensitizing potency of furocoumarins (psoralens) and related compounds. *J. Invest. Derm.* 48: *103-118* (1967).

PIRIE, A. Color and solubility of the proteins of human cataract. *Invest. Ophth.* 7: *634-650* (1968).

PIRIE, A. Formation of N'-formylkynurenine in proteins from lens and other sources by exposure to sunlight. *Biochem. J.* 125: *203-208* (1971).

PIRIE, A. Photo-oxidation of proteins and comparison of photo-oxidized proteins with those of the cataractous human lens. *Israel. J. Med. Sci.* 8: *1567-1573* (1972).

REGNAULD, J. Sur la fluorescence des milieux de l'oeil chez l'homme et quelques mammiferes. *L'Institut* 26: *410* (1858).

RUSSELL, G.A. Electron spin resonance in organic chemistry. *Science* 161: *423-433* (1968).

SATO, K., BANDO, M. & NAKAJIMA, A. Fluorescence in human lens. *Exp. Eye Res.* 16: *167-172* (1973).

SCHACHAR, R.A. & SOLIN, S.A. The microscopic protein structure of the lens with a theory for cataract formation as determined by Raman spectroscopy of intact bovine lenses. *Invest. Ophth.* 14/5: *380-396* (1975).

259

SHIELDS, H. & HAMRICH, P.J., Jr. Relative stability of the characteristic sulfur and doublet resonances in x-irradiated native proteins as measured with ESR. *Radiation Res.* 41: *259-267* (1970).

SPECTOR, A., ROY, D. & STAUFFER, J. Isolation and characterization of an age-dependent polypeptide from human lens with non-tryptophan fluorescence. *Exp. Eye Res.* 21: *9-24* (1975).

TAN, K.E.W.P. Vision in the ultraviolet. Cited by Wolbarsht. *Fed. Proc.*, 1976, 35: *44-50* (1971).

TAPPEL, A.L. Lipid peroxidation damage to cell components. *Fed. Proc.* 32: *1870-1874* (1973).

TEALE, F.W.J. Structural dependence of protein ultraviolet fluorescence. *Biochem. J.* 80: 14p (1961).

TEALE, F.W.J. The ultraviolet fluorescence of proteins in neutral solution. *Biochem. J.* 76: *381-388* (1960).

TOTH, L.Z.J., BALAZS, E.A. & HOWE, A.F. Biophysical and biochemical changes in irradiated vitreous body. *Invest. Ophth.* 1: *797* (1962).

VAN HEYNINGEN, R. Assay of fluorescent glucosides in the human lens. *Exp. Eye Res.* 15: *121-126* (1973a).

VAN HEYNINGEN, R. Fluorescent derivatives of 3 hydroxy-l-kynurenine in the lens of man, the baboon and the grey squirrel. *Biochem. J.* 123: *30-31* (1971).

VAN HEYNINGEN, R. The glucoside of 3-hydroxykynurenine and other fluorescent compounds in the human lens. Ciba Symp. 19. The human Lens in Relation to Cataract. Elsevier/Amsterdam (1973b).

WALD, G. Alleged effects of the near ultraviolet on human vision. *J. Opt. Soc. Amer.* 42: *171-177* (1952).

WALLS, G.L. & JUDD, H.D. Intra-ocular colour filters of vertebrates. *Brit. J. Ophth.* 17: *641-705* (1933).

WEALE, R.A. The effects of the aging lens on vision. Ciba Symp. 19. The Human Lens in Relation to Cataract. pp. 7-19 (1973).

WEBER, G. Fluorescence-polarization spectrum and electronic-energy transfer in proteins. *Biochem. J.* 75: *345-352* (1960).

WEITER, J.J. & FINCH, E.D. Paramagnetic species in cataractous human lens. *Nature* 254: *536-537 (1975)*.

WOLBARSHT, M.L. The function of intra-ocular color filter. *Fed. Proc.* 35: *44-50* (1976).

YU, N-T & EAST, E. Laser Raman spectroscopic studies of ocular lens and its isolated protein fraction. *J. Biol. Chem.* 250: *2196-2202* (1975).

ZIGMAN, S. Eye lens color formation and function. *Science* 171: *807-809* (1971).

ZIGMAN, S., GRIESS, G., YULO, T. & SCHULTZ, J. Ocular protein alteration by near UV light. *Exp. Eye Res.* 15: *255-264* (1973).

ZIRLIN, A. & KAREL, M.J. Oxidation effects in a freeze dried gelation-methyl linoleate system. *Journal of Food Sci.* 34: *160-164* (1969).

Keywords:

lens fluorescence
lens fluorogens
tryptophan
tryptophan free radical
lens-aging
nuclear cataract (brown cataract)
intrinsic protein fluorescence

Author's address:

Department of Ophthalmology
Emory University
30322 Atlanta, Georgia, USA

EFFECT OF LONG-WAVE ULTRAVIOLET LIGHT ON THE LENS
II. METABOLIC INHIBITORS SYNERGISTIC WITH UV IN VITRO

JOHN F.R. KUCK, JR., PH.D.

(Atlanta, Georgia)

INTRODUCTION

That long wave ultraviolet light (UV) may injure the lens is an old idea (BELLOWS, 1972) based on clinical experience and some experimental evidence (BACHEM, 1956, ZIGMAN, 1974). UV plus photosensitizers produces definite cataractous changes in vivo (CLARK, 1961; CLOUD et al., 1960 & 1961; and FREEMAN, 1969) but such chronic responses are of little utility for screening suspected potentiating agents for UV. This investigation employed the irradiation apparatus previously described by which an effective dose can be imposed on a lens in vitro in a few hours (KUCK, 1976). The typical photosensitizer tested, trimethylpsoralen, proved too insoluble for in vito work but metabolic poisons, beginning with the catalase inhibitor 3-aminotriazole (AT), were tested for synergistic action with UV. AT was used to enhance the accumulation of hydrogen peroxide (H_2O_2) in the lens to reduce the level of glutathione (GSH), a known scavenger of H_2O_2 and other active species produced by irradiation and oxidation. The oxidation of GSH to GSSG by H_2O_2 and GSH-peroxidase in the lens was noted by PIRIE (1965). Further evidence for H_2O_2 toxicity in the lens was provided by BHUYAN et al. (1973) who produced cataracts in AT-fed rabbits which developed high levels of H_2O_2 in the aqueous humor (BHU-YAN et al., 1974). Since this procedure did not involve light, it appeared that UV with AT would affect the lens in a shorter perioa of time. This action of AT plus UV was reported previously (KUCK, 1976); this report concerns tests of compounds similar to AT, and other metabolic inhibitors acting on different enzymes. The identification of such agents promoting the action of UV on the lens is of interest in determining those environmental factors which may be involved in senile cataractogenesis.

This report concerns a variety of metabolic inhibitors, most of which affect the UV-irradiated rat lens with the same apparent end results, although the known actions of the inhibitors embrace a diversity of mechanisms. In many cases an inhibitor could be used at a concentration which little affected the shielded lens but which in combination with about 18 hours exposure to UV caused a significantly depressed accumulation of the non-metabolizable α-aminoisobutyric acid (α-AIB). This change was correlated with later inhibition of water, loss of lens GSH and eventually the appearance of subcapsular vacuolization.

Table I. Effect on CL/CM for α-AIB of several metabolic inhibitors under UV or in the dark

Inhibitor	CL/CM, UV	CL/CM, Dark
AT, 10. mM	.46 ± .02	13.53 ± 1.86
CyS, 10.	.47 ± .09	10.7 ± 0.7
NaN$_3$, 1.0	.45 ± .09	22.2 ± 1.0
CBZ, 10.	.57 ± .07	6.2 ± 1.7
NH$_2$OH, 0.5	.49 ± .04	7.79 ± 2.1
(NH$_2$)$_2$, 1.0	.38 ± .06	14.8 ± 1.2
SCZ, 5.0	.44 ± .08	21.3 ± 1.4
ADC, 0.1	.41 ± .07	18.1 ± 3.5
KCNO, 1.0	.48 ± .07	38.8 ± 6.8
t-BHP, 1.0	.61 ± .06	.43 ± 0.04
IAc, 0.1	.56	.4
NEM, 1.0	.58 ± .07	.46 ± 0.05
NBS, 1.0	.46 ± .07	1.53 ± 0.1
NaF, 5.0	.49 ± .07	6.6 ± 0.5
NaCN, 10	.47 ± .03	17.9 ± 0.2
Ouabain, 0.5	.40 ± .04	.98 ± 0.17
Arsenite, 0.5	.36 ± .05	1.82 ± 0.44
5BDU, 5.0	.47 ± .10	25.9 ± 1.1
DMSO, 10	.51	17.6

CL/CM = Concentration of ^{14}C in lens water

Concentration of ^{14}C in incubation medium

Preincubation with inhibitor ± UV lasted 18 hours followed by a further incubation with tracer α-AIB for 6 hours. Each value is the mean for usually 4 rat lenses weighing 45-50 mg each. The mM concentration appears after each inhibitor.

AT: 3-aminotriazole, CyS: cycloserine, CBZ: carbohydrazide, SCZ: semicarbazide, t-BHP: tert-butylhydroperoxide, IAc: iodoacetate, NEM: N-ethylmaleimide, NBS: N-bromosuccinimide, 5BDU: 5-bromo-2-deoxyuridine, DMSO: dimethylsulfoxide, ADC: azodicarbonimide.

METHODS

The UV irradiation bath was that described previously (KUCK, 1976), having a 'black light' lamp immersed in the water so that incubation tubes above and in contact with the lamp held lenses about 2-3 mm from the lamp. The flux intensity at the level of the lens was about 2 mwatts/cm^2. A 50 ml round-bottom centrifuge tube held a pool of 7 lenses so that each received about the same amount of light. The incubation medium was that used previously and the tracer uptake was conducted as described there. In general the incubation was carried out for 24 hours with a transfer to fresh medium containing the tracer at the 18 hour point. The experiments to determine the length of the irradiation period needed to produce detectable damage was carried out in a similar fashion except that the total incubation time was a lesser amount and the tracer was added only during the latter hours of incubation.

RESULTS

In Table I are given values of CL/CM for α-AIB obtained when rat lenses were incubated in the inhibitor with or without exposure to UV. In some cases the effect of the inhibitor was so marked that the additional imposition of UV gave no further reduction in CL/CM; among these are iodoacetate, N-ethylmaleimide and t-butyl-hydroperoxide. Fluoride, which acts only by precipitating Mg ion, has an effect significantly enhanced by UV. DMSO which has unknown effects on metabolism also enhanced the effect of UV. Many inhibitors, including AT in particular, act on Fe-containing enzymes such as catalase and are very potent in enhancing the effect of UV.

In Table II are results showing that the duration of irradiation is an important factor for imposing UV injury on a lens. Up through 16 hours of exposure there is no effect of UV but at 18 hours the effect becomes significant.

In Table III are the results for several different tracers which show that UV + AT does not alter the mannitol space, does not affect transport by

Table II. Effect of AT ± UV on lens accumulation of α-AIB (CL/CM) as a function of exposure duration

Exposure, Hours	UV	Dark	% Water Gain
4	.15 ± .03	.17 ± .04	1.13
6	.18 ± .04	.17 ± .06	.81
8	.16 ± .04	.17 ± .04	.58
12	.14 ± .07	.22 ± .05	.70
16	.17 ± .04	.21 ± .07	2.06
18	.15 ± .03	.23 ± .05	8.78
20	.13 ± .04	.21 ± .03	11.92

45-50 mg rat lenses were incubated for the indicated number of hours with tracer added 1 hour before the end of the experiment. Contralateral lenses were divided between the UV and Dark pools giving greater precision in measuring water gain. Each value is the mean for 7 lenses.

Table III. Effect of AT ± UV on the accumulation of several different tracers, expressed as CL/CM

Tracer	Rad. Hrs.	Tra. Hrs.	CL/CM, UV	CL/CM, Dark
Mann	18	8	.58 ± .11	.60 ± .09
Thiou	23	1	.32 ± .06	.37 ± .07
α-AIB	19	8	.74 ± .21	1.45 ± .57
Gal	19	8	1.01 ± .48	1.08 ± .18

Tracers were: mannitol-U-^{14}C, thiourea-^{14}C, α-AIB-1-^{14}C and galactose-U-^{14}C. Lenses were irradiated for the indicated time (Rad. Hrs.) then placed in tracer and incubated further for the indicated time (Tra. Hrs.). Each value is the mean for 6 rat lenses: 45-50 mg for Mann and Thiou, 25 mg for α-AIB and Gal.

Table IV. Effect of AT and UV on levels of GSH in chick lenses

	Lens GSH (mg%)	Lens Weight (mg)
UV only	28.6 ± 10.3	42.1 ± 2.5
UV + AT	19.7 ± 9.1	43.6 ± 2.4
Control in Dark	66.1 ± 8.7	35.6 ± 2.2
AT in Dark	70.2 ± 18.1	35.6 ± 1.7

Fresh lenses (35 mg) had a level of about 120 mg%. The incubation in 10 mM AT lasted 20 hours. The UV only values are not significantly different from the UV + AT values. The GSH was determined by Ellman's method on trichloroacetic acid extracts of lenses.

passive diffusion (thiourea) nor by facilitated transport (galactose) but does depress active transport of α-AIB.

In Table IV it is shown that for a 20 hour incubation using chick lenses (28 day) the effect of UV is marked enough that little enhancement is produced by AT. The loss of GSH is accompanied by an 18% uptake of water in the UV-only lenses.

SUMMARY

These experiments show that many different metabolic inhibitors may potentiate the toxicity of UV for the lens. The similarity in the effect of quite different inhibitors and the pronounced depression of amino acid uptake suggest that the injury interferes with energy generation in the lens. Normally the lens seems to have some resistance to UV and an appreciable capacity for repair. However, on long irradiation during depressed metabolism, this resistance is lowered. It appears that the maintenance of the lens GSH level is a good index of lens viability and this level falls in the course of injury before water uptake is observed. Under the conditions of these experiments water uptake and the formation of cortical opacities with vacuolization are a later result of UV-induced damage. Thus the possibility exists that the action of the UV of sunlight over many decades, potentiated by environmental toxicants, is a factor in human senile cataractogenesis.

ACKNOWLEDGEMENT

This work was supported by NIH Grant EY 00260.

REFERENCES

BACHEM, A. Ophthalmic ultraviolet action spectra. *Amer. J. Ophthalmol.* 4: *969-975* (1956).

BELLOWS, J.G. Ultraviolet light and the crystalline lens. *Ann. Ophthalmol.* 4: *11-12* (1972).

BHUYAN, K.C., BHUYAN, D.K. & KATZIN, H.M. Amizol-induced cataract and inhibition of lens catalase in rabbit. *Ophthalmic Res.* 5: *236-247* (1973).

264

BHUYAN, K.C., BHUYAN, D.K. & TURTZ, A.I. Aminotriazole-effect on the ocular tissues in rabbit. *Inter. Res. Comm. System.* 5: *1594* (1974).

CLARK, J.H. Photosensitization by 8-methoxypsoralen. *J. Invest. Dermatol.* 37: *171-174* (1961).

CLOUD, T.M., HAKIM, R. & GRIFFIN, A.C. Photosensitization of the eye with methoxsalen. I. Acute effects. *Arch. Ophthalmol.* (Chicago) 64: *346-351* (1960).

CLOUD, T.M., HAKIM, R. & GRIFFIN, A.C. Photosensitization of the eye with methoxsalen. II. Chronic effects. *Arch. Ophthalmol.* (Chicago) 66: *689-694* (1961).

FREEMAN, R.G. & TROLL, D. Photosensitization of the eye by 8-methoxypsoralen. *J. Invest. Dermatol.* 53: *499-553* (1969).

KUCK, J.F.R. Effect of long-wave ultraviolet light on the lens. I. Model system for detecting and measuring effect on the lens in vitro. *Invest. Ophthalmol.*, 15: *405-407* (1976).

PIRIE, A. Glutathione peroxidase in lens and a source of hydrogen peroxide in aqueous humor. *Biochem. J.* 96: *244-253* (1965).

ZIGMAN, S, YULO, T. & SCHULTZ, J. Cataract induction in mice exposed to near UV light. *Ophthalmic Res.* 6: *259-270* (1974).

Keywords:

Catalase inhibitors
Long-wave ultraviolet
Rat lens
Cataract
Amino acid uptake

Author's address:

Laboratory for Ophthalmic Research
Department of Ophthalmology
Emory University
Atlanta, Georgia, USA

265

TRYPTOPHAN EXCITED STATES IN THE LENS

SEYMOUR ZIGMAN, PH.D.*

(Rochester, New York)

ABSTRACT

Calf aqueous humor, whole rat lenses, and solutions of purified calf lens gamma crystallin were exposed to near UV-light in the presence and absence of tryptophan. ESR signals of these preparations demonstrated excited state species similar to the signals of whole dried normal human lenses. The findings support a theory that such excited state species can accumulate in the lens by binding to its proteins. A positive relationship between lens color and ESR signal intensity was also found. The near-UV light induction of stable colored excited state species from tryptophan that become associated with the lens proteins may thus be one means by which lens pigmentation is enhanced.

INTRODUCTION

Recent literature has provided evidence that the state of human lens is influenced by exposure to near-UV light (ZIGMAN, 1971; ZIGMAN, et al., 1972; KURZEL et al., 1973; WEITER & FINCH, 1975; ZIGMAN et al., 1976). During our studies of the possible roles of near-UV light in cataractogenesis samples were also collected for ESR studies. Such data provides further evidence in support of the theory that near-UV light exposure is a real factor in cataractogenesis.

MATERIAL AND METHODS

Details of the ESR determinations and the spectra of other standard amino acids may be found in Forbes and SULLIVAN (1967).

Human lens studies

Fresh normal human lenses obtained from the Rochester Eye and Human Parts Bank, Inc., within 24 hrs of death were used exclusively. These were dried in an evacuated dessicator over solid KOH for 8 weeks and then were subjected whole and dry to ESR spectral analysis in Quartz tubes at 22 °C. using a JEOLCO ESR Spectrometer (Model JES 3 BX). The machine was operated under the conditions detailed in the legends of the figures.

* Supported by the National Eye Institute (Research No. EY 00459) of the P.H.S.

Table I. ESR Values and Color Densities of Normal Human Lenses

Age of Donors years*	Optical Density[+] at 440 nm	g value	Line half-width (Gauss)	Relative signal Intensity
57	.395	2.0040	9.2	0.42
53	.460	2.0045	9.8	0.44
63	.420	2.0045	9.2	0.28
65	.445	2.0035	9.8	0.34
67	.520	2.0050	9.4	0.63
69	.540	2.0040	8.8	0.65
82	1.050	2.0020	9.3	1.00
UV-exposed poly-L-tryptophan in air		2.0043	13.1	
UV-exposed poly-L-tyrosine in air		2.0041	9.3	

* Two lenses of the same individual were analyzed separately and the values averaged.
[+] Corrected for scattering.

Calf aqueous humor studies

Fresh samples of calf aqueous humor were obtained at the local meat packing plant and were kept on ice until use. Samples of 10 ml each were incubated for 24 hrs at 22 °C. as follows:
a) in darkness
b) exposed to 3 mW/cm^2 of near-UV light (320 to 400 nm, peak at 365 nm);
c) with 1 mg/ml of L-tryptophan in darkness; and
d) with 1 mg/ml of L-tryptophan and exposed to near-UV light.
The samples were then evacuated at room temperature until dry and subjected to ESR analysis as above.

Rat and mouse lens studies

Lenses of freshly sacrificed Holtzmann Albino rats were extracted and incubated in Earle's BSS solutions at 37 °C. for 24 hrs under the same conditions used in the calf aqueous humor studies (see ZIGMAN et al., 1972). These lenses were then washed extensively in Earle's balanced salt solution, rinsed with distilled water, and then evacuated until dry. Fresh lenses of mice maintained either in normal room light or in black light (450 μW/cm^2 at 365 nm; 12 hrs a day; 70 weeks) were extracted, washed and dried as above, and then studied in the same way. The whole dried mouse lenses were subjected to ESR analysis as above.

Calf purified gamma crystallin I. studies

Calf lens γ-I crystallin prepared by isoelectric focusing (see ZIGMAN et al., 1973) was dissolved in water at 1 mg/ml and parts of the solution were either exposed to near-UV light or kept in darkness with and without added tryptophan (at 1 mg/ml) for 24 hrs at 22 °C. The solutions were then extensively dialyzed and lyophilized to dryness. These samples were then subjected to ESR analysis, using irradiated and lyophilized L-tryptophan as a standard. The ESR signals observed resemble these described earlier for lens proteins exposed to near-UV light (see LERMAN et al, 1968).

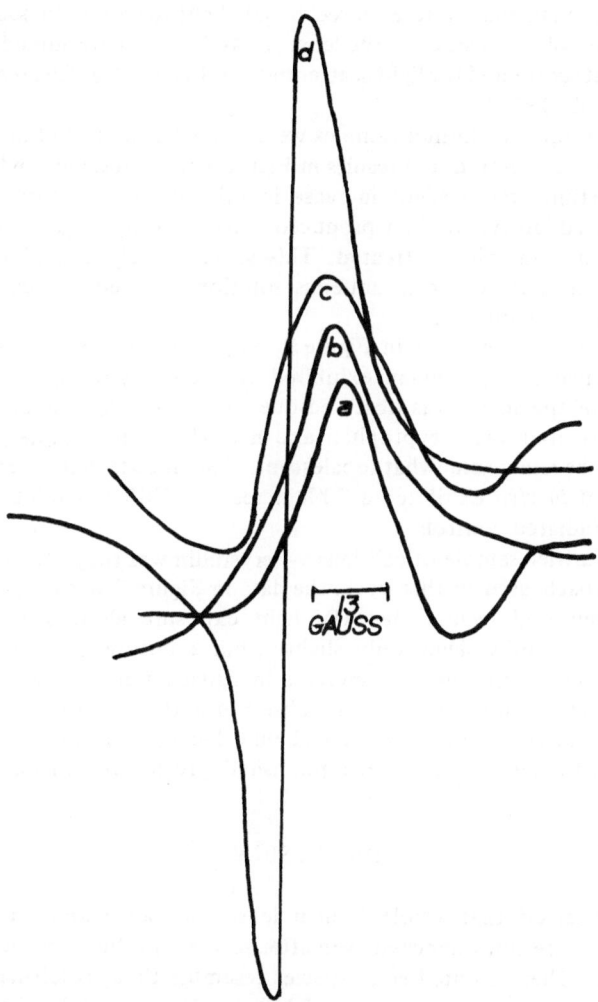

Fig. 1 ESR spectra of calf aqueous humor. a) untreated; b) near-UV irradiated for 24 hrs at 22 °C. at 3 mW/cm² with no additive c) plus 0.1% tryptophan; d) plus 0.1% tryptophan and near-UV irradiated for 24 hrs. at 22 °C. ESR spectrometer settings: power, 10 mW; crystal 0.5 mA; field, 3288± 100 G; gain, 10,000; response, 0.3 sec., modulation, 6.3; phase 8 o'clock; frequency, 9.24 GH2; Temperature, R.T.; sweep 10 mm; no irradiation.

RESULTS

Table I summarizes the data for the human lenses subjected to ESR analysis. No special relationship was noted between the relative intensities of the signals and the age of the lens donors, but all lenses examined exhibited an ESR signal. Also included are the values for UV irradiated standards of poly-L-tyrosine, and poly-L-tryptophan. The data does not presently allow us to identify the free radicals present, but they are not sulfur-related. The signals appear to be intermediate between those of poly-L-tyrosine and poly-L-tryptophan that were exposed to UV light for 5 hrs. Included in the table are the color densities of the lenses at 440 nm as determined by direct measurement (corrected for light scattering; see GROVER & ZIGMAN, 1972; ZIGMAN et al., 1976).

When calf aqueous humor samples were treated as indicated in the methods and materials section, the results in Figure 1 were obtained. While N-UV light alone stimulated a slight increase in ESR signal intensity, N-UV exposure with added tryptophan produced a significantly larger signal in the aqueous humor sample so treated. This signal closely resembles that of tryptophan in agar gel or in aqueous solution exposed to near-UV light under the same conditions.

For *in vitro* rat lenses, as in Figure 2, only those exposed to N-UV light in the presence of tryptophan exhibited an intense ESR signal. Little enhancement of the signal was observed due to near-UV light exposure only. The lenses treated with tryptophan and near-UV light became pigmented brown and became somewhat opalescent. The mouse lenses exposed to near-UV light *in vivo* exhibited a 20% increase in ESR signal intensity over that of unirradiated controls.

When a purified sample of calf lens γ-I crystallin was subjected the experimental approach used in this work, the data in Figure 3 was obtained. As in the other reported results, near-UV light exposure alone stimulated the intensity of the ESR signal only slightly, but exposure in the presence of tryptophan led to the greatest increase in signal intensity. Here again, the presence of brown pigment was only observed in the tryptophan plus N-UV treated protein. The alterations in the chemical and physical properties of γ-I due to this procedure have been published previously (ZIGMAN et al., 1973).

DISCUSSION

We have observed that whole human lenses contain stable excited state species which are not quenched even after several months of drying at room temperature. These excited state species resemble those resulting from the exposure of free tryptophan to near-UV light. Using entirely different procedures, WEITER & FINCH (1975) have alo concluded that stable triplet state species of tryptophan were present in the nuclei of human lenses.

A point that is difficult to discuss at this time is the apparant lack of a relationship between the intensity of the ESR signal and the age of the lens. WEITER & FINCH (1975) also found no difference in line width or signal intensity of the tryptophan triplet state between normal and cataractous lenses. This may be the result of the formation of both stable excited states and unstable free radicals. When several of the human lenses were re-exposed to UV-light, the ESR signal intensity was increased and exhibited a rapid decay within several hours, indicating stimulation of an unstable radical specie. The intensity of the unstable radical species may be positively related to the age of the lens, or the presence of cataracts, but these species could not be observed in our studies. If these unstable radicals were quenched, only the stable excited state species would remain after a length of time, thereby giving the constant ESR signal observed.

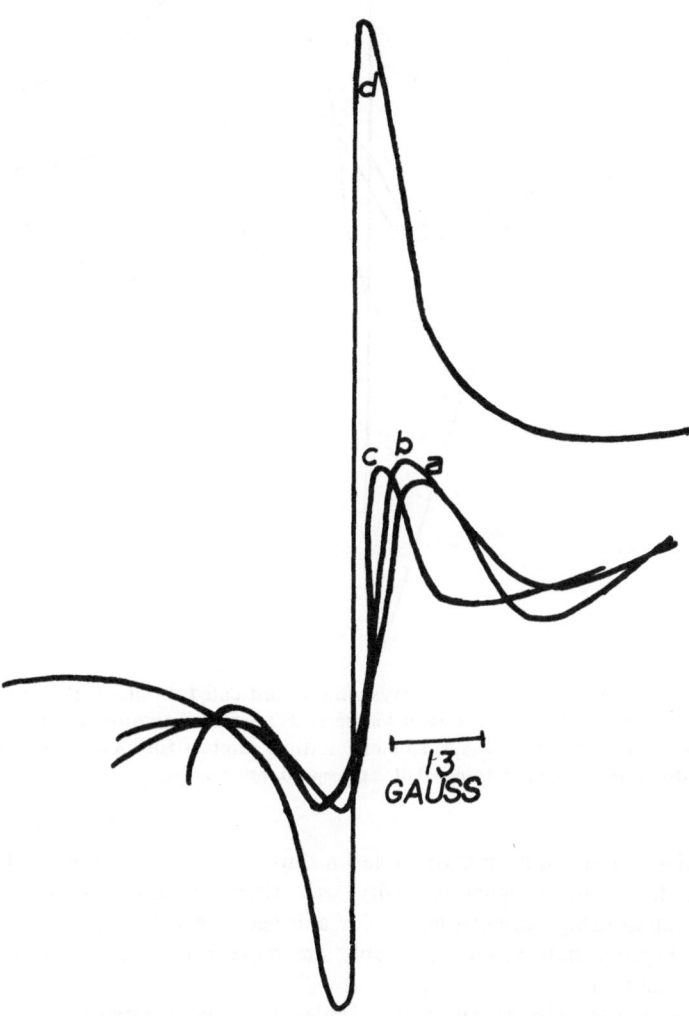

Fig. 2. ESR spectra of rat lenses maintained in Earle's balanced salt solution. a) untreated; b) plus 0.1% tryptophan; c) near-UV irradiated as in Figure 1; d) plus 0.1% tryptophan and near-UV irradiated as in Figure 1. ESR spectrometer settings as in Figure 1.

271

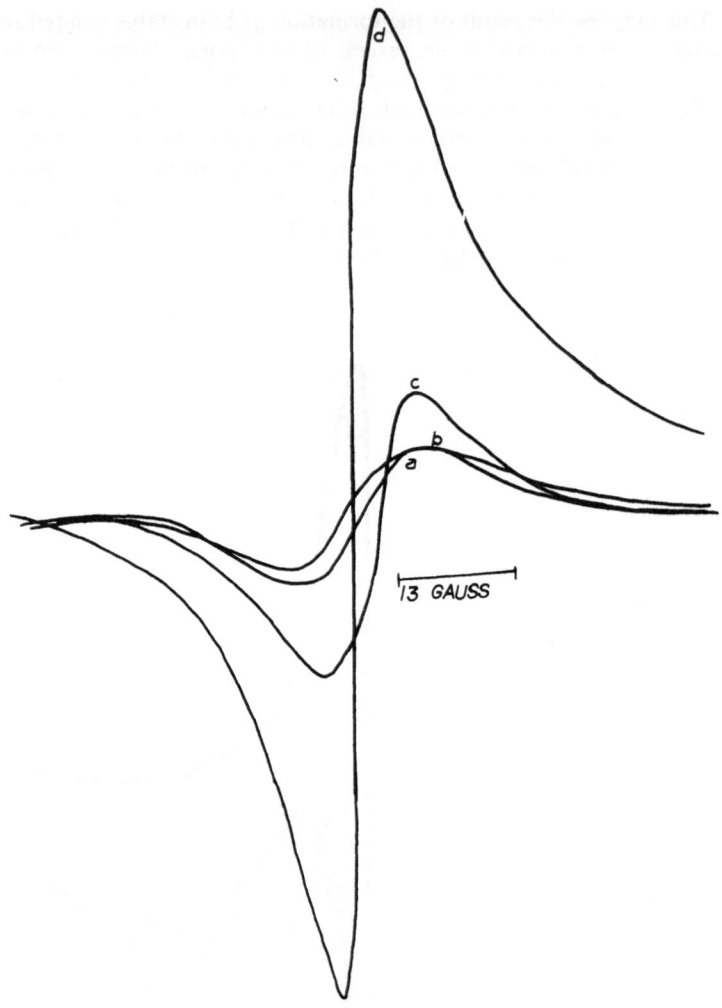

Fig. 3. ESR spectra of calf lens γ-I crystallin; a) untreated; b) plus 0.1% tryptophan; c) near-UV irradiated for 24 hrs as in Figure 1. d) plus 0.1% tryptophan and near-UV irradiated as in Figure 1. ESR spectrometer settings same as for Figure 1. except gain, 100; modulation, 5; temperature, 10 °C.; sweep 50 mm.

However, a generally positive relationship between the color of the lens and the free radical signal intensity was observed. Since there is not a perfect relationship between lens color and age, the color density and content of excited state species probably are more related to environmental factors than to age.

Other results seem to support the idea that the pigmented species are also the excited state species. This idea is upheld by the data obtained for near-UV irradiated calf aqueous humor and *in vitro* rat lenses. In these results an enhanced ESR signal and an increased pigmentation were only observed when tryptophan was present. Examination of excited states of tryptophan induced by exposure to near-UV light has also shown that they are pigmented. The relationship between color of biomolecules and their excited state characteristics has been described previously by SZENT-GYORGYI (1974, 1975; unpublished data presented at The Marine Biological Laboratory). When a purified gamma crystallin was exposed to near-UV light in the presence of tryptophan, pigmented tryptophan photoproduct(s) was bound to this protein. The protein subsequently was found to exhibit an ESR signal not previously present having characteristics in common with pigmented and excited state tryptophan photoproduct(s). The ESR characteristics of the human lenses examined and reported above have much in common with the tryptophan excited states artificially produced in the aqueous humors, rat lens proteins and pure calf lens gamma crystallin.

The lenses of living mice exposed to near-UV light over a long period of time (in this case for 70 weeks and 12 hrs a day; see ZIGMAN et al., 1974) also exhibited an enhanced signal over controls even without any additional tryptophan present. However, no visible pigment was observed in these lenses. The ESR signals in the mouse lenses were much less intense than those found in normal human lenses or the near-UV light artificially-produced tryptophan excited states.

This report then presents additional data to support the idea that near-UV light entering the eye can excite such molecules as tryptophan, possibly in the aqueous humor so that photoproducts can enter the lens, and bind to and alter lens proteins. The question of whether the source of these pigmented excited states in human lenses is free tryptophan or the tryptophan present in peptide linkage in the lens proteins still remains to be answered. The results of other workers (STEIN et al., 1976) and those of ours referred to above seem to support the idea that free tryptophan is the most probable source.

ACKNOWLEDGEMENT

I gratefully thank Dr. William Frobes and his associates at Waterloo University, Ontario, Canada for carrying out the ESR analysis.

REFERENCES

GROVER, D. & S. ZIGMAN. Coloration of human lenses by near ultraviolet photo-oxidized tryptophan. *Exp. Eye Res.* 13: *70-76* (1972).

FORBES, W.F. & P.D. SULLIVAN. Free radicals of biological interest. *Canadian J. Biochem.* 45: *1831-1839* (1967).

KURZEL, R.B., M.L. WOHLBARSHT & B.S. YAMANASHI. Spectral studies on normal and cataractous intact human lenses. *Exp. Eye Res.* 17: *65-71* (1973).

LERMAN, S., W.F. FORBES, S. ZIGMAN & J. KIRMAN. A study of gamma crystallin derived from the rat and dogfish lens. Proc. Symp. Biochem. of the Eye, Tutzing Castle, pp. *292-300* (Karger, Basel/New York) (1968).

STEIN, P., S. ZIGLER, B.S. YAMANASHI, J.B. SIDBURY, R.W. HENKENS & M.L. WOHLBARSHT. Fluorescence of normal and cataractous lens protein (accepted for publication, *Ophthal. Res.*) (1976).

WEITER, JOHN J. & E.D FINCH. Paramagnetic species in cataractous human lenses. *Nature* 254: *536-537* (1975).

ZIGMAN, S. Eye lens color: formation and function. *Science* 171: *807-809* (1971).

ZIGMAN, S., J. SCHULTZ, T. YULO & D. GROVER. Effects of near-UV irradiation on lens and aqueous humor proteins. *Israel J. Med. Sci.* 8: *1590-1595* (1972).

ZIGMAN, S., J. SCHULTZ & T. YULO. Binding of near-UV light photoproduct of tryptophan to a purified calf lens gamma crystallin. *Exp. Eye Res.* 15: *201-208* (1972).

ZIGMAN, S., T. YULO & J. SCHULTZ. Cataract induction in mice exposed to near-UV light. *Invest. Ophthal.* 6: *159-270* (1974).

ZIGMAN, S., J. GROFF, T. YULO & G. GRIESS. Light extinction and protein profiles in human lenses (accepted for publication, *Exp. Eye Res.*) (1976).

Keywords:

Excited states
Free radicals
Near-UV light
Tryptophan
Lens
Aqueous humor

Author's address:

Opthalmology Research Laboratory
Division of Ophthalmology
Department of Surgery
University of Rochester School of
Medicine and Dentistry
601 Elmwood Avenue
Rochester, New York 14642, USA

ON THE INDEPENDENT ACTION OF CATARACTOGENIC AGENTS
X-RAYS AND GALACTOSE*

W. MANSKI, A.T. YORK, G.R. MERRIAM, Jr., B.V. WORGUL
& A. SZECHTER

(New York, U.S.A.)

There is considerable information concerning genetic, environmental, toxic and other factors which induce loss of lens transparency (FRANCOIS, 1963; MANN, 1966; NORDMANN, 1972; PIRIE, 1972). Cataracts occur in a variety of patterns, many of which are sufficiently characteristic to allow an etiologic diagnosis to be made clinically (DUKE-ELDER, 1969). Many studies of the mechanism of cataractogenesis have pointed to a close relationship between different inducing factors and various specific metabolic pathways of the lens epithelium (VAN HEYNINGEN, 1969).

In contrast to the great variability of etiologic and morphologic patterns in cataracts, immunochemical studies from this laboratory have shown that the structural lens proteins of transparent and cataractous lenses do not exhibit significant differences (YORK, HAMADA & MANSKI, 1971a; YORK, MARTINEZ & MANSKI, 1971b). Antigenically, no new 'pathological' lens proteins were found to occur nor native ones to be completely lost. As compared to normal lenses, lesser amounts of pre-alpha and a decrease of at least one specific beta crystallin were apparent in lenses with galactose cataract in inbred rats (YORK et al., 1971a) and a decrease of at least one specific beta crystallin similarly located in immunoelectrophoresis was also observed in human senile cataract crystallins, usually more difficult to resolve by this technique (YORK et al., 1971b).

These observations led to the hypothesis (MANSKI, 1973) that the similarity of involvement of specific lens proteins in various cataracts may be the result of their response to a departure from cellular homeostasis. The sequence in which the individual lens proteins become affected by changed cellular conditions appears to be independent of the inducing factor, resulting in the similarity of lens protein changes in etiologically different cataracts. The diversity of clinical patterns in cataract, on the other hand, may be an expression of the different distribution of cells primarily responding to the particular cataractogenic agent.

This hypothesis was tested by two types of experiments presented in this report. In the first experiment, X-ray cataract lens proteins of rats were compared to galactose cataract and to normal ones by immunochemical

* This investigation was supported by U.S.P.H.S. Research Grant EY 00189 and a grant from the Skerryvore Foundation.

analysis. As will be shown, lens proteins similar to those in galactose cataract are involved in X-ray cataract.

In the other experiments these two cataractogenic agents (X-rays and galactose), which produce clinically distinct patterns, were applied at the same time. The independent origin and progression of the specific clinical cataract patterns found in such double stress experiments as well as the similarity of X-ray and galactose lens protein changes found are in agreement with the stated hypothesis.

MATERIALS AND METHODS

Animals

Columbia-Sherman, male and female rats (CAMM, Wayne, N.J.) and Fisher 344 male rats (Microbiological Associates, Bethesda, Md.) were used in the experiment.

Experimental Cataracts

The animals were two weeks old at the time of irradiation. 184 kVp X-rays filtered by 0.55 mm Cu and 0.5 mm of Al (HVL = 1 mm of Cu) were used. A circular field 16 mm in diameter enabled treatment of one eye only. The fellow eye received less than 2% of the dose to the treated eye. In the X-ray set up the plexiglass cone, 16 mm in diameter, assured a reproducible source-skin distance of 21 cm. Either one eye was irradiated, the other serving as a control, or both eyes were treated one at a time and a separate untreated control group was included. Single doses of 400, 600, 1000 and 1400 rads were used. The 50% or 35% galactose diet according to Z. Dische (Microbiological Associates, Bethesda, Md.) was started four weeks after irradiation when the animals were six weeks old. At this time, clinical radiation cataracts were not observed. The diet was continued for a period of four weeks by which time the animals had developed complete opacification. The control irradiated and the control normal animals were kept on a regular diet (Purina Rabbit Chow, Vincentown, N.J.). At the end of each week from the onset of the experiment, one or two rats from each group were sacrificed and the eyes removed for histological study.

Clinically, the eyes were examined weekly with the corneal microscope (slit lamp) and the cataracts graded according to the degree of opacity. The clinical grading system for radiation cataracts has been described in more detail elsewhere (MERRIAM & FOCHT, 1962). Essentially it is as follows:
Grade 1+ Clusters of vacuoles and opaque dots, centrally in the posterior and subcapsular region.
Grade 2+ Moderately dense posterior cortical opacity, early opacifications of anterior cortex.
Grade 3+ Posterior cortex very opaque and anterior cortex moderately opaque.
Grade 4+ Lens completely opaque.

The grading system for galactose cataracts used in this report may be summarized as follows:
Grade 1+ Incomplete circle of subcapsular vacuoles anteriorly in the pre-

equatorial zone. Slight haziness in the posterior cortex or no visible changes.
Grade 2+   More extensive changes anteriorly extending centrally. Circle of subcapsular vacuoles closer to the posterior pole. Beginning anterior cortical changes and some early opacities posteriorly.
Grade 3+   Extensive anterior subcapsular opacities with only a small transparent area at the anterior pole plus extensive cortical changes. An increase in posterior cortical opacities.
Grade 4+   Lens completely opaque.

From the clinical standpoint stages 3+ and 4+ in both cataract classifications mean significant visual impairment.

Histology

The rats were sacrificed by decapitation at intervals according to protocol. Following enucleation the posterior portion of each eye was incised prior to immersion in Carnoy's solution (glacial acetic acid: absolute ethanol, 1 : 3) for 24 hours. After an additional 24 hours in 70% ethanol, the eyes were paraffin-embedded as described elsewhere (WORGUL, MERRIAM, SZECHTER & SRINIVASAN, 1976) and sectioned at $10 \mu m$ thickness. The sections were then routinely stained with PAS and hematoxylin.

Lens Proteins

Immediately after decapitation the lenses were dissected and kept on ice. They were washed in ice cold saline and rolled over filter paper in order to free them from vitreous, aqueous and other tissue material. X-ray cataract lenses were collected from animals which developed a 4+ cataract after 1000 r. Completely opaque galactose cataract lenses were collected after four weeks of galactose diet. Normal lenses of corresponding age were also collected.

The crystallin fraction was obtained from normal or cataract rat lenses by homogenization in a Ten Broeck Teflon-glass homogenizer with 15X weight of H_2O at 4°C and centrifugation at 15,000 rev/min for 30 min in a Servall PR centrifuge.

The albuminoid fraction was purified by extraction at 20 °C with 10X volume of H_2O. After each extraction, the albuminoid was centrifuged at 15,000 rev/min for 30 min in a Servall PR centrifuge. The above procedure was repeated 15-20 times. At this time the protein content in the supernatant was less than 0.01 mg/ml. Both the crystallin and albuminoid fractions were kept lyophilized.

Solubilization of albuminoid was done according to RUTTENBERG (1965) by exposure of an albuminoid suspension to pH 10.5 (NaOH) for 30 min. The pH was then reduced to 7.4.

Estimation of Protein Concentration

Absorption measurements were done at 280 and 260 mμ wavelength in a 1 cm silica cell in a Beckman DU 2 spectrophotometer. The concentrations were estimated according to KALCKAR (1947) by the formula $1.45 D_{280} - 0.75 D_{260} = $ protein mg/ml.

277

Normal three- to four-week old rats were immunized with normal, X-ray or galactose cataract rat lenses. 1.5 mg of lyophilized lenses in complete Freund's adjuvant (with *M. tuberculosis*) per animal was used for each immunization. The first 3 immunizations were given in the footpad and subcutaneously in the back at two-week intervals. The booster immunizations were administered at monthly intervals for six to eight months.

In addition to the above isoantisera, heterologous antisera were prepared. For this, five to six pound chinchilla rabbits were used. 15 mg of lyophilized rat normal, X-ray or galactose cataract lenses in complete Freund's adjuvant per animal were injected subcutaneously at four to six sites. The time schedule of immunization was the same as for rats.

All immune sera were collected twelve days after the last immunization and stored at $-65\,^{\circ}$C.

For absorption, the antiserum was gently homogenized with the lyophilized and powdered lens in a proportion of 2 mg/ml. The absorption mixture was kept at 4°C, shaken twice daily and kept for 2-3 days and then centrifuged at $4\,^{\circ}$C for 30 minutes at 3,000 rev/min (International Centrifuge Rotor 269, International Equipment Company, Needham Heights, Mass.). The absorption procedure was repeated two more times.

Immunoelectrophoresis

The micromethod by SCHEIDEGGER (1955) was used. Microscopic slides were covered with 1.5% agar in Veronal buffer (pH 8.2). The antigen well was 1.5 mm in diameter, the serum trench was 2.0 x 64.5 mm and the distance between the edges of the two was 2.0 mm. The potential difference of 5.0 V/cm was applied for 90 min. The equipment was manufactured by L.K.B. (Stockholm, Sweden). The development of precipitin lines was carried out at 4°C.

The relative content of different lens antigens in the normal or cataractous lenses was established by comparing the persistence on serial dilution of total lens proteins of particular precipitin lines in immunoelectrophoresis. The concentration range of lens proteins studied was 1.25 to 40 mg/ml. The precipitin lines were permitted to develop for 72 hours at $4\,^{\circ}$C at which time photographs were taken under uniform condition.

Passive Hemagglutination

Passive hemagglutination was carried out according to BOYDEN (1951) with formalized sheep erythrocytes (Bacto-Formo cells, Difco Laboratories, Detroit, Mich.) using the microtiter system (Cooke Engineering Company, Alexandria, Va.).

RESULTS

The antigenic similarity or difference between X-ray cataract and normal as well as between X-ray and galactose cataract lens proteins was investigated

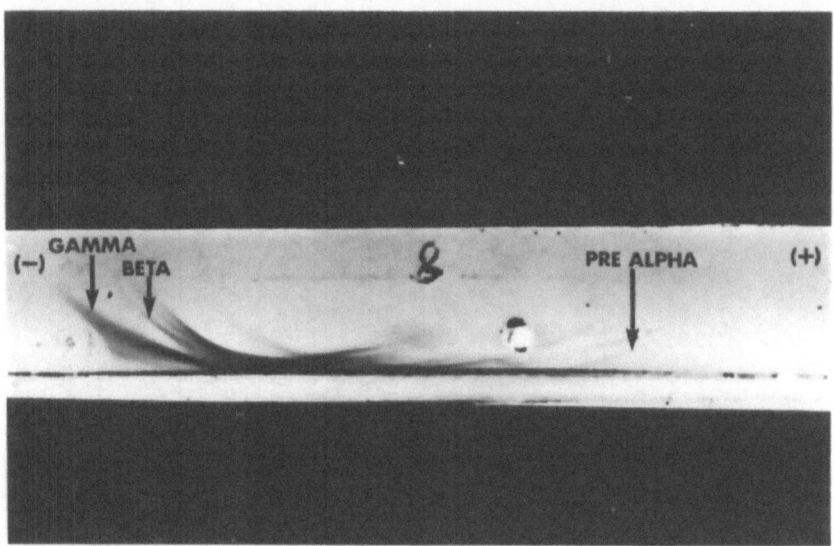

Fig. 1. Immunoeletrophoretic pattern of rat lens crystallins (20 mg/ml) developed with rabbit anti-normal rat lens serum. Arrows indicate the pre-alpha, beta and gamma crystallin decrease in cataractous lenses.

by absorption experiments. Samples of the different antisera were absorbed separately by each of the lens proteins studied and then reacted with the homologous lens proteins used to obtain the particular immune serum. The presence of residual antibodies was tested by passive hemagglutination and used as an indication of the presence or absence of antigenic differences between lens proteins used for immunization and absorption.

It was found that absorption of rabbit or rat anti-rat X-ray cataract lens serum with normal rat lens proteins as well as of rabbit or rat anti-normal rat lens sera with rat X-ray cataract lens proteins completely removed reactivity with the homologous lens crystallins or solubilized albuminoids. The same was true for rabbit or rat anti-rat X-ray cataract lens sera absorbed with rat galactose cataract lens proteins as well as for rabbit or rat anti-rat galactose cataract lens sera absorbed with rat X-ray cataract lens proteins. No antigenic differences were found between the Fisher or Columbia-Sherman rat lens proteins when used for immunization or testing. The antisera in the above experiments were absorbed with ca 6 mg lens protein/ml antiserum.

The negative reactions of the absorbed antisera are an indication that formation of X-ray cataracts is not associated with the induction of new antigenic determinants absent in normal lens proteins. The negative reactions are also an indication that all the antigenic determinants of normal lens proteins are still present in X-ray cataract lens proteins. Similar results were obtained for lens proteins from galactose cataract rat lenses (YORK et al., 1971a).

The lack of qualitative immunochemical differences between normal and

Table I. Lens changes specific of X-ray (X) or galactose (G) cataract in rats:
I: exposed to **400** rads and 29 days later started on a 50% galactose diet.
II: exposed to **400** rads.
III: on a 50% galactose diet.
IV: normal

Experimental Group	No. Animals	400 rad irradiation (both eyes)	Galactose diet started 29 days after irradiation with 400 rads	Days after irradiation	Biomicroscopic observation
I	20	+	+	52	Appearance of small opacities in a few animals, characteristic for 1+ radiation cataracts. Prominent posterior sutures visible. In one animal, anterior radial lines were observed. Twelve animals showed no changes.
				59	1+ to 2+ galactose cataracts, 1+ radiation cataracts in some animals
				66	3+ galactose cataracts. Posterior changes hard to observe through a small opening at the anterior pole. Posterior changes classified as 2+ radiation cataracts.
				73	3+ to **4**+ galactose cataracts. Anterior completely opaque, no longer possible to grade radiation changes.

II	15	+	–	52	1+ radiation cataracts in some animals. In 5 animals no changes.
				59	1+ radiation cataracts in some animals.
				66	1+ radiation cataracts in 50% of animals.
				73	1+ to 2+ radiation cataracts.
III	15	–	+	52	Many tiny, radial, white, anterior cortical opacities.
				59	Changes not prominent enough to be classified as 1+ galactose cataract.
				66	2+ to 3+ galactose cataracts.
				73	3+ to 4+ galactose cataracts.
IV	10	–		52	–
				59	–
				66	No changes.
				73	–

cataract lens proteins raised the question of potential quantitative differences between them. To answer this question, serial dilutions of normal and cataract lens crystallins were electrophoresed and their precipitin patterns were developed with the same antiserum. The immunoelectrophoretic titrations of crystallins from normal and X-ray cataract lenses were done using both anti-normal and anti-cataract lens serum. With both antisera the same precipitin lines of lens crystallins from irradiated eyes tended to disappear earlier on serial dilution, than the ones of normal lens crystallins at equal total protein concentrations. The proteins whose amount appeared thus decreased in X-ray cataracts are marked by arrows in Fig. 1. As in the rat galactose cataract lens, a beta crystallin was the one which showed the most marked decrease in comparison to the normal lens crystallins. Also, similar to galactose cataract lens proteins, a pre-alpha crystallin was involved in X-ray cataracts. The immunoelectrophoretic pattern of X-ray cataract lens crystallin differed from the galactose cataract as well as the normal crystallins by an additional decrease of a gamma crystallin line.

Two series of cataract experiments were performed in which a galactose diet was given to animals whose eyes had been previously irradiated. In the first series 60 rats were used. At age two weeks 35 Fisher rats were given 400 rads in a single dose to both eyes. Four weeks after irradiation, when all animals were six weeks old, 20 of the irradiated rats and 15 non-irradiated animals were started on a galactose diet. The remaining irradiated and non-irradiated animals were kept on a regular diet of Purina pellets. In this way, groups with only X-ray or galactose or both and one group of normal animals were formed. The galactose diet was continued for a period of four weeks by which time the animals had developed complete opacification. The clinical course of lens changes in these animals is summarized in Table 1. The clinical observations were started 52 days after irradiation and four days after the start of galactose feeding.

As can be seen during the first two weeks of galactose feeding, the changes produced by galactose and those produced by irradiation progressed independently in the animals exposed to both stresses. The rate of progression of radiation changes in animals which were on a galactose diet appeared accelerated, especially in the anterior cortex, in comparison to animals on a normal diet. Also there was some acceleration of specific galactose cataract changes observed in the irradiated animals. At 66 days after irradiation alone (group II), half of the animals developed just a 1+ cataract, whereas in group I (X-ray and galactose) many animals showed 2+ specific X-ray cataract changes. In animals which received galactose alone (group III) at day 59, the animals just started to develop a 1+ specific galactose cataract. On a similar galactose diet, animals which also received X-ray (group I) showed more pronounced 1+ to 2+ specific galactose induced changes.

In view of the comparatively faster progress of galactose than X-ray cataract, five animals from group I and group III were switched to a regular diet eleven days after the beginning of the galactose feeding and observed for the next two weeks. When the change to a regular diet was made, the animals were at stage 2+ of galactose cataracts. It was found in group I, those animals which received both X-ray and galactose that in one animal cataractous changes progressed and complete opacities developed in both eyes.

Two animals regressed, however, to 1+ galactose cataracts but still progressed to 3+ radiation cataracts. In two animals it was difficult to grade the galactose cataracts, since the radiation changes were at stage 2+ in one and 3+ in another. In group III with animals on a galactose diet alone, all animals progressed to 2-3+ cataracts, most of the changes being anterior.

In the subsequent series of experiments in which Columbia-Sherman rats were used, the dose of radiation was increased in the expectation that the radiation opacities would accelerate to rates corresponding more closely to those produced by the galactose diet. For the same reason the galactose diet was lowered to 35% galactose. It was observed in independent experiments used for histology that Columbia-Sherman rats do not show any deviation from the well established X-ray or galactose lens pathologies. Because of this, the observations in experiments II-IV were restricted to the study of specific X-ray or galactose cataract changes in the same eye. The data summarized in Tables II-IV.

As can be seen by comparing Tables II, III and IV, a decrease of the galactose diet from 50% to 35% and an increase of the radiation dose to 600, 1000 and 1400 r caused a change in the relative progression of galactose specific and X-ray specific changes in the same eye. After 600 r, 50% of the animals developed a 2+ X-ray cataract at 49.5 days after irradiation. By comparison, a 2+ galactose cataract developed in 50% of animals of the same group at 43.7 days. After 1000 r, it took 42.5 days for 50% of the animals to develop a 2+ radiation cataract, and 41.1 days for 50% of the animals to develop a 2+ galactose cataract. After 1400 r the corresponding times needed to develop 2+ specific cataract changes in 50% of the animals was 36.3 days for X-ray and 41.2 days for galactose. In all the experiments, the galactose diet was started on day 29. The above data were calculated assuming that within a short time interval, e.g. 40 to 45 days, the progression of cataract changes is linear. Thus, significantly in all the experimental groups put on a galactose diet after 600, 1000 or 1400 r, it was possible to

Table II. Lens changes specific of X-ray (X) or galactose (G) cataract in rats exposed to 600 rads and 29 days later started on a 35% galactose diet.

Days after radiation with 600 rads	No. animals	Biomicroscopic observation: X-ray (X) and galactose (G) cataract changes in the same eye									
		0*		1+		2+		3+		4+	
		X	G	X	G	X	G	X	G	X	G
29	20	20	20	0	0	0	0	0	0	0	0
40	18	9	6	9	12	0	0	0	0	0	0
45	15	0	0	11	5	4	10	0	0	0	0
54	15	0	0	4	0	11	11	0	4	0	0
59	14	0	0	0	0	14	9	0	4	0	1

* 0 = no cataract

283

Table III. Lens changes specific of X-ray (X) or galactose (G) cataract in rats exposed to 1000 rads and 29 days later started on a 35% galactose diet.

Days after irradiation with 1000 rads	No. Animals	0*		1+		2+		3+		4+	
		X	G	X	G	X	G	X	G	X	G
29	18	15	18	3	0	0	0	0	0	0	0
40	14	0	0	13	9	1	5	0	0	0	0
45	14	0	0	1	0	13	14	0	0	0	0
54	14	0	0	0	0	9	6	5	8	0	0
59	12	0	0	0	0	5	0	7	7	0	5

Biomicroscopic observation: X-ray (X) and galactose (G) cataract changes in the same eye

* 0 = no cataract

Table IV. Lens changes specific of X-ray (X) or galactose (G) cataract in rats exposed to 1400 rads and 29 days later started on a 35% galactose diet.

Days after irradiation with 1400 rads	No. Animals	0*		1+		2+		3+		4+	
		X	G	X	G	X	G	X	G	X	G
29	10	0	10	7	0	3	0	0	0	0	0
40	10	0	0	4	6	6	4	0	0	0	0
45	10	0	0	0	0	5	8	5	2	0	0
54	10	0	0	0	0	0	5	1	5	9	0

Biomicroscopic observation: X-ray (X) and galactose (G) cataract changes in the same eye

* 0 = no cataract

distinguish the initiation and progression of changes typical of radiation cataract and galactose cataract in the same lens for up to 59 days post-irradiation or 29 days after the start of galactose feeding. This distinction became difficult to observe as the changes advanced beyond stage 2+.

The following histology is from normal rats as well as from animals which were sacrificed 45 days after unilateral irradiation (1000 rads to the right eye). These included animals which were on a regular diet and animals which were maintained on a galactose diet. The animals were nine weeks old at time of sacrifice.

Fig. 2 shows the anterior pole and Fig. 3 the posterior pole of a normal rat lens. The microscopic magnification in these and the following pictures

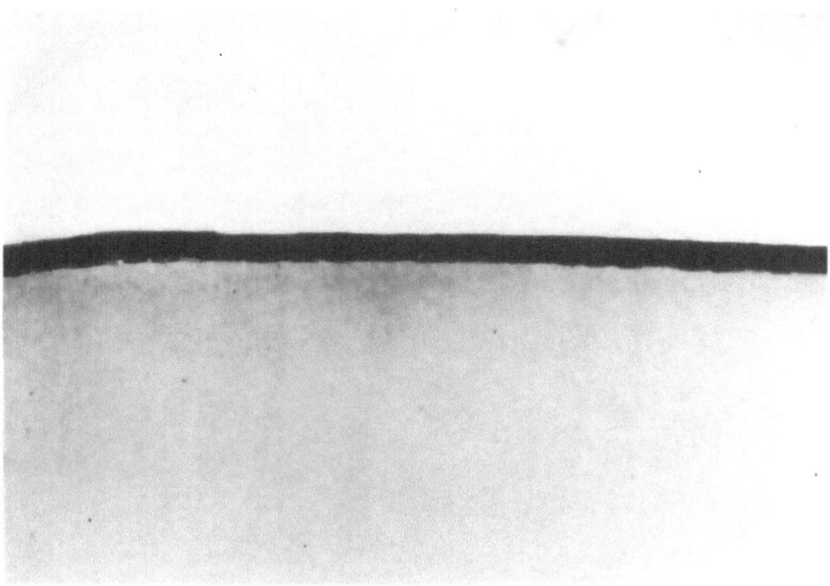

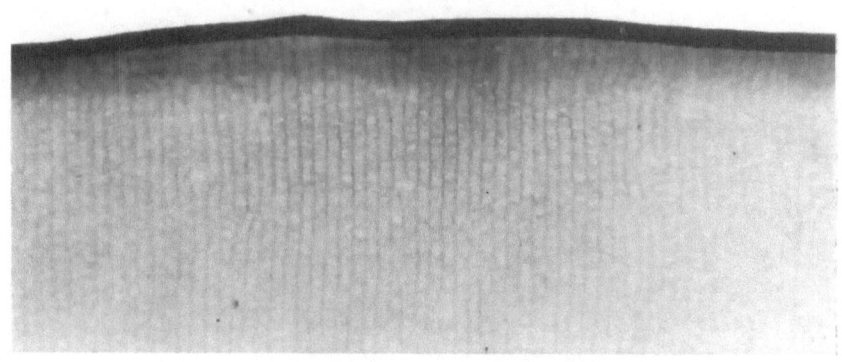

Figs. 2 & 3.   Anterior and posterior pole of a normal lens.

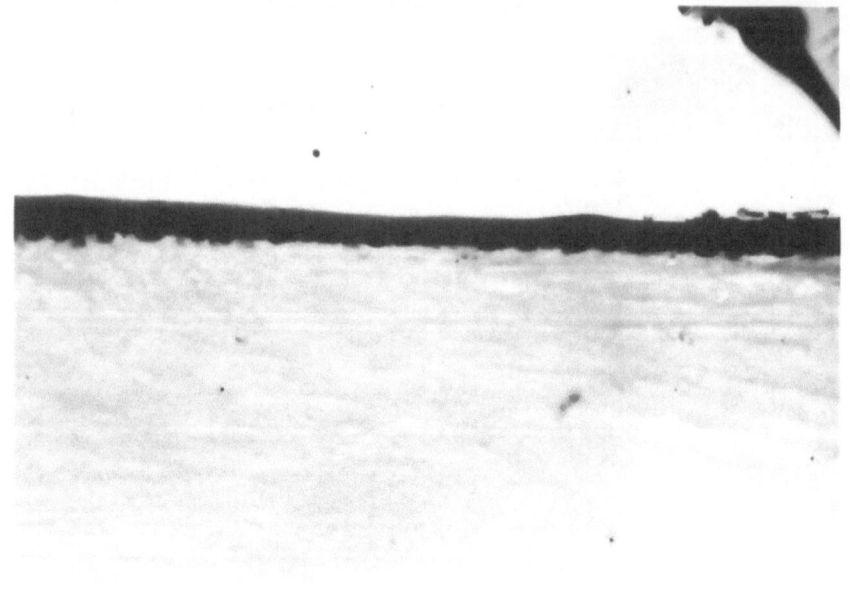

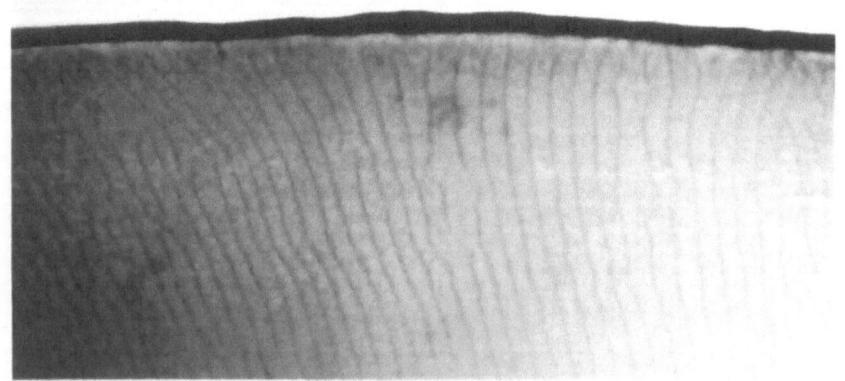

Figs. 4 & 5. Anterior and posterior pole of a galactose induced cataract lens.

is 500X. The hexagonal shape and tight packing of normal superficial fibers are readily seen. The anterior pole of an unirradiated lens from an animal kept on a galactose diet for two weeks is shown in Fig. 4. The typical swelling of the underlying cortical fibers and an altered intercellular spacing can be observed. A different histologic picture is seen in Fig. 5 which shows the posterior cortex of the same lens. The appearance of this area is normal except for a slight swelling of the fibers and some loss of definition.

The situation is reversed in irradiated lenses. Fig. 6 shows the anterior pole of an irradiated lens of an animal on a regular diet. Excepting some irregularity in the subepithelial layer, the cytoarchitecture is normal. In this case it is the posterior pole of the same lens which is principally involved (Fig. 7). The presence of nuclei in normally non-nucleated fibers and changes in fiber morphology are typical. In addition, vacuoles, which may actually represent swollen fibers, are evident.

Fig. 8 shows the anterior pole and Fig. 9 the posterior pole of an irradiated lens from an animal which was on a galactose diet for two weeks. As can be seen, particularly the anterior and to a lesser degree, the posterior portion of the lens are affected to a greater degree than if either radiation or galactose were applied alone. The anterior cortex (Fig. 8) shows some nucleated cells while such cells are not shown in Fig. 9. Some were found in other sections but interestingly fewer than when X-rays alone were applied. However, the overall damage posteriorly is similar to that produced by radiation alone.

DISCUSSION

The sensitive passive hemagglutination technique showed that anti-normal lens serum could be completely absorbed by the cataractous lens and conversely anti-cataract lens serum could be completely absorbed by normal lens. These absorption experiments thus proved that specific cataract lens proteins were not formed nor was there a complete loss of normal lens proteins in X-ray cataract formation.

Comparison of serial dilutions of normal and cataract lens proteins by immunoelectrophoresis revealed that a pre-alpha and a beta crystallin were present in relatively lesser amounts in the X-ray cataract than in the normal lens. A similar observation was made in galactose cataracts. The X-ray cataract lens proteins differ, however, from the galactose cataract proteins by a relative decrease of a gamma crystallin. This difference may be related to the differences in time involved in the formation of these two types of cataracts. Under the experimental conditions chosen, a 1+ galactose cataract developed in all animals in about one week after initiation of the galactose diet and a 4+ cataract developed in all animals about three weeks later. In X-ray cataracts the time involved in the progression from 1+ to 4+ changes was usually much greater even when 1400 rads were applied. This difference suggests the possibility that there is a sequence in which lens crystallins become affected by abnormal cellular conditions. Independent of the specific factors (DISCHE, 1968; KINOSHITA, 1974; NORDMANN, 1972) which may have initiated the cellular pathology, the pre-alpha and beta crystallins appear to be more readily affected than the gamma crystallin. In view of

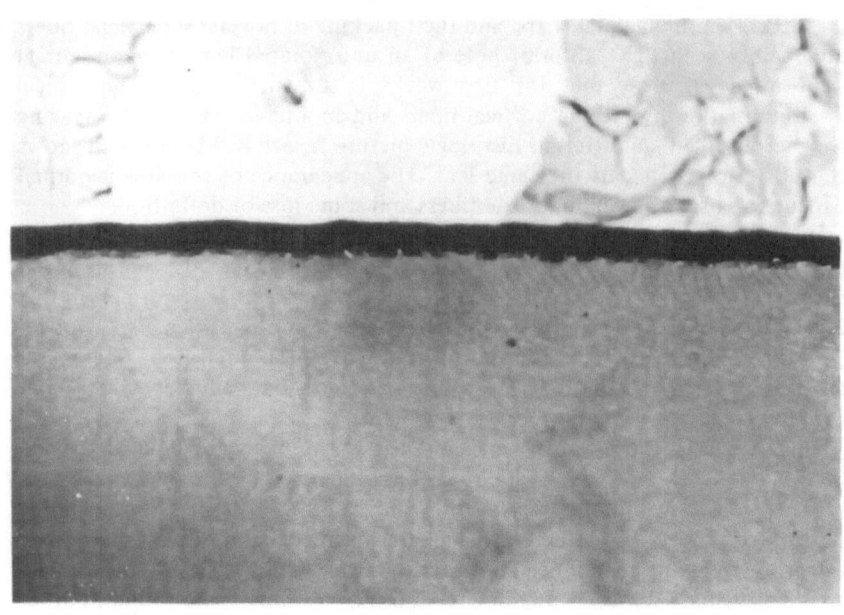

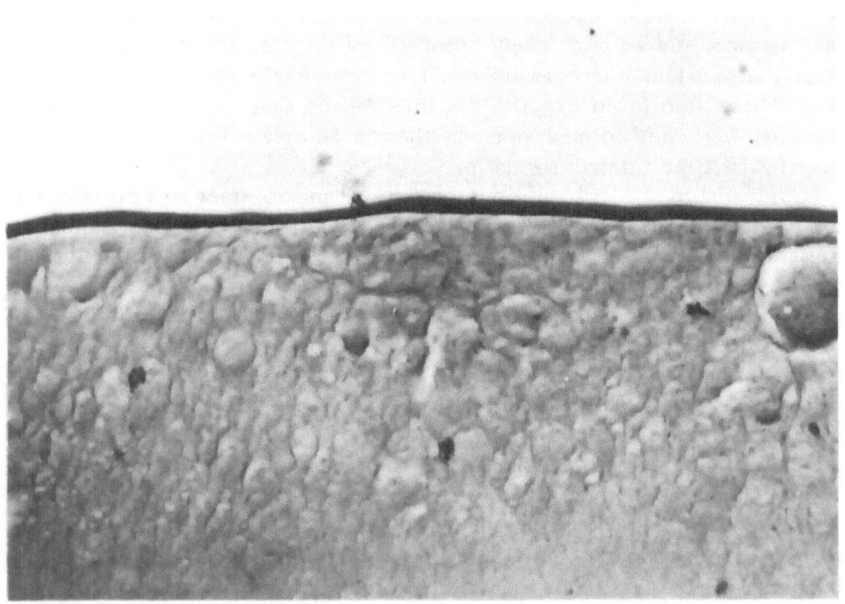

Figs. 6 & 7 Anterior and posterior pole of an X-ray induced cataract lens.

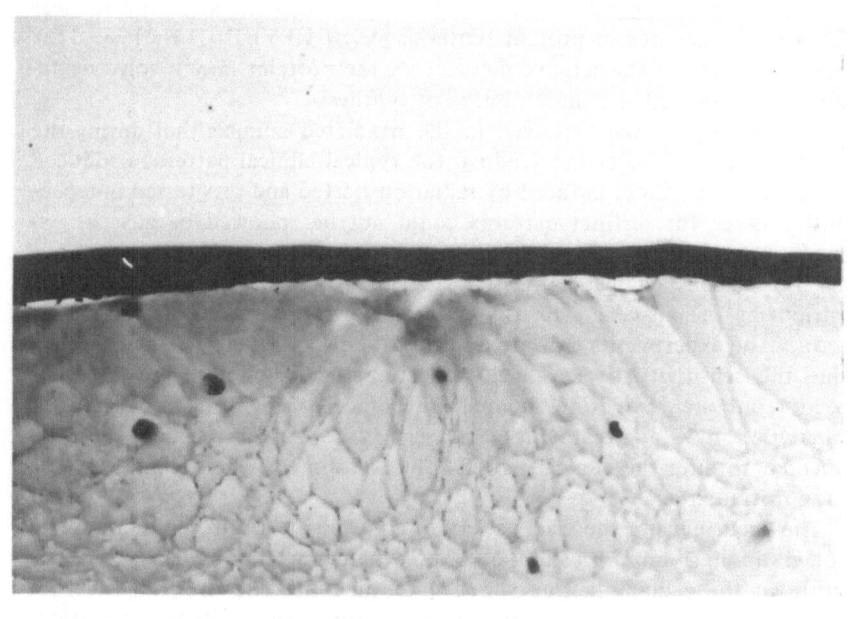

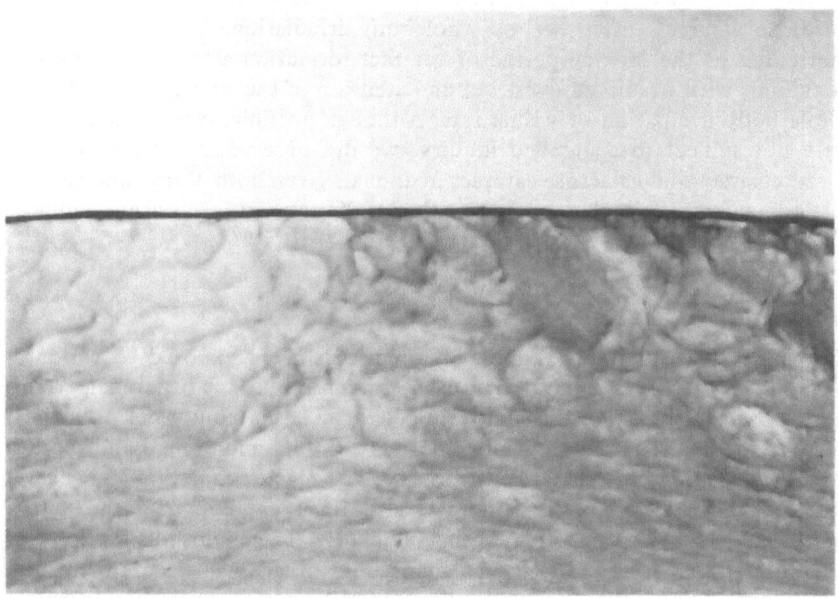

Figs. 8 & 9. Anterior and posterior pole of a simultaneously induced galactose and X-ray cataract lens.

the fact that in normal lenses transparency is maintained in the nuclear region in the absence of protein synthesis (VAN HEYNINGEN, 1969), the above sequence of the relative decrease of the proteins may involve degradative processes rather than inhibition of synthesis.

Significantly, it was observed in the irradiated animals that during the first two weeks of galactose feeding, the typical clinical patterns produced by galactose and those induced by radiation started and progressed independently. Later the distinct patterns could not be followed because of extensive opacification. These results are in agreement with the hypothesis that the various clinical patterns in cataracts may be a reflection of the distribution of lens cells primarily sensitive to the particular cataractogenic factors. The experiments indicate also that the factor or factors which determine the sensitivity of lens cells to cataractogenic factors are not only specific but are also quite independent of other environmental changes. Otherwise, an X-ray treatment of a lens before a galactose diet could be expected to alter the clinical pattern of development when compared to a lens not irradiated.

The occurrence of the wide variety of clinical patterns in cataract may be looked upon as an expression of a large heterogeneity of lens cells. The nature of the cellular factors which determine the selective sensitivity of some lens cells to specific cataractogenic factors needs further exploration.

Reports in the literature on the simultaneous application of cataractogenic agents have dealt basically with the occurrence of synergistic effects (HOCKWIN, OKAMOTO, BERGEDER, KLEIN, FERRARI & STREIT, 1969/1970). HOCKWIN, BERGEDER & KAISER (1967) and HOCKWIN, BERGEDER, NINNEMANN & FINK (1974) studied the development of galactose cataracts after eye or wholebody irradiation. They reported a shortening of the latency period of cataract formation after galactose diet in animals with irradiated eyes, but an extension of the latency period after whole body irradiation of young rats. Although possible, synergistic effects were not subject to a detailed inquiry, we did observe an acceleration of X-ray cataract and galactose cataract in animals given both X-rays and galactose compared to animals exposed to either of the cataractogenic agents alone.

SUMMARY

Eyes of two week old Columbia-Sherman rats were exposed to varying single doses of X-rays. Four weeks after irradiation groups of animals were started on a 35% or 50% galactose diet which lasted four weeks. Ocular changes in these animals were followed with the biomicroscope and representative samples were taken for histology. The specific radiation and galactose induced changes in the same eye of animals exposed to both agents were found to begin and progress independently. The clinical distinction of galactose versus X-ray induced lens changes in these animals could be made clearly for incipient opacities and followed until cataracts became extensive.

By immunochemical analysis the similarity of normal, X-ray and galactose cataract rat lens proteins was proven by complete cross-absorption of anti-normal lens sera with cataractous lenses and of anti-cataract lens sera with normal lenses. A decrease of a pre-alpha and of at least one beta crystallin was observed in both forms of cataract. In addition, in the X-ray cataract lenses a decrease of at least one gamma crystallin was observed.

These results are compatible with the hypothesis that the clinical patterns of various cataracts may be an expression of a different topographical distribution of the cells primarily responsive to the particular cataractogenic agent. The similarity of lens proteins involved in different cataracts may reflect a constant sequence in which individual lens proteins are affected by changes in cellular homeostasis.

REFERENCES

BOYDEN, S.V. The absorption of proteins on erythrocytes treated with tannic acid and subsequent hemagglutination by antiprotein sera. *J. Exp. Med.* 93: *107* (1951).

DISCHE, Z. Alterations of lens proteins as etiology in cataracts. In: *Biochemistry of the Eye*, Symposium, Tutzing Castle, p. 413-428, Dardeene, M.U. and Nordmann, J., eds., Karger, Basel/New York (1968).

DUKE-ELDER, S. Diseases of the lens and vitreous; glaucoma and hypotony. In: *System of Ophthalmology*, Vol. XI, p. 152-165, C.V. Mosby Co., St. Louis (1969).

FRANCOIS, J. *Congenital Cataracts*, Charles C. Thomas, Royal Van Gorcum, Assen, Netherlands (1963).

HEYNINGEN, R. VAN. The lens: metabolism and cataract. In: *The Eye*, Vol. 1, p. 381-488, Davson, H., ed., Academic Press, New York (1969).

HOCKWIN, O., BERGEDER, H.D. & KAISER, L. Über die Galactose-Katarakt junger Ratten nach Ganzkörper-Röntgenbestrahlung. *Ber. Dtsch. Ophth. Ges.* 68: *135-139* (1967).

HOCKWIN, O., BERGEDER, H.D., NINNEMAN, V. & FINK, H. Untersuchungen zur Latenzzeit der Galaktosekatarakt von Ratten. *Albrecht v. Graefes Arch. klin. exp. Ophthal.* 189: *171-178* (1974).

HOCKWIN, O., OKAMOTO, T., BERGEDER, H.D., KLEIN, W., FERRARI, L. & STREIT, A. Genesis of cataracts, cumulative effects of subliminal noxious influences. *Ann. Ophthalmol.* 1: *321-325* (1969/1970).

KINOSHITA, J.H. Mechanisms initiating cataract formation. Proctor Lecture. *Invest. Ophthal.* 13: *713-724* (1974).

MANN, I. Culture, Race, Climate and Eye Disease: An Introduction to the Study of Geographical Ophthalmology, p. 316-317 Charles C. Thomas, Springfield, Ill. (1966).

MANSKI, W. Immunological studies on normal and pathological lenses. In: The Human Lens – in Relation to Cataract, Ciba Foundation Symposium, Elliott, K. and Fitzsimons, D.W., eds., p. 227-248, Excerpta Medica, Elsevier, North-Holland, Amsterdam (1973).

MERRIAM, G.R., Jr. & FOCHT, E.F. A clinical and experimental study of the effect of single and divided doses of radiation on cataract production. *Trans. Am. Ophthal. Soc.* 60: *35-52* (1972).

MERRIAM, G.R., Jr. & SZECHTER, A. The relative radiosensitivity of rat lenses as a function of age. *Rad. Res.* 62: *488-497* (1975)

NORDMANN, J. Problems in cataract research. *Ophthalmic Res.* 3: *323-359* (1972).

PIRIE, A. An Introduction in Causes and Prevention of Blindness, Michaelson, C. & Berman, E.R., eds., p. 530-536, Academic Press, New York/London (1972).

RUTTENBERG, G. The insoluble proteins of bovine crystalline lens. *Exp. Eye Res.* 4: *18-23* (1965).

SCHEIDEGGER, J.J. Une micro-methode de l'immuno-electrophorese. *Int. Arch. Allergy* 7: *103-110* (1955).

WADSWORTH, C. A microplate technique employing a gel chamber compared with other micro- and macroplate techniques for immune diffusion. *Int. Arch. Allergy* 21: *131-137* (1962).

WORGUL, B.V., MERRIAM, G.R., Jr., SZECHTER, A. & SRINIVASAN, B.D. The lens epithelium and radiation cataract. I. Preliminary studies. *Arch. Ophthal.* 94: *996-999* (1976).

YORK, A.T., HAMADA, S. & MANSKI, W. Immunochemical studies on crystallins and albuminoids in galactose cataracts of inbred rats. *Ophthal. Res.* 2: *273-284* (1971a).

YORK, A.T., MARTINEZ, C. & MANSKI, W. Immunochemical studies on crystallins and albuminoids in human senile cataracts. *Ophthal. Res.* 3: *183-191* (1971b).

Keywords:

Galactose cataract
X-ray cataract
double stress cataract
anti-normal lens antiserum
anti-cataract lens antiserum
immunological cross reaction
immunoelectrophoresis
histopathology of cataract

Authors' addresses:

W. Manski & A.T. York
Immunology Laboratory
The Edward S. Harkeness Eye Institute
Columbia University/Presbyterian Hospital
New York, N.Y., USA
G.R. Merriam, Jr. & B.V. Worgul
Radiation Biology Laboratory
The Edward S. Harkness Eye Institute
Columbia University/Presbyterian Hospital
New York, N.Y., USA
A. Szechter
Department of Radiation Therapy
St. Vincent's Hospital and Medical Center
New York, N.Y., USA

NAPHTHALENE CATARACTS IN RATS.
ASSOCIATION OF EYE PIGMENTATION AND
CATARACT DEVELOPMENT*

HANS-REINHARD KOCH, KATRIN DOLDI & OTTO HOCKWIN

(Bonn, W. Germany)

ABSTRACT

The development of naphthalene cataracts was studied in 5 strains of *rattus norvegicus* of different pigmentation. Whereas all animals of the pigmented strains (E3, BDE, DA) developed zonular cataracts after latencies of 20 to 28 days, only some of the albinos (Wistar, Sprague Dawley) exhibited less pronounced changes after longer latencies of 32 to 61 days. The possible importance of the melanin-synthetizing enzyme phenol oxidase (tyrosinase) of the iris for the formation of the cataractogenic substance 1,2-naphthodiquinone is discussed.

INTRODUCTION

In 1886 naphthalene, then widely used as a therapeutic agent for many diseases, was found by BOUCHARD & CHARRIN to cause cataracts in rabbits. For half a century this substance remained the favorite experimental cataractogenic of investigating ophthalmologists, although clinical observations of naphthalene cataracts were extremely scarce (LEZENIUS, 1902).

VAN DER HOEVE reported in 1902 clinical and experimental results indicating that β-naphthol was also cataractogenic, even after topical administration. According to him the similarity of naphthalene and β-naphthol cataracts results from a biological conversion of naphthalene to the better soluble α- and β-naphthols. The biotransformation of naphthalene was then elaborately studied by EDLEFSEN (1905), who found β-naphthol as well as several conjugated compounds.

During the years to come many theories were proposed to explain the cataractogenic action of naphthalene. It was soon realized that the tissues surrounding the lens must have some bearing on cataract development. Thus a cyclitis, hyperemia or toxic changes of the ciliary body were accused as primary lesions.

Both UYAMA et al. (1955) and PIRIE & VAN HEYNINGEN (1966) were then able to show that 1,2-naphthodiquinone is responsible for cataract formation. This highly reactive compound is formed within the body after naphthalene intoxication. It will interfere with the proteins, coenzymes, amino acids, and other constituents of the lens (REES & PIRIE, 1967; PIRIE, 1968). Based on investigations of BOYLAND and his group

---

* A preliminary report of these results has been presented to the Association for Eye Research by KOCH & DOLDI in 1974.

(1956-1964) they proposed a scheme according to which naphthalene is converted into the quinone (VAN HEYNINGEN & PIRIE, 1967).

Both from earlier experimental observations of our own and from data in the literature we were struck by several peculiarities of naphthalene opacities:

— first by the affinity of the *pigmented* tissues of the eye to toxic naphthalene changes,

— secondly by the *varying susceptibility* of rabbits to naphthalene, first reported by KOLINSKI (1889) and well known to everybody who worked in this field, and

— thirdly by the fact that only GOLDMANN (1929) was able to induce naphthalene cataracts in *rats*, while more recent experiments with that species proved futile.

A possible answer would be that the occurance of experimental naphthalene cataracts is correlated with the pigmentation of the test animals. For GOLDMANN's experiments were performed at a time, before the inbred albino strains revolutionized rat experimentation, and at least part of the animals used by GOLDMANN were pigmented (H. GOLDMANN, pers. comm., 1974). Interesting results supporting this theory were brought forward by LINDBERG (1922), who found in rabbits that the parts of the lens adjacent to the iris were opacified first. No opacities occured in the region of iris colobomas (Fig. 1a), and anisocoria after sympathectomy lead to opacities differing in size (Fig. 1b).

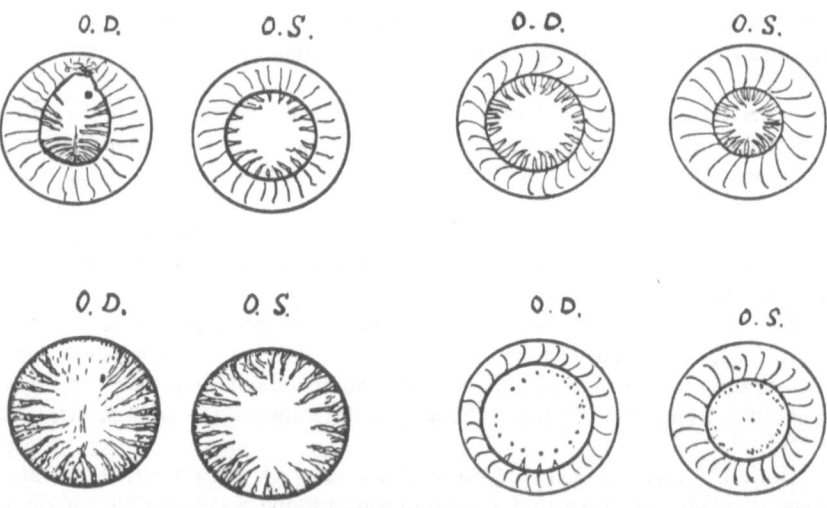

Fig. 1. Importance of the iris in naphthalene cataract development, reproduced from J.G. LINDBERG (1922) with kind permission of Ferdinand Enke Verlag, Stuttgart. a.) Effect of iris coloboma on the formation of spokes, 2 days after naphthalene administration (top), and appearance of dissected lenses 24 days after onset of feeding (bottom); b) effect of anisocoria due to sympathectomy on the formation of spokes 12 h after naphthalene ingestion (top) and on the location of vacuoles 3 days later (bottom).

Table I. Pigmentation of 5 different strains of *rattus norvegicus*, used for the experiment

	1 Wistar	2 Sprague Dawley	Strain 3 E 3	4 B D E	5 D A
Coat pigmentation	albino	albino	light (hooded)	dark (hooded)	dark (agouti)
Eye pigmentation	absent	absent	light	dark	dark
Color genes*	ccPpAaHh	ccPpAaHh	CCppaahh	CCPPaahh	CCPPAAHH

(*: Cc - albino: Pp - pink-eyed: Aa - agouti; Hh - hooded)

Table II. Experimental set-up and sizes of groups

		1. Wistar	2. Sprague Dawley	Strain 3. E 3	4. B D E	5. D A
Treatments	·0 solvent	group 10 (n=6)	group 20 (n=6)	group 30 (n=4)	group 40 (n=6)	group 50 (n=6)
	·1 naph- thalene	group 11 (n=6)	group 21 (n=6)	group 31 (n=3)	group 41 (n=6)	group 51 (n=6)

To test our hypothesis we investigated whether rats of different pigmentation would react differently to a naphthalene intoxication.

MATERIAL AND METHODS

We used 5 differently pigmented strains of the brown rat (*rattus norvegicus*), all aged 7 weeks at the beginning of the experiment. They were supplied by Zentralinstitut für Versuchstierzucht, Hannover (Table 1).

Naphthalene was dissolved in liquid paraffine and administered by stomach tube every second day to groups of 6 animals of each strain (1 g/kg

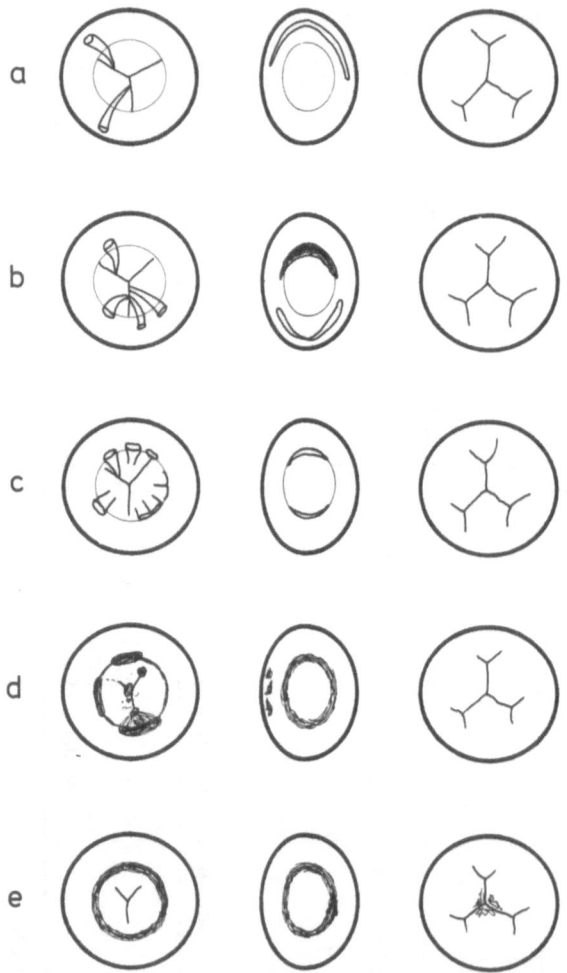

Fig. 2. Naphthalene cataract development in rats. Schematic drawings in three levels: anterior cortex (left), optical section (middle), and posterior cortex (right). a.) and b.) formation of water clefts, c.) movement of clefts to the supranuclear layer, d.) collaps of waterclefts, and e.) transformation into supranuclear zonular opacity.

296

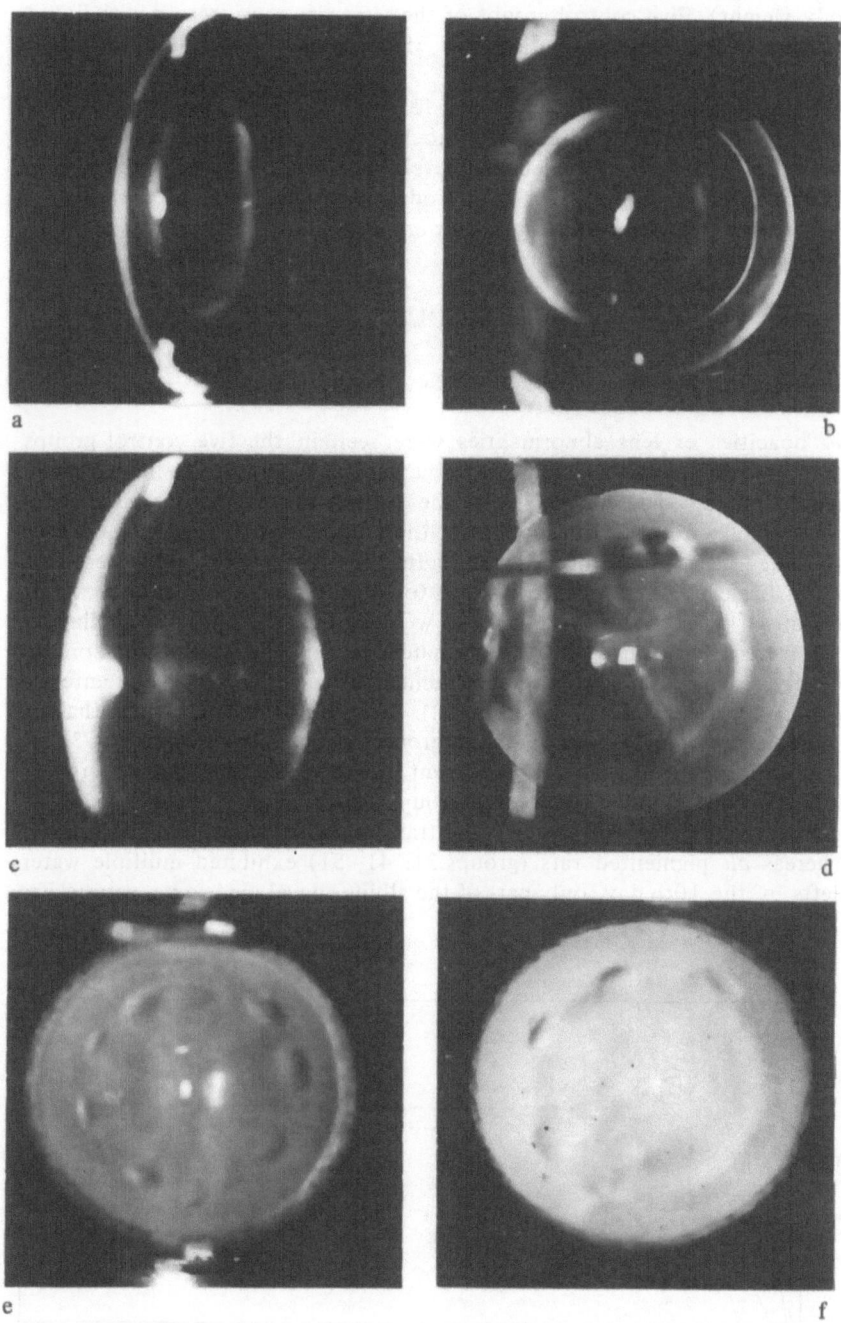

Fig. 3. Naphthalene cataract formation in an animal of group 51 (DA); a.), b.) formation of water clefts after 8 and 12 days, respectively; c.), d.) collaps of water clefts
after 16 days, retroillumination and focal illumination; e.), f.) zonular opacity after
28 days.

body weight). Five control groups of the same size were treated with liquid paraffine only. The test period was 75 days. The experimental set-up is shown in Table 2.

Development of lens changes was followed up by regular examinations with a photo slit lamp (Zeiss, Oberkochen). Results were routinely documented by drawings of the lens in 3 levels (cf. Fig. 2). Typical findings were photographed on Kodak Plus-X or Kodak Highspeed Ektachrome 135/36.

After the test period the animals were killed and lens fresh weights were measured with a Mettler microbalance.

RESULTS

Morphologic findings

No opacities or lens abnormalities were seen in the five control groups treated with the solvent alone. Opacities occured only in the naphthalene-treated groups. These began with the formation of large cortical water clefts, which followed the course of the cortical lens fibres. As the lenses continued to grow during the test period and new fibre layers were laid down, the clefts were pushed inwards towards the supranuclear layer. After this initial phase no new water clefts were formed, the older ones collapsed and were transformed into a supranuclear homogenous whitish zonular opacity. In some animals the development of vacuoles within the anterior Y-shaped suture was observed (Fig. 2). The typical course of naphthalene cataract development in an animal of group 51 (BDE) is shown in Fig. 3.

With respect to cataract development there were considerable differences between the 5 naphthalene-treated groups (11-51). This applies both to the formation of water clefts and to the transformation into zonular opacities. Whereas *all* pigmented rats (groups 31, 41, 51) exhibited multiple water clefts by the 10th day, only part of the albinos developed some water clefts

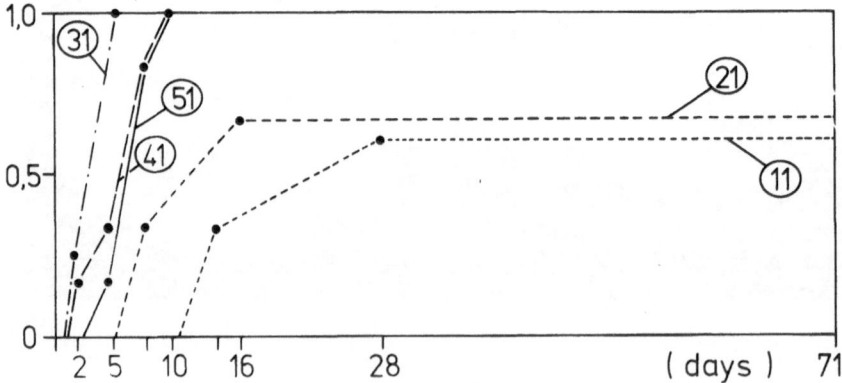

Fig. 4. Relative frequency (i.e. affected number by total number) of the onset of water cleft formation in the 5 naphthalene-treated groups in the course of the experiment.

after much longer latencies. Fig. 4 shows the relative frequencies of water cleft formation in the animals of the 5 test groups.

The transformation into a zonular cataract also occured after different latencies. Whereas *all* animals of the pigmented strains had developed such cataracts after 20-28 days, only some of the albino rats had reached that stage after 61 days (Fig. 5).

Fig. 6 gives an impression of typical lens findings in animals of 3 different groups on the 32nd day. An oildroplet-like demarcation of the nucleus can be observed in one of the affected albinos (Sprague Dawley), whereas a less pronounced and a marked zonular cataract can be seen in the lenses of E3 and DA animals, respectively.

This difference remained visible until the end of the experiment. At a later stage, however, there was also a difference between the less affected two albino strains. On the 62nd day only one of the remaining 5 Wistars exhibited minor lens changes, while 3 of 5 Sprague Dawley rats had now developed zonular opacities, which were considerably less pronounced than the ones in the pigmented strains (Fig. 7).

Lens wet weights

Lens wet weights had been measured at the end of the experiment. Results and statistical evaluations are given in Table 3. Although the animals were of the same age, lens wet weight was significantly influenced by the strain. Their was neither a significant effect of the treatment, nor an interaction between strains and treatment.

DISCUSSION

Our results confirm a suspected interrelation between eye pigmentation and naphthalene cataract in rats. They are in agreement with the observations of LINDBERG (1922), who observed an effect of the iris on the development of naphthalene opacities (Fig. 1).

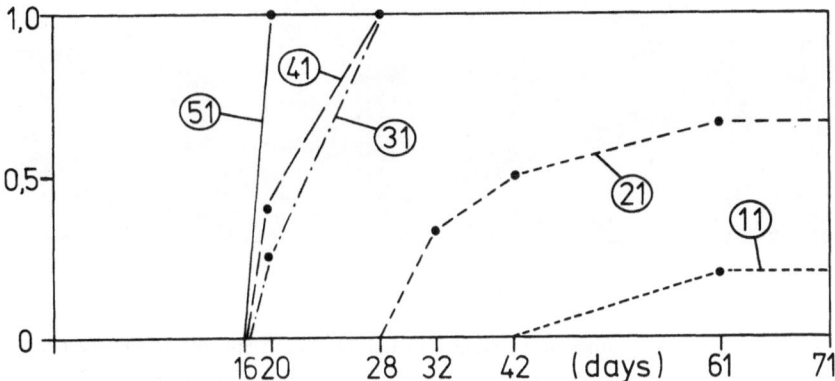

Fig. 5. Relative frequency of the occurrance of zonular cataracts in the 5 naphthalene-treated groups in the course of the experiment.

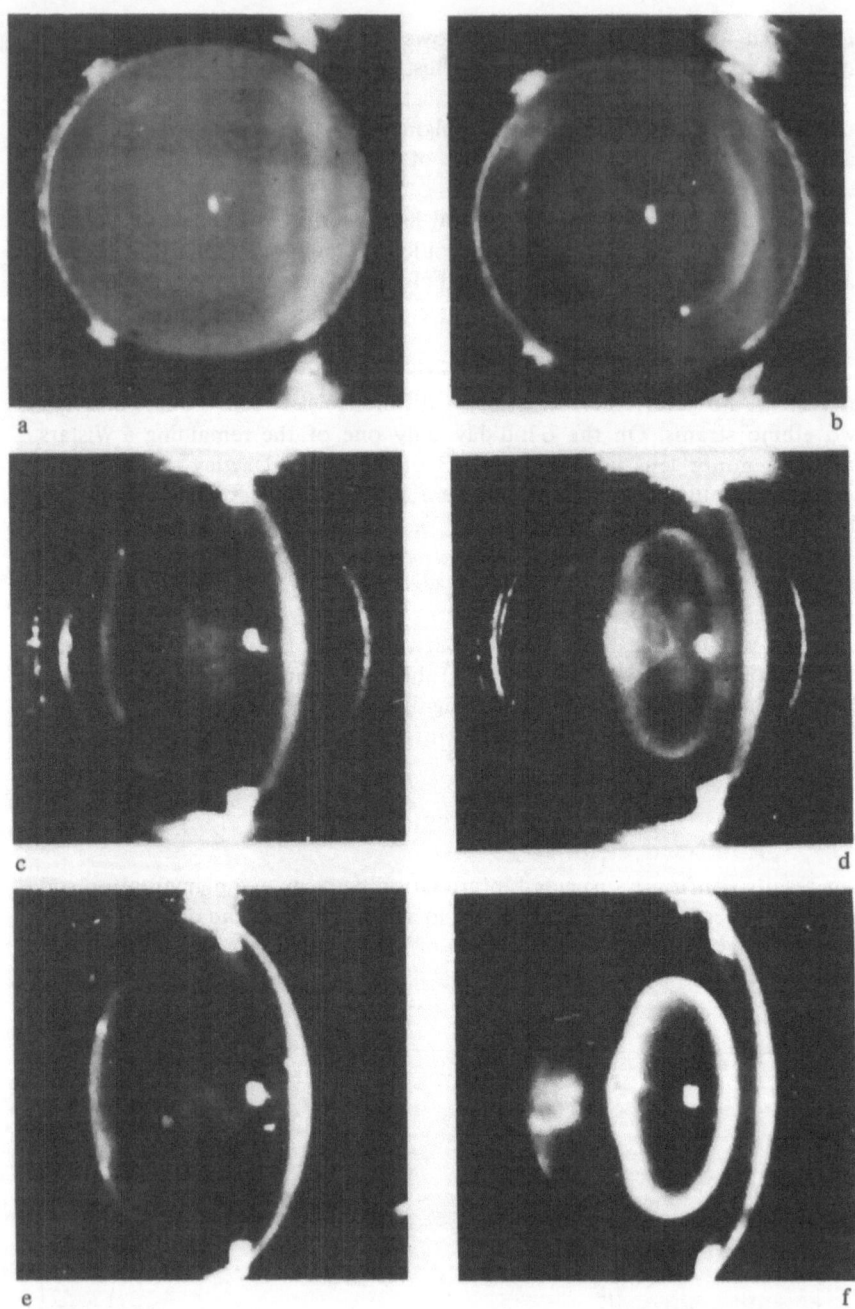

Fig. 6. Typical lens findings in 6 animals on the 32nd day; Sprague Dawley; a.) control (group 20), b.) oildroplet-like demarcation of the nucleus after naphthalene feeding (group 21); E3-strain: c.) control (group 30), d.) zonular opacity in naphthalene-fed rat (group 31); DA-strain: e.) control (group 50), f.) pronounced zonular opacity after naphthalene feeding (group 51).

300

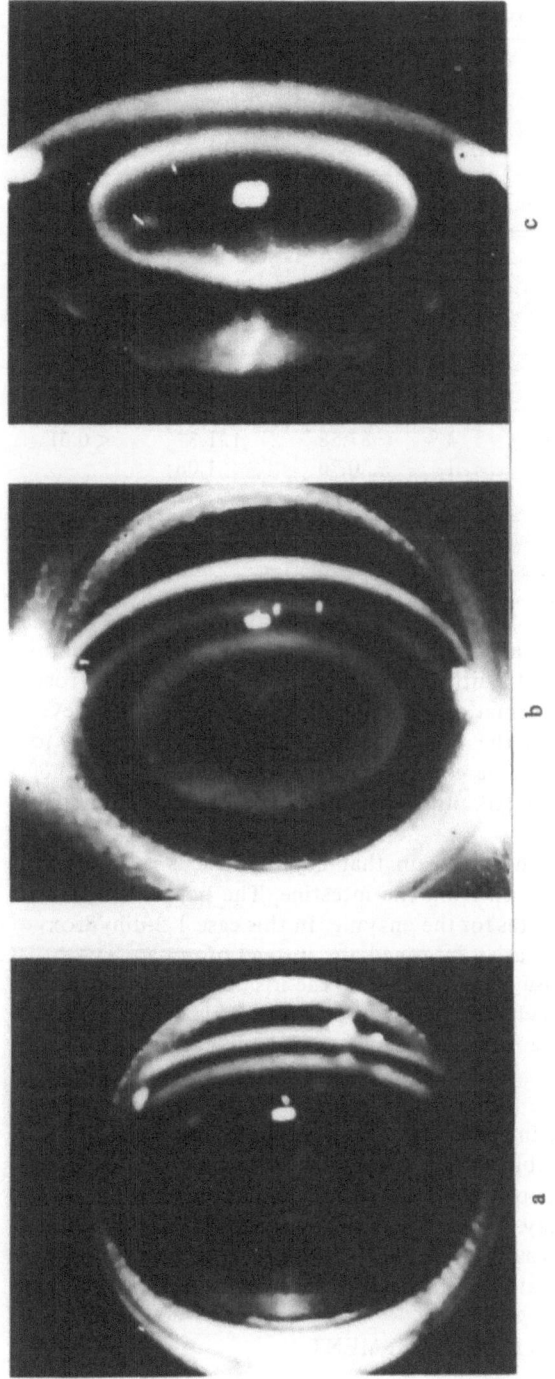

Fig. 7. Lens findings after 62 days: a.) discrete changes in 1 of 5 Wistar rats (group 11); b.) less pronounced zonular cataract in 3 of 5 Sprague Dawley rats (group 21); c.) marked opacity in DA-strain (group 51).

Table III. Lens fresh weights. Means and standard deviations. Statistical analysis with two factor anova (fixed effects, unweighted-means solution).

		Factor A: strains				
		1.	2.	3.	4.	5.
			Sprague			
		Wistar	Dawley	E 3	B D E	D A
Factor B: treatments	·0 solvent	43.0 ± 0.7	39.6 ± 0.7	34.8 ± 0.8	39.7 ± 1.0	39.6 ± 0.7
	·1 naph-thalene	43.9 ± 1.2	38.8 ± 1.5	34.5 ± 0.6	39.1 ± 0.7	39.1 ± 0.3

Source	SS	df	MS	$\hat{F}$	p
A (strains)	350.32	4	87.58	121.37	< 0.01
B (treatments)	0.76	1	0.76	1.06	–
AB (interaction)	4.09	4	1.02	1.42	–
ϵ (error)	36.70	37	0.72		

A possible reason for such an interaction of naphthalene and pigmentation could be that the pigment-synthetizing enzyme phenol oxidase (tyrosinase) is responsible for the formation of 1,2-naphthodiquinone in the eye. Under physiologic conditions the enzyme converts tyrosine via dopa to dopaquinone, a precursor of melanin. The enzyme is known to be rather unspecific and can convert a large number of other phenolic compounds to analogous orthodiquinones.

It has been reported again and again that naphthalene is oxidized to α- or β-naphthol after absorption from the intestine. The naphthols would possibly be appropriate substrates for the enzyme. In this case 1,2-dihydroxy-naphthalene would be formed as an intermediate, instead of dopa.

It is known that tyrosinase is most active in the iris of young animals, in which the synthesis of iris melanine is still in progress. This would explain, why after an initial phase the formation of water clefts in our animals came to a standstill.

There may of course be other routes by which the cataractogenic quinone can also be formed in the body. This is suggested by the fact that, after longer latencies, our albinos also developed less severe lens changes. Here the metabolic route adapted by VAN HEYNINGEN & PIRIE (1967) from BOYLAND (1963) may be responsible for an oxidation of naphthalene to the quinone. Our results indicate, however, that a conversion by phenol oxidase is the major pathway in the eyes of pigmented animals.

ACKNOWLEDGEMENT

We should like to express our thanks to Mr. Viorel Dragomirescu for valuable assistance.

REFERENCES

BOUCHARD, C.J. & A. CHARRIN. La cataracte arteficielle du lapin. *C. r. Soc. Biol.* 8: *614-615* (1886).

BOYLAND, E. The biochemistry of bladder cancer. Thomas: Springfield, Ill. (1963).

BOYLAND, E. & P. SIMS. The conversion of naphthalene into 2-hydroxy-1-naphthylsulfate in the rabbit. *Biochem. J.* 66: *38-40* (1959).

BOYLAND, E. J.B. SOLOMON. Estimation of metabolites of naphthalene by paper chromatography. *Biochem. J.* 63: *679-683* (1956).

BOYLAND E., M. KIMURA, & P. SIMS. The hydroxylation of some aromatic hydrocarbons by the ascorbic acid model hydroxylating system and by rat liver microsomes. *Biochem. J.* 92: *631-638* (1964).

EDLEFSEN, G. Untersuchung über die Ausscheidung und den Nachweis des β-Naphthols im Harn nach Einführung kleiner Dosen von Naphthalin, Benzonaphthol und β-Naphthol. *Arch. exper. Pathol. Pharmakol.* 52: *429-458* (1905).

GOLDMANN, H. Experimentelle Supranukleärkatarakt und Kernsklerose. *Klin. Mbl. Augenheilk.* 83: *433-438* (1929).

KOCH H.-R. & K. DOLDI. Naphthalene cataracts in rats of differently pigmented strains. 15th Meeting, Association for Eye Research, Würzburg, 1974. *Exp. Eye Res.* 20: *180* (1975).

KOLINSKI, J. Zur Lehre von der Wirkung des Naphthalins auf das Auge und über den sogenannten Naphthalinstar. *Graefes Arch. Ophthal.* 35, II: *29-50* (1889).

LEZENIUS, A. Ein Fall von Naphthalinkatarakt beim Menschen. *Klin. Mbl. Augenheilk.* 40: *129-141* (1902).

LINDBERG, J.G. Ueber die Initialstadien des Naphthalinstares im Kaninchenauge. Spielt die Iris eine Rolle bei der Ausbreitung des Stars im vorderen Linsenkortex? *Klin. Mbl. Augenheilk.* 68: *527-533* (1922).

PIRIE, A. Pathology in the eye of the naphthalene-fed rabbit. *Exp. Eye Res.* 7: *354-357* (1968).

PIRIE, A. & R. VAN HEYNINGEN. Naphthalene Cataract (2). In: Biochemistry of the eye. Symp., Tutzing, 1966, p. *410-412* (M.U. DARDENNE & J. NORDMANN, editors). Karger: Basel & New York (1968)

REES, J.R. & A. PIRIE. Possible reactions of 1,2-naphthoquinone in the eye. *Biochem. J.* 102: *853-863* (1967).

UYAMA, Y., S. OGINO & T. ICHIHARA. The cataractogenic substance excreted in the urine of rabbits treated with naphthalene. *Med. J. Osaka Univ.* 6: *229-239* (1955).

VAN DER HOEVE, J. Über die schädliche Wirkung des β-Naphthols in therapeutischen Dosen auf das menschliche Auge. *Graefes Arch. Ophthal.* 53: *74-78* (1902).

VAN HEYNINGEN, R. & A. PIRIE. The metabolism of naphthalene and its toxic effect on the eye. *Biochem. J.* 102: *842-852* (1967).

Keywords:

Cataract
Lens fresh weight
Naphthalene
Pigmentation
Rat
Slit lamp follow-up
Phenol oxidase

Authors' address:

Klinisches Institut für experimentelle Ophthalmologie
Abbestrasse 2
5300 Bonn-Venusberg, W. Germany

TOPICAL TREATMENT OF GALACTOSE CATARACTS

SHAMBHU D. VARMA & JIN H. KINOSHITA

(Bethesda, U.S.A)

SUMMARY

In experimental galactosemia, topical administration of aldose reductase inhibitor, 1,3-dioxo-1H-benz-[de]-isoquinoline-(3H)-acetic acid (Alrestatin) was observed to decrease the level of dulcitol accumulated in the lens as compared to that in the control lens of the contralateral eye receiving the placebo only. In addition, topical application of Alrestatin led to a significant delay in the appearance of nuclear cataracts in eyes of galactosemic rats. The results are thus in conformity with the concept that aldose reductase plays a key role in initiating the formation of galactose cataracts and suggest the possibility of the usefulness of aldose reductase inhibitors in therapeutic ocular treatment of sugar cataracts.

The formation of cataracts in galactosemia is initiated by accumulation of excessive dulcitol (galactitol) in the lens (KINOSHITA, MEROLA, SATOH & DIKMAK, 1962). Dulcitol, which is a hexahydric sugar alcohol, is formed in the lens by the reduction of galactose catalyzed by the enzyme aldose reductase (VAN HEYNINGEN, 1959). Previous studies have demonstrated that the cataractous changes can be attenuated, both in vitro (KINOSHITA, DVORNIK, KRAML & GABBAY, 1968) and in vivo (DVORNIK, DUQUESNE, KRAML, SESTANJ, GABBAY, KINOSHITA, VARMA & MEROLA, 1973) by the use of compounds which inhibit aldose reductase. The obvious next step in the treatment of this form of cataract is to develop means of administering aldose reductase inhibitor directly in the eye in the form of aqueous drops or ointment. These studies may not only be of practical importance but can also serve to substantiate the findings of the earlier feeding experiments which required that control animals form a separate group. In the present studies, the experimental design was considered to be more ideal with one eye serving as a control while the contralateral eye is treated with aldose reductase inhibitor in the same galactosemic rat.

MATERIALS AND METHODS

Sprague dawley rats weighing about 60-80 gms were used in all the experiments. The inhibitor used was AY-22,284 (Alrestatin), chemically known as 1,3-dioxo-1H-benz-[de]-isoquinoline-(3H)-acetic acid supplied through the courtesy of Ayerst Chemical Company of Montreal, Canada. Methyl cellulose 4000 c.p.s. was obtained from Dow Chemical Company, U.S.A.

The inhibitor was applied to the eyes in the form of drops or ointment.

Table 1. Effect of AY-22,284 applied as eye drops on dulcitol content of lenses of rats fed 50% galactose diet

Animal No.	Treated Eye	Untreated Eye	% decrease in dulcitol accumulation
1	285	522	45
2	242	351	30
3	190	765	75
4	440	750	41
5	217	650	34
6	456	674	32
7	287	360	20
8	143	230	38
9	184	323	43
10	50	371	86
11	157	290	56
12	13	130	90
13	195	372	48
14	46	384	88
15	63	215	70
16	206	335	38
17	142	268	47
18	121	250	52
19	160	710	77
20	442	750	41
21	217	650	67
22	447	1000	55

Mean Decrease   53 (4.2)

Values are nanomoles/lens
Figure in bracket is standard error of the mean

A 10% solution of AY-22,284 adjusted to pH 6.8 and thickened with 0.3% methyl cellulose 4000 c.p.s. was used as eye drop. Benzalkonium chloride (1:50,000) was used an antiseptic. Control (untreated eye) was treated with saline containing methyl cellulose and benzalkonium chloride in concentration used as above. The drops were administered every two to three hours. The animals were fed regular lab chow for the first three days and a 50% galactose diet for the last 2 days. Following this the animals were sacrified and lens dulcitol determined.

The drop preparation was made by dissolving the sodium salt of AY-22,284 in water and adjusting the pH to 6.8. Methyl cellulose was added in required concentrations (0.3% in eye drop preparation and 2% in ointment) and the solution warmed to 70° for 2 minutes. It was left to clarify in the refrigerator overnight. The placebo was prepared in a similar way from saline without the inhibitor. Benzalkonium chloride (1:50,000) was used as antiseptic in all the preparations.

    Diet consisted of purina lab chow pellets or purina lab chow powdered and mixed with equal weight of galactose.

Following the experimental periods, eyes were enucleated and lenses dissected out for polyol determination. The freshly dissected lens was homogenized in 1 ml of 5% ZnSO4, $7H_2O$ solution following which 1 ml or equivalent of barium hydroxide solution 0.3N was added. The contents were rehomogenized, centrifuged, and an aliquot lyophilized. The residue was silylatated and analyzed for dulcitol by gas liquid chromotography on 3% SE-30 column maintained at $150°$ as described previously (Varma & Kinoshita, 1974).

RESULTS AND DISCUSSION

The possibility of affecting the level of polyol accumulation in the lens of galactose fed rats by topical application of AY-22,284 in the form of drops was first studied. Table 1 described the results of such experiments. One eye of the animals received the drops containing the inhibitor and the control eye was treated with the same vehicle without the inhibitor (placebo). Since the rats are nocturnal and consume most of their food during the night, it was essential to continue to administer the drops during the night. The

Table 2. Effect of AY-22,284 applied topically as ointment on dulcitol content of lenses of rats fed 50% galactose diet

Animal No.	Treated	Untreated	% decrease in dulcitol accumulation
1	490	787	38
2	275	734	62
3	426	650	35
4	190	437	56
5	234	390	40
6	356	600	41
7	67	531	87
8	547	800	32
9	460	753	39
10	313	1041	70
11	324	517	38

Mean Decrease   48.9 (5)

Values are nanomoles/lens
Figure in bracket is standard error of the mean

Animals 1-6. A 10% ointment of AY-22,284 containing 2% methyl cellulose (4000 c.p.s.) and 1:50,000 dilution of benzalkonium chloride was used. One eye of the animals received the ointment every 2-3 hrs for 5 days. The other eye was given the placebo. The animals were given lab chow for the first three days and 50% galactose on the last two days. Following this the animals were sacrificed and their lenses analyzed for dulcitol by G.L.C.
Animals 7-11 were treated the same way as 1-6, but were given food as well as the ointment only during the day time (8 a.m. 6 p.m.). The animals were pretrained to eat during the day before starting the experiment.

Table 3. Days taken for nuclear opacity to appear after starting the rats on galactose diet

Animal No.	Control Animals (Both Eyes)	Experimental Animals		Delay in experimental animals
		Untreated Eye	Treated Eye	
1	13	15	25	10
2	12	14	21	7
3	14	14	20	6
4ç	13	15	20	5
5	13	16	23	7
6	14	17	23	6
7	13	19	27	10
8	13	17	25	8
9	13	18	26	8
10	12	18	23	5
Mean	13.1 (.7)	16.3 (1.67)	23.5 (2.19)	7.2 (1.7)

Figures in brackets are standard deviations of the means

In experimental group one eye of the animal was treated with ointment as described in table 2 containing AY-22,284 and other eye received the placebo. Preparation was instilled every two hours between 8:30 a.m. and 6 p.m. Food was allowed only during the day time. Animals trained to eat during the day were used.

protocol of treatment is described in the legends. By reviewing the data in Table I it becomes obvious that the lens of the inhibitor treated eye without exception had a lower content of dulcitol than that of lens of the contra-lateral eye receiving the placebo in all the twenty two galactosemic rats studied. The decrease varied between 20-90%. Overall it appears that there was a 50% lowering of lens dulcitol in the treated eye as compared to the contralateral control. The rather wide fluctuation observed in the level of dulcitol from one animal to the other is probably related to variation in consumption of the galactose diet and other physiological forces. However, the dulcitol contents of the contralateral lenses of the same animal not receiving any treatment was found essentially the same. Therefore the results obtained in experiments treating the contralateral eye as controls in the individual animals provide more conclusive evidence about the efficacy of aldose reductase inhibitors in reducing the polyol accumulation.

The effect of applying AY-22,284 in the form of ointment rather than drops on the dulcitol level of the lenses of galactose fed animals is described Table 2. The results are similar to those described in Table 1 showing that ointment had no great advantage over the drops. As in the previous group, the data again indicate that without exception the lens of the eye treated with the aldose reductase inhibitor accumulates much less dulcitol than that of the contralateral control receiving the placebo only, the decrease in level being about 50%.

The next step was to continue the topical application experiments until the appearance of nuclear cataracts. The results of this series of experiments are summarized in Table 3. Nuclear cataracts in control animals fed 50% galactose diet appeared on about 13th day. The cataracts appeared in both eyes almost simultaneously, the difference in time being not more than 24 hrs. In experimental animals, it appeared on about the 16th day in placebo treated and 23rd day in ointment treated eyes. Thus, there was a delay in appearance of nuclear cataracts in eyes receiving the inhibitor considering as controls either the eyes of separate animals or the contralateral eyes. The delay was unambiguously observed in all the animals. That the slight delay in the appearance of nuclear cataracts in placebo treated eyes as compared to controls is caused by cross circulation of the inhibitor from the contralateral eye cannot be ruled out.

The results thus clearly show that aldose reductase inhibitor applied topically is effective in reducing the polyol accumulation in the lens as well as in delaying the cataractous process. The effectiveness of these topical experiments provides more direct evidence that the observed decrease in polyol accumulation and the delay of the cataractous process is specifically a result of the inhibitory activity of AY-22,284 on aldose reductase and not a nonspecific or systemic effect of this compound or its metabolite, a possibility which could not be ruled out by oral feeding experiments. Thus the observations lend further support to the theory that aldose reductase initiates the process of cataract formation in galactosemia. In addition, the results offer the possibility of a more practical way of delaying the formation of sugar cataracts. What is obviously needed is an inhibitor of aldose reductase that would be more potent so that it is effective therapeutically (VARMA, MIKUNI & KINOSHITA, 1975). Work in this direction is in progress in this laboratory.

REFERENCES

DVORNIK, D., SIMARD-DUQUESNE, N., KRAMI, M., SESTANJ, K., GABBAY, K.H., KINOSHITA, J.H., VARMA, S.D. & MEROLA, L.O. Polyol accumulation in galactosemic and diabetes rats: Control by an aldose reductase inhibitor. *Science* 182: *1146-1148* (1973).

KINOSHITA, J.H., DVORNIK, D., KRAHML, M. & GABBY, K.H. The effect of an aldose reductase inhibitor on the galactose-exposed rabbit lens. *Biochim. Biophys. Acta* 158: *472-475* (1968).

KINOSHITA, J.H., MEROLA, L.O., SATOH, K. & DIKMAK, E. Osmotic changes caused by the accumulation of dulcitol in lenses of rats fed with galactose. *Nature* (London) 194: *1085-1087* (1962).

VAN HEYNINGEN, R. Formation of polyols by lens of rats with sugar cataracts. *Nature* (London) 184: *194-195* (1959).

VARMA, S.D. & KINOSHITA. J.H. Sorbitol pathway in diabetic and galactosemic rat lens. *Biochim. Biophys. Acta,* 338: *632-640* (1974).

VARMA, S.D., MIKUNI, I. & KINOSHITA, J.H. Flavonoids as inhibitors of lens aldose reductase. *Science* 188. *1215-1216* (1975).

Authors' address: Laboratory of Vision Research
National Eye Institute
National Institutes of Health
Department of Health, Education and Welfare
Bethesda, Maryland 20014. USA

STUDIES ON THE CRYSTALLINE LENS.
XXIV. BICARBONATE CONTENT AND FLUX DETERMINATIONS *

V. EVERETT KINSEY

Considerable uncertainty exists concerning the bicarbonate content of the ocular lens. To the author's knowledge, there are no published data on the rate of exchange of bicarbonate between the lens and the aqueous and vitreous humors, even though bicarbonate is a major anionic constituent of these fluids. Information about its concentration in the lens is needed in order to estimate the number of unbalanced cations in the intracellular fluid of the lens, which, in turn, is a measure of the magnitude of the unbalanced anionic charges on the non-diffusible molecules in the intracellular fluid of this organ. It is important to know how many of these fixed charges are present since, as a result of the Gibbs-Donnan effect, they establish the ionic gradients that exist between intracellular fluid of lens fibers and the ocular humors and, thus, are responsible for the osmotic influx of water. In other words, the fixed charges are intimately involved in the control of lens hydration.

NORDMANN (1954), in his excellent treatise on the crystalline lens, points out that the process of ashing commonly employed in preparing lens tissue for electrolyte analysis frees CO_2 from carbonates, and additional loss of CO_2 from lenses occurs from handling prior to incineration, both of which lead to an underestimate of the bicarbonate-carbonate present in the lens. On the assumption that carbonate represents the difference in weight between ash and the total of all other ions present, SALIT, SWAN & PAUL (1942) found that normal rat lenses contained 0.023 percent carbonate (wet weight) or 5.2 millimoles per liter. A considerably higher concentration of CO_2 from the ash of calf lenses was reported by MANDEL, NORDMANN & BLOCH (1953) who found 30 mg of CO_2 per 100 grams of fresh lens (10 millimolar), assuming a water content of 65 percent. A somewhat lower value (6.4 millimolar) for equivalent bicarbonate was cited by NORDMANN (1962) for analyses made by AURICCHIO (1956). Using the direct manometric method of Warburg, which consists of acidifying lenses in Warburg flasks, CHRISTIANSEN & LEINFELDER (1952) found what appeared to be an unusually low level of bicarbonate, equal to 20 to 25 microliters of CO_2 per 100 grams fresh weight (rabbit lenses), which, using a mean value

* Supported in part by Research Grant No. EY00483 from the National Institutes of Health, United States Public Health Service, and by the USERDA, Contract No. AT(11-1)-2012-31.

of 22.5 microliters, is equivalent to 1.54 millimolar HCO_3, again based on a water content of 65 percent.

In addition to possible species variations, the extraordinarily wide range of values for bicarbonate in the lens reported in the literature is probably a reflection of the numerous technical difficulties involved in the chemical analyses of bicarbonate. Major emphasis in the present work was devoted to developing procedures for bicarbonate determinations that would overcome these problems and at the same time be suitable for both chemical analyses and quantitative assay of radioactively labelled bicarbonate. While the War-burg method of bicarbonate analysis which involves direct manometric deter-minations of the CO_2 liberated upon addition of acid to the tissue or fluid being analyzed is a convenient and accurate means of estimating bicarbonate chemically, freed $^{14}CO_2$ gas must be collected when assaying carbon labelled bicarbonate ($H^{14}CO_3$) in order to perform an assay of the ^{14} carbon.

Both of these objectives are realized by the procedures outlined in this paper.

MATERIAL & METHODS

Culture Technique

Lenses from albino rabbits weighing approximately 2 kilograms were removed from the posterior portion of enucleated eyes after cutting the zonules close to the ciliary body. The procedures for culturing the lenses in the absence of radioactive bicarbonate were similar to those described previously (WACHTL & KINSEY, 1958 and KINSEY & REDDY, 1965) except that culture tubes were pregassed with the usual CO_2 mixture, after which the outlets were sealed with rubber injection vial stoppers. Lenses were weighed only before culture to minimize loss of CO_2, the assumption being that no significant changes in weight occurred during culture.

The rate of exchange of $H^{14}CO_3$ between lens and culture fluid was deter-mined in lenses cultured in media pregassed to a pH of 7.55 and then sealed. One hundred microliters of a solution of 5 microcuries/ml of $NaH^{14}CO_3$ were injected through the rubber seal. The culture tubes were not gassed after adding radioactive HCO_3 because such an addition would lead to the rapid loss of $^{14}CO_2$ by exchange with nonlabelled CO_2.

For the experimental determination of efflux, lenses were cultured for an hour in the presence of $H^{14}CO_3$ in sealed culture tubes to accumulate radio-active bicarbonate. At the end of this time, the media were analyzed for $H^{14}CO_3$ and the lenses were removed and placed in individual sealed culture tubes that contained tracer-free media that had been pregassed. They were then cultured for varying periods during which time $H^{14}CO_3$ was diffused out of the lens. Lenses were removed and analyzed for $H^{14}CO_3$ content by the procedure outlined below.

The concentration of radioactive bicarbonate initially, i.e. one hour after culture in the presence of $H^{14}CO_3$, was assumed to be identical with that obtained from experiments involving determination of the rate of accumu-lation of $H^{14}CO_3$ at one hour (Fig. 3).

311

Immediately following removal from the eye or culture tube, lenses were gently blotted on filter paper, moistened with aqueous humor or culture media, weighed and then introduced quickly into empty culture tubes with sealed gas outlets.

A small glass vial containing 0.5 ml of known concentration $Ba(OH)_2$ was held in a small basket formed of stiff steel wire and suspended from a silicone stopper inserted into the main opening of the tube (Fig. 1). The $Ba(OH)_2$ was employed to absorb CO_2 which was liberated from bicarbonate by the injection of 2 ml of $1N$ H_2SO_4 through one of the two rubber stoppers. Tubes were shaken at $37°C$ at the same rate as used in the culture procedure over a five hour period to allow time for the complete absorption of the CO_2. This technique was essentially the same as that described by REDDY et al. (1975).

The concentration of CO_2 was determined by comparing the difference in normality of the $Ba(OH)_2$ before and after absorption by titrating with $0.025N$ $HC1$ using phenol red → yellow endpoint. Control analyses without a lens were performed under identical conditions in order to allow for the small amount of CO_2 in the air contained in the culture tube. This blank was subtracted in calculating the CO_2 evolved from the lens.

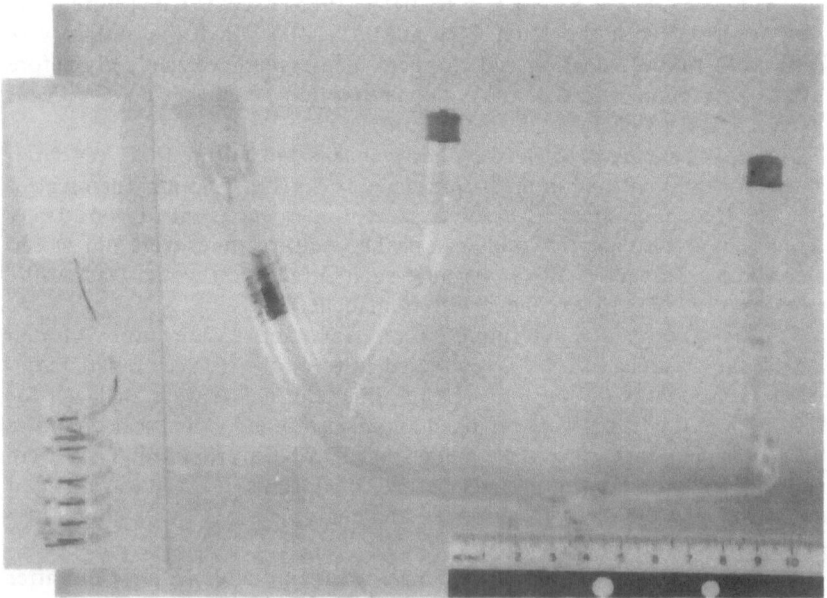

Fig. 1. A lens culture tube with sealed gas outlets containing a small glass vial (inset) to hold absorbent alkali. $Ba(OH)_2$ or hydroxide of Hyamine is suspended from a silicone stopper

Radioactive Assay, $H^{14}CO_3$ in Lenses

Lenses containing $H^{14}CO_3$ were quickly removed from the tubes, rapidly blotted on filter paper moistened with the culture fluid containing $H^{14}CO_3$ and the amount of $H^{14}CO_3$ in the lens was determined by assaying the $^{14}CO_2$ formed upon addition of 2 ml of 1N H_2SO_4 using the procedure described above for chemical determination of CO_2 except that 0.5 ml of hydroxide of Hyamine was substituted for $Ba(OH)_2$ to absorb the $^{14}CO_2$. The small glass vials containing Hyamine were introduced into bottles containing 15 ml of scintillation fluid and the radioactivity was determined in a scintillation counter. Lenses cultured in radioactive bicarbonate were also weighed before culture to prevent loss of $^{14}CO_2$ and this weight was employed in calculating concentrations.

Radioactive Assay, $H^{14}CO_3$ in Media

The concentration of labelled bicarbonate in the culture media was determined by removing 100 microliters of media at the end of a culture period and adding it quickly to a culture tube containing 100 microliters of 0.01N NaOH which had been introduced into the pit of the tube that ordinarily holds the lens (to prevent loss of CO_2) then sealing the tube with a rubber vial stopper. Two ml of 1N H_2SO_4 were then injected into the solution to liberate $^{14}CO_2$ which was absorbed in Hyamine in the course of five hours, during which time the tubes were rocked and maintained at $37°C$. At the end of this time the radioactivity in the Hyamine was assayed in the usual manner. This indirect technique was used because of experimental difficulties encountered in obtaining consistent results when known amounts of media containing $NaH^{14}CO_3$ were added directly to scintillation fluid and assayed for radioactivity. The cause of the inconsistent results seemed to be associated with both variations in quenching and the presence of water added to the scintillation fluid.

RESULTS

The concentration of bicarbonate is shown plotted in Figure 2 for lenses cultured in a complete medium (KEI-4) for various periods up to 24 hours. The concentration of the only major non-organic anion present in the lens, chloride, cultured under the same conditions, is shown at each time for comparison.

The bicarbonate level (16.8±3.3 (25)) of lenses initially (freshly removed) is only slightly less than that of chloride (17.6±2.0 mM (13)) for lenses similarly removed from the globe and otherwise treated identically. Chloride analyses were performed using a newly developed analytical procedure in which glutathione, which titrates as chloride electrometrically, is eliminated before titration by oxidation of lens homogenates (in water) with diamide.

The rate of accumulation of $H^{14}CO_3$ in lenses cultured with and without 10^{-3} M Diamox is shown in Figure 3, plotted as a ratio of concentration in lens water to that in the media (C_L/C_M). Accumulation up to a concentration

313

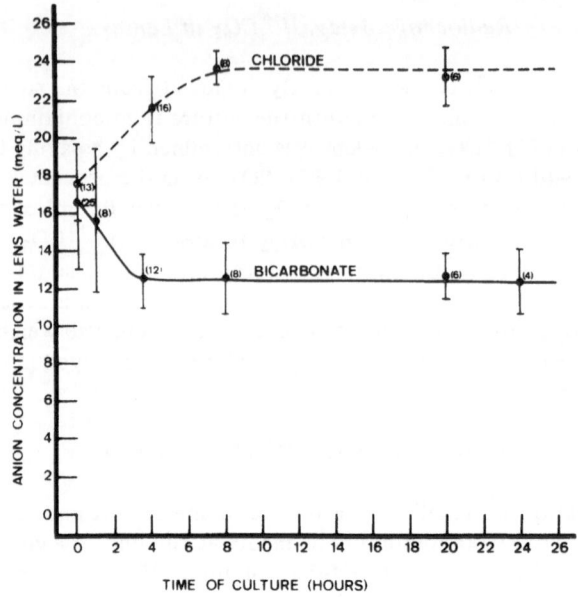

Fig. 2. Concentration of HCO_3^- and Cl^- in rabbit lenses cultured for varying periods.

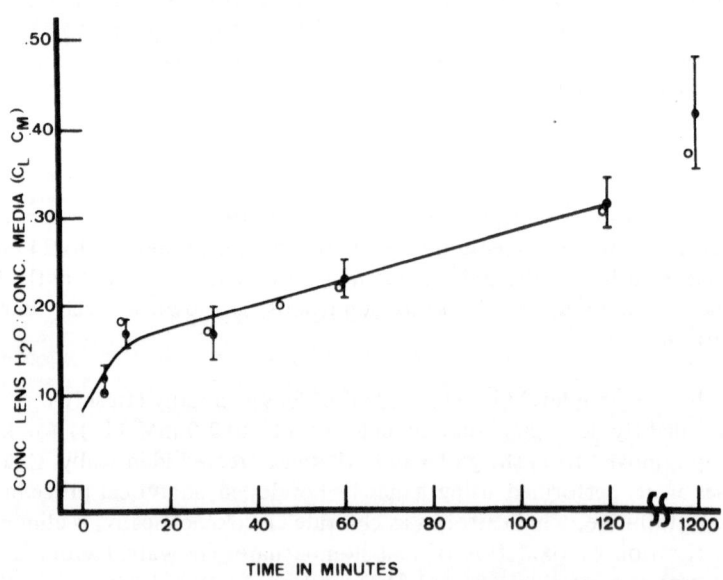

Fig. 3. Rate of accumulation of $H^{14}CO_3$ in rabbit lenses cultured with (filled circles) and without (open circles) 10^{-3} M Diamox. Bars indicate one standard deviation.

314

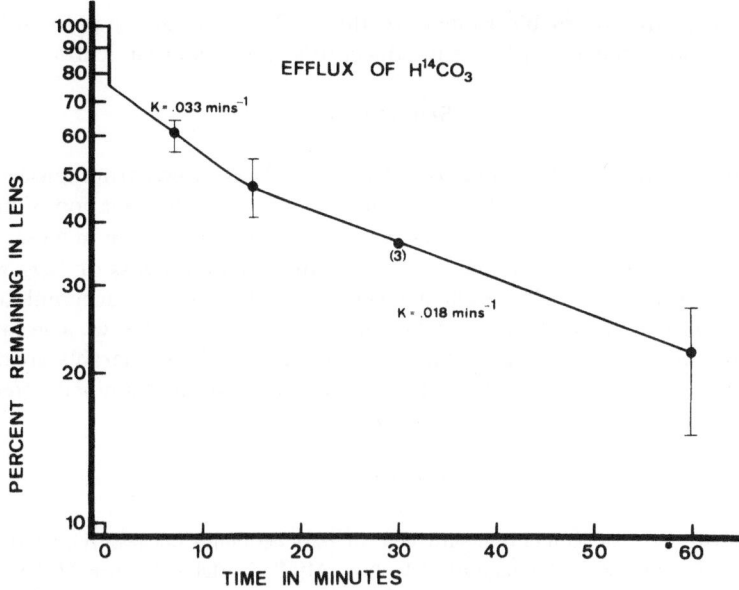

Fig. 4. Semi-log plot of the rate of efflux of $H^{14}CO_3$ from cultured rabbit lenses. Bars indicate one standard deviation.

of 0.07 is extremely rapid. This value is probably due to bicarbonate entering the capsule and is almost identical with that found for sodium (KINSEY, 1973) and chloride (KINSEY & HIGHTOWER, 1976). Subsequent accumulation, assuming exponential approach to a steady state ratio of 0.41, is biphasic; the rates corresponding to values of K_{in} equal to 0.154 and 0.033 mins^{-1} for periods of zero to five, and five to sixty minutes, respectively. These rates of accumulation are much greater than those found by the author for any other substance except water (KINSEY & REDDY, 1965) and are presumed to be due to the rapid penetration of CO_2 as postulated to occur in the transport of bicarbonate between blood and aqueous humors (KINSEY & REDDY, 1959).

Diamox, even at the relatively high concentration employed, appears to be without effect on the rate of accumulation suggesting that the transport of bicarbonate is not cell mediated.

The rate of efflux of $H^{14}CO_3$, as shown in Figure 4, is also biphasic after an initial extremely rapid loss (from the capsule) of approximately 25 percent of the radioactive bicarbonate. The apparent K_{out} of the first phase is 0.033 mins^{-1} and the second 0.018 mins^{-1}. These rates are probably significantly lower than the corresponding ones for accumulation and may reflect the effect of differences in viscosity of the lens compared with the bathing fluid, in which case the rate of diffusion through the comparatively viscous lens would be expected to occur more slowly than through the culture medium bathing the lens.

The higher bicarbonate content of the lenses observed in the present investigation compared with those found in previous studies may result from better conservation of CO_2.

315

The contribution of bicarbonate to the total anionic charge in the intracellular fluid of the lens will be the subject of a future communication.

SUMMARY

Procedures involving the collection of CO_2 or $^{14}CO_2$ freed from lenses by acidification have been developed for the quantitative determination of normal or radioactive bicarbonate. The concentration of this anion in lenses removed from rabbit eyes under conditions that minimize loss of CO_2 was found to be 16.8 mM. Measurements were made of the rate of accumulation and efflux of radioactive labelled bicarbonate from rabbit lenses. The turnover rates observed were triphasic in both directions and considerably greater ($t_{\frac{1}{2}}$ approximately 20 minutes) than for any other substance studied heretofore except water.

REFERENCES

AURICCHIO, G.: Sul comportamento dell' anidrasi carbonica dei tessuti oculari nel corso di un processo infiammatoria dell' uvea; Atti Soc. oftal. ital. *15*:66 (1956).

CHRISTIANSEN, G.S. & LEINFELDER, P.J.: A critical study of lens metabolism. I. Nonenzymatic 'respiration'; Amer. J. Ophthal. *35*(Pt. II): 21 (1952).

KINSEY, V.E.: Studies on the crystalline lens. XIX. Quantitative aspects of active and passive transport of sodium. Exp. Eye Res. *15*:699 (1973).

KINSEY, V.E. & HIGHTOWER, K.R.: Studies on the crystalline lens. XXII. Characterization of chloride movement based on the pump-leak model. Exp. Eye Res. (1976) (in press).

KINSEY, V.E. & REDDY, V.N.: Turnover of total carbon dioxide in the aqueous humors and the effect thereon of acetazolamide. Arch. Ophthal., Chicago *62*:78 (1959).

KINSEY, V.E. & REDDY, V.N.: Studies on the crystalline lens. XI. The relative role of the epithelium and capsule in transport; Invest. Ophthal. *4*:104 (1965).

MANDEL, P., NORDMANN, J. & BLOCH, R.: Les electrolytes in cristallin; Compt. Rend. Soc. Biol. *147*:1285 (1953).

NORDMANN, J.: Biologie du Cristallin; Masson et Cie, edit., Paris (1954).

NORDMANN, J.: Biologie du Cristallin, Part 2; Karger, Basel, New York (1962).

REDDY, V.N., CHAKRAPANI, B., RATHBUN, W.B. & HOUGH, M.M.: Evidence for lens oxyproline, an enzyme of the gamma glutamyl cycle; Invest. Ophthal. *14*:228 (1975).

SALIT, P.W., SWAN, K.C. & PAUL, W.D.: Changes in mineral composition of rat lenses with galactose cataract; Amer. J. Ophthal. *25*:1482 (1942).

WACHTL, C. & KINSEY, V.E.: Studies on the crystalline lens. VIII. A synthetic medium for lens culture and the effects of various constituents of cell division in the epithelium; Amer. J. Ophthal. *46*(Pt. II):288 (1958).

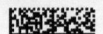